TREATING TOURETTE SYNDROME AND TIC DISORDERS

Treating Tourette Syndrome and Tic Disorders

A Guide for Practitioners

Edited by

DOUGLAS W. WOODS
JOHN C. PIACENTINI
JOHN T. WALKUP

Foreword by Peter Hollenbeck

THE GUILFORD PRESS
New York   London

©2007 The Guilford Press
A Division of Guilford Publications, Inc.
72 Spring Street, New York, NY 10012
www.guilford.com

Printed in the United States of America

This book is printed on acid-free paper.

Last digit is print number: 9 8 7 6 5 4 3 2 1

The authors have checked with sources believed to be reliable in their efforts to provide information that is complete and generally in accord with the standards of practice that are accepted at the time of publication. However, in view of the possibility of human error or changes in medical sciences, neither the authors, nor the editor and publisher, nor any other party who has been involved in the preparation or publication of this work warrants that the information contained herein is in every respect accurate or complete, and they are not responsible for any errors or omissions or the results obtained from the use of such information. Readers are encouraged to confirm the information contained in this book with other sources.

Library of Congress Cataloging-in-Publication Data

Treating Tourette syndrome and tic disorders : a guide for practitioners / edited by Douglas W. Woods, John C. Piacentini, and John T. Walkup.
        p. ; cm.
  Includes bibliographical references and index.
  ISBN-13: 978-1-59385-480-5 (hardcover : alk. paper)
  ISBN-10: 1-59385-480-3 (hardcover : alk. paper)
  1. Tourette syndrome—Treatment.   2. Tic disorders—Treatment.   I. Woods, Douglas W.,
1971–   II. Piacentini, John C.   III. Walkup, John T.
  [DNLM: 1. Tourette Syndrome—psychology. 2. Tourette Syndrome—therapy.
3. Psychotherapy—methods.   4. Social Support.   5. Tics—psychology.
6. Tics—therapy.   WM 197 T782   2007]
  RC375.T74   2007
  616.8′3—dc22

                                                                    2007000535

To my family, Laurie, Sullivan, and Zachary—DWW

To my family, Caroly, Nick, James, Laura, and Eric—JCP

To my loving wife, Jennifer—JTW

About the Editors

Douglas W. Woods, PhD, is Associate Professor of Clinical Psychology and Director of Clinical Training at the University of Wisconsin–Milwaukee. He received his doctorate in clinical psychology from Western Michigan University in 1999. Dr. Woods is a recognized expert in the assessment and treatment of tic disorders and trichotillomania. He has written or cowritten over 90 articles and book chapters on these topics and has presented his work nationally and internationally at numerous conferences and invited talks. Dr. Woods is a member of the Tourette Syndrome Association Behavioral Sciences Consortium and its Medical Advisory Board, and serves on the Scientific Advisory Board of the Trichotillomania Learning Center. He has been funded by the Tourette Syndrome Association Grants Program and the Trichotillomania Learning Center Grants Program, and is currently funded by the National Institutes of Health as part of two separate multisite research projects investigating the efficacy of behavior therapy for children and adults with Tourette syndrome.

John C. Piacentini, PhD, is Professor of Psychiatry and Biobehavioral Sciences in the David Geffen School of Medicine at the University of California at Los Angeles, and Director of the UCLA Child OCD, Anxiety, and Tic Disorders Program in the Semel Institute for Neuroscience and Human Behavior. He received his doctorate in clinical psychology from the University of Georgia and completed postdoctoral research training at the New York State Psychiatric Institute at Columbia University, where he was a faculty member prior to moving to UCLA in 1995. Dr. Piacentini has written over 125 articles, book chapters, and books, and is the recipient of multiple National Institutes of Health and other grants pertaining to the etiology, assessment, and treatment of Tourette disorder, obsessive–compulsive disorder, and other child anxiety disorders. He is the Chair of the Tourette Syndrome Association Behavioral Sciences Consortium and the Comprehensive Behavioral Intervention for Tics Studies Steering Committee, a Founding Fellow of the Academy of Cognitive Therapy, and a member of the American Board of Clinical Child and Adolescent Psychology. Dr. Piacentini serves on the editorial boards of several leading mental health journals and is actively involved in national and international efforts to promote evidence-based practice methods for the care of child mental health problems.

John T. Walkup, MD, is Associate Professor of Psychiatry and Behavioral Sciences and Deputy Director of the Division of Child and Adolescent Psychiatry, Johns Hopkins University School of Medicine. He is the Principal Investigator of the National Institute of Mental Health-funded Johns Hopkins' Research Unit of Pediatric Psychopharmacology and Psychosocial Interventions and has been the Principal Investigator on a number of large-scale, federally funded clinical trials evaluating both pharmacological and psychosocial treatments for childhood depression, anxiety, bipolar disorder, teen suicide, and tic disorders. Dr. Walkup is Chair of the Medical Advisory Board of the Tourette Syndrome Association and past chair of the National Institutes of Health Initial Review Group—Child Psychopathology and Developmental Disabilities. For the past 3 years, he has been honored by the American Academy of Child and Adolescent Psychiatry as a "Master Clinician." He is the author of a number of articles and book chapters on Tourette syndrome, obsessive–compulsive disorder, other anxiety disorders, and psychopharmacology.

Contributors

Ulrike Buhlmann, PhD, Obsessive–Compulsive Disorder Clinic and Research Unit, Massachusetts General Hospital, Boston, Massachusetts

Susanna Chang, PhD, UCLA Child OCD, Anxiety, and Tic Disorders Program, Semel Institute for Neuroscience and Human Behavior, University of California at Los Angeles, Los Angeles, California

Susan Conners, MEd, Tourette Syndrome Association, Bayside, New York

Laura Cook, BA, Obsessive–Compulsive Disorder Clinic and Research Unit, Massachusetts General Hospital, Boston, Massachusetts

Thilo Deckersbach, PhD, Obsessive–Compulsive Disorder Clinic and Research Unit, Massachusetts General Hospital, Boston, Massachusetts

Christopher A. Flessner, MS, Department of Psychology, University of Wisconsin–Milwaukee, Milwaukee, Wisconsin

Golda S. Ginsburg, PhD, Division of Child and Adolescent Psychiatry, Johns Hopkins University School of Medicine, Baltimore, Maryland

Joyce N. Harrison, MD, Division of Child and Adolescent Psychiatry, Johns Hopkins University School of Medicine, Baltimore, Maryland

Michael B. Himle, MS, Department of Psychology, University of Wisconsin–Milwaukee, Milwaukee, Wisconsin

Hayden O. Kepley, PhD, Division of Child and Adolescent Psychiatry, Johns Hopkins University School of Medicine, Baltimore, Maryland

Robert A. King, MD, Yale Child Study Center, Yale University, New Haven, Connecticut

Julie Newman Kingery, PhD, Division of Child and Adolescent Psychiatry, Johns Hopkins University School of Medicine, Baltimore, Maryland

Jana Leary, MD, Division of Child and Adolescent Psychiatry, Johns Hopkins University School of Medicine, Baltimore, Maryland

Brook A. Marcks, MS, Department of Psychology, University of Wisconsin–Milwaukee, Milwaukee, Wisconsin

Amanda J. Pearlman, BA, Division of Child and Adolescent Psychiatry, David Geffen School of Medicine at the University of California at Los Angeles, Los Angeles, California

Tara S. Peris, PhD, Division of Child and Adolescent Psychiatry, David Geffen School of Medicine at the University of California at Los Angeles, Los Angeles, California

Alan L. Peterson, PhD, Behavioral Wellness Center for Clinical Trials, Department of Psychiatry, University of Texas Health Science Center at San Antonio, San Antonio, Texas

John C. Piacentini, PhD, Division of Child and Adolescent Psychiatry, David Geffen School of Medicine at the University of California at Los Angeles, Los Angeles, California

Tyler Reimschisel, MD, Department of Pediatric and Developmental Neurology, Washington University School of Medicine, St. Louis, Missouri

Lawrence Scahill, PhD, Yale Child Study Center, Yale University, New Haven, Connecticut

Benjamin Schneider, MS, Division of Child and Adolescent Psychiatry, Johns Hopkins University School of Medicine, Baltimore, Maryland

Harvey S. Singer, MD, Division of Child and Adolescent Psychiatry, Johns Hopkins University School of Medicine, Baltimore, Maryland

Denis G. Sukhodolsky, PhD, Yale Child Study Center, Yale University, New Haven, Connecticut

John T. Walkup, MD, Division of Child and Adolescent Psychiatry, Johns Hopkins University School of Medicine, Baltimore, Maryland

Sabine Wilhelm, PhD, Obsessive–Compulsive Disorder Clinic and Research Unit, Massachusetts General Hospital, Boston, Massachusetts

Douglas W. Woods, PhD, Department of Psychology, University of Wisconsin–Milwaukee, Milwaukee, Wisconsin

Foreword

You are fortunate to have picked up this particular volume on the management of Tourette syndrome (TS). Our view of TS as a disorder, as a subject for diagnosis, and as a focus for integrated clinical care has advanced rapidly in recent years. The professional view of TS has undergone a sea change, from being considered an idiosyncratic and rare disorder to being recognized as a more common, model neuropsychiatric disorder. This is nowhere truer than in the theme of this volume: comprehensive, multidisciplinary treatment. TS, like most neuropsychiatric disorders, cannot be cured at present, and so the goal is to bring all available approaches to bear to promote the best possible function and healthy development in patients. Even this collection will be superseded some day, but for now it is the most timely and comprehensive compendium of what we know about managing TS. The questions will remain the same whatever the status of the field: What exactly is TS? What are its related problems? How is it assessed? How, and by whom, should it be managed?

Since TS was recognized and named by Gilles de la Tourette and Jean-Martin Charcot in the late 19th century, its diagnosis and treatment have followed an awkward trajectory. Its conception by Gilles de la Tourette as a neurological disorder with organic origins contrasted with the psychological view of many other disorders that was promulgated in that era. But this conception did not persist for long. In fact, until recent years TS had been abandoned in turns by both biologically and psychologically oriented clinicians, whose divergent approaches to treatment rarely intersected in the clinic. In the 1970s the dramatic results of haloperidol treatment for severe TS provided a triumph for the biological view of the disorder and at last placed TS firmly in the realm of neurological disease. Work on the biological origins and medical treatment of Tourette has proceeded apace since then and has included clinical trials of other medications, neuroimaging, neurophysiological, and neuropathological studies, and gene hunting. More recently, insights about the brain's motor circuitry have given rise to a promising behavioral approach to TS. We are now poised to reject the old dichotomy between neurology and behavioral science and recognize a wide range of useful approaches. This volume lays out a new synthesis: the knowledge and expertise of neurologists, psychiatrists, psychologists, educators, social workers, and parents can—and should—be brought to bear to ameliorate the effects of TS and its comorbid disorders.

What about those with comorbid disorders? During most of the past century TS was recognized only in its most extreme manifestations, such as florid or self-injurious motor tics and coprolalia. This narrow perspective placed the focus entirely on the observable tics (while also erroneously consigning TS to the status of being a very rare disorder). Work in recent years has yielded two important insights: First, we recognize that the premonitory urges that precede and perhaps impel the tics are sometimes as great a burden for patients as the tics themselves. Second, TS has been recognized as a complex phenotype that includes not just tics but also one or more disorders that often occur in association with it. The most common comorbid conditions are attention-deficit/ hyperactivity disorder, obsessive–compulsive disorder, and a handful of other behavioral and affective disorders. In order to select appropriate treatment for a patient, it is essential to discern accurately between TS alone and TS accompanied by one or more of these comorbid disorders. It may be the tics that bring patients with TS into the clinic, but when comorbid disorders are present, they may result in more functional impairment than the tics themselves. As a result, the comorbid disorders will often be the major focus of treatment. The extent to which tics alone impair functioning is difficult to estimate, as is the related question of exactly how often TS is accompanied by comorbid disorders. The population that presents in the specialty clinic will obviously be self-selected for greater impairment. Although this self-selection process hinders accurate estimates of the prevalence of different phenotypes, it is clear that a significant part of the total disability burden of TS derives from comorbid disorders and not from tics alone. Thus, accurate evaluation and successful management of patients with TS can be very challenging, and the complexity of the phenotype demands the sort of multidisciplinary treatment described in this volume.

The relatively recent behavioral addition to the tool kit for treating TS is habit reversal therapy (HRT). In this approach, the therapist first works with the patient with TS to develop fine awareness of premonitory urges and tics: When do they occur most, and what are the cues that can make the patient aware that they are coming? Then the patient is instructed to practice a competing response, an action that is usually opposite to, or in some manner incompatible with, the tic. This practice is generalized into everyday situations and may provide a significant reduction in tic severity and functional impairment. It should come as no surprise that a behavioral approach of this kind has emerged during the heyday of the biological approach to TS. After all, the groundwork for HRT came from several decades of basic neuroscience studies on the basal ganglia, from the cellular level up through neuroimaging. These studies revealed that the basal ganglia encode motor sequences, and that they can change and modify their circuitry in response to appropriate types of conditioning. But medical treatment and behavioral therapy do not end the list: psychosocial management of comorbid disorders and family issues and support of patients in the school and work environments are also part of a comprehensive model of TS treatment. All of these modalities are addressed in this volume, because each contributes to the desired result: reduced impairment and enhanced personal development for patients with TS.

Multidisciplinary approaches have long held promise for complex neuropsychiatric disorders. My own experience is perhaps instructive: As an undiagnosed boy with TS in the 1960s, I nonetheless received a combination of ineffective but benign medication, excellent psychosocial support, and effective advocacy, all from my neurologist. This was nothing if not a broad, albeit one-doctor, approach! But the current synthesis of diverse approaches to TS did not originate in one mind, nor did it arrive by chance. Since the 1970s, the Tourette Syndrome Association (TSA), a patient- and family-based organization, has supported a broad program of research into the causes and treatments of TS. The TSA believes strongly in the comprehensive approach to treatment detailed in this volume and has supported many of the approaches described herein. Over the years the TSA has harnessed the best available scientific and medical expertise to identify opportunities for progress on TS, to fund promising work, and to establish collaborative groups of investigators and clinicians to tackle large problems and undertake clinical trials. An example is the TSA's Behavioral Sciences Consortium, whose members are developing HRT for both child and adult patients with TS, and several of whom have authored chapters here.

Along with the authors, I hope that this volume will serve the needs of a wide range of professionals charged with the clinical care and education of individuals with TS.

PETER HOLLENBECK, PHD
Co-chairman, Tourette Syndrome Association
Scientific Advisory Board
Professor of Biological Sciences, Purdue University

Acknowledgments

First, we would like to thank the children and adults with Tourette syndrome and their families who have taught us so much about this disorder and what is required to live with it day in and day out. They have shaped our view of what TS is and isn't and have sharpened the focus of our treatment efforts. We would also like to thank all of the contributors for their hard work and patience with the editorial process. Our sincere appreciation goes to Sue Levi-Pearl, Neil Swerdlow, Judith Ungar, Jonathan Mink, Peter Hollenbeck, and the Tourette Syndrome Association for what they have done to improve the lives of people with TS and for the professional support and encouragement they have given us. Last, we would like to thank Kitty Moore and the staff at The Guilford Press; without their vision and diligence, this volume would not exist.

Contents

III. CLINICAL MANAGEMENT OF SECONDARY PROBLEMS

CHAPTER 1

Introduction to Clinical Management of Tourette Syndrome

Douglas W. Woods
John C. Piacentini
John T. Walkup

In recent years there has been an explosion of interest in Tourette syndrome (TS). Not only has TS captured the attention of researchers and clinicians, but the popular media has begun to focus on the disorder, by including people with TS as characters in movies, guests on talk shows, and as the focus of cable documentaries. Despite this increased attention and the growing scientific knowledge about TS, there are limitations in our knowledge and understanding of what causes the disorder and how to cure it. In this book we take advantage of what is known about TS to describe a comprehensive, multidisciplinary approach to its management in children and adults. This volume focuses primarily on children and adolescents because TS presents early in life, usually from age 4 to 6, and peaks in adolescence. For some, it dissipates, but for others, it persists into adulthood. Several chapters consequently look beyond childhood and into adulthood in order to convey a more complete understanding of the disorder.

Although multidisciplinary care has become increasingly popular for many neuropsychiatric disorders, multidisciplinary care for TS is a relatively recent development. To appreciate the evolving nature of treatment approaches in TS, a brief discussion of the history of the disorder, its conceptualization, and treatment is warranted.

Tic disorders have been recognized in humans throughout recorded medical history, but it was not until 1885 that Gilles de la Tourette, a French neurologist, identified a cluster of behaviors as the syndrome that would eventually bear his name. Given Tourette's training as a neurologist, it is not surprising that he viewed the disorder as a hereditary, biologically based condition. However, with the lack of effective treatments in neurology at that time and the early successes of psychoanalysis (e.g., with hysteria) in the early 20th century, the initial biological conceptualizations quickly gave way to a primarily psychoanalytic explanation, wherein tics were viewed as a result of underlying psychic conflicts or repressed sexual or aggressive impulses (e.g., Ferenczi, 1921; Kushner, 1999). The lack of other effective treatments and the rising interest in psychoanalysis and psychotherapeutic approaches, in general, in the first half of the 20th century resulted in a psychological model for TS and psychotherapy as the treatment of choice. One unfortunate complication of this initial psychological conceptualization of TS was the implication that those with tics lacked willpower or had a deficit in character. Even now, patients who in their late 50s or older often report a very difficult time trying to reconcile their personal experience with TS with the psychological model that was operative when they were first diagnosed.

The psychological conceptualization of TS held fast until the mid-1960s, when a combination of factors—including basic brain research on movement processes (i.e., the role of the basal ganglia and dopamine in movement control), the discovery that antipsychotic medications could effectively reduce tics, and the growing influence of practitioners such as Arthur and Elaine Shapiro in championing the biological model—coalesced and resulted in more effective TS management strategies. Since that time, the biological/neurological conceptualization of TS has become dominant; it has fostered an explosion of research on the etiology and treatment of TS and an expanding armamentarium of new medically based treatment options (Kushner, 1999).

In the 1970s–1980s the biological nature of the disorder was no longer in question, but the historical battles between biological and psychological conceptualizations had taken their toll. As the pendulum swung to the biological model, the reaction against psychology in the understanding and treatment of TS was significant. With the growing understanding of TS's neurological underpinnings as well as the emergence of medications as an effective management strategy, it became unpopular to consider the possibility that psychological science—and beyond that, psychological treatment—may be useful in understanding and treating TS symptoms. Within the TS community researchers and practitioners began to recommend against the use of nonpharmacological treatments for tics, although largely supportive psychological interventions were still seen as useful in learning to cope with the disorder (e.g., Bruun, 1984; Comings, 1990).

The negative reactions to psychological conceptualizations and treatment alternatives for TS were at least partly the result of the negative effects of the early psychological conceptualizations of TS. Invoking the unconscious in the etiology of TS, blaming early parent–child interactions, and simplistically holding patients accountable for an inability to control themselves was an unfortunate result of these early psychological theories.

Ironically, concurrent with the development of medical approaches to TS in the late 1960s, psychological and early genetic studies suggested that environmental factors were involved in tic severity and that psychiatric comorbidity in TS was common (e.g., Doleys & Kurtz, 1974). In addition, a number of small but carefully controlled studies showed that the use of primarily behavioral psychological approaches (as opposed to psychodynamic approaches) could be effective in reducing tic severity (e.g., Azrin, Nunn, & Frantz, 1980). Regrettably, this newer psychological understanding of TS and approach to treatment did not take hold until more recently (as reviewed in Himle, Woods, Piacentini, & Walkup, 2006).

Care for those with TS may have been restricted to medical practitioners had it not been for the work of Leckman and Cohen (1999), who highlighted the importance of an integrated approach to the understanding and treatment of individuals with TS. Perhaps it was the shift to an integrated approach that once again opened the door for psychology to become involved in the development of a more comprehensive understanding and treatment of TS. Indeed, since 1999, there has been a renaissance in the psychology of TS, with the creation of a comprehensive model that integrates neurobiological and environmental factors in the understanding and treatment of this disorder. Modern psychological approaches focus more on the here and now than the past, expect progress to occur over briefer treatment periods, and emphasize improved functioning and behavior change rather than the development of insight.

Based on this evolving integrated conceptual model of TS, the Tourette Syndrome Association formed the Behavioral Sciences Consortium (BSC) in 2002. Founding members of the BSC included Drs. John C. Piacentini (UCLA), John T. Walkup (Johns Hopkins University), Douglas W. Woods (University of Wisconsin—Milwaukee), Sabine Wilhelm (Massachusetts General Hospital—Harvard University), Alan Peterson (University of Texas Health Sciences Center—San Antonio), Lawrence Scahill (Yale University Child Study Center), Susanna Chang (UCLA),

Thilo Deckersbach (MGH/Harvard), and Golda Ginsburg (Johns Hopkins University). The BSC was charged with developing and researching an integrated model of TS and conducting research to evaluate the model and resulting psychosocial treatment options. Two large-scale clinical trials funded by the National Institutes of Health are now underway by BSC members to address these aims.

The purpose of this book is to give practitioners a guide on how to comprehensively treat those with TS. The approach to treatment outlined in this book is influenced by our emerging integrated model. A complete understanding of the model is not necessary to competently implement treatment, but a general understanding of the integrated model, especially the behavioral component, will put the assessment and treatment recommendations in this volume into an appropriate context.

OVERVIEW OF THE COMPREHENSIVE, INTEGRATED MODEL OF TS

The comprehensive, integrated model (CIM) suggests that the complex presentation of TS commonly observed in clinical settings is the result of two interacting forces. First, tics and associated features (e.g., premonitory urges) have a neurobiological substrate; tics emerge because of abnormal genetic and/or neurological factors. Second, tics do not occur in a vacuum; they occur in the world, and as a result, tic symptom expression reflects an underlying neurobiology that both influences and is influenced by a person's external and internal (i.e., inside the person's body) environments. Essentially, the *environment* in interaction with the underlying *neurobiology* shape tic expression in a context-dependent fashion, and it is this interaction that serves to shape the often complex and at times baffling presentation of some people with TS.

In the following chapters the authors describe tic disorders and their treatment across a wide array of domains. Each chapter offers something unique and important in the treatment of children and adults with tic disorders. Indeed, each chapter in this book could be pulled out and used in isolation, but we encourage you to refrain from this approach. The book was designed to be consulted/read as a whole, because we believe that the integrated approach to treating tic disorders is the best approach.

Chapter 2 provides an overview of tic disorders and their phenomenology. Chapter 3 addresses the assessment of tic disorders and Chapter 4, the assessment of comorbid conditions. Meaningful and ongoing assessment is critical to a comprehensive management of tic disorders. Chapter 5 provides an in-depth look at the genetic and neurological factors underlying tic disorders, and this discussion is extended in Chapter

6 by Chang's description of the cognitive manifestations of these neurological factors.

Comprehensive management strategies are described next. After a discussion in Chapter 7 of general medication strategies for tics and related conditions, nonpharmacological treatment options for tics are described in Chapter 8, nonpharmacological options for common co-morbid conditions are described in Chapter 9 and the management of disruptive behavior disorders is described in Chapter 10.

Recognizing that the tic disorders impact more than just the person with tics, and that the contexts in which tics occur can have a tremendous impact on their expression, chapters are devoted to strategies for managing tic disorders and related problems in family settings (Chapter 11), in a variety of different environments, including school (Chapter 12), and in social and occupational settings (Chapter 13).

Of course, not all individuals with a tic disorder diagnosis will demonstrate impairment across all domains addressed in this book, nor will all need treatment for all of the issues described here. Nevertheless, the astute clinician, after reading this book, should be able to understand how tic disorders can impact the client's life, what issues should be assessed, and generally how tics should be managed. It is our hope that this book facilitates the comprehensive, integrated care of persons with TS and related tic disorders.

REFERENCES

Azrin, N. H., Nunn, R. G., & Frantz, S. E. (1980). HR vs. negative practice treatment of nervous tics. *Behavior Therapy, 11,* 169–178.

Bruun, R. D. (1984). Gilles de al Tourette's syndrome: An overview of clinical experience. *Journal of the American Academy of Child Psychiatry, 23,* 126–133.

Comings, D. E. (1990). *Tourette syndrome and human behavior.* Duarte, CA: Hope Press.

Doleys, D. M., & Kurtz, P. S. (1974). A behavioral treatment program for the Gilles de la TS. *Psychological Reports, 35,* 43–48.

Ferenczi, S. (1921). Psychoanalytic observations on tic, tic convulsif. In *Further contributions to the theory and technique of psychoanalysis.* New York: Basic Books.

Gilles de la Tourette, G. (1885). Etude sur une affection nerveuse caracterisée par de l'incoordination motrice, acompagnée d'echolalie et de coprolalie (jumping, lata, myriachit). *Archives of Neurology (Paris), 9,* 158–200.

Himle, M. B., Woods, D. W., Piacentini, J. C., & Walkup, J. T. (2006). Brief review of habit reversal training for Tourette syndrome. *Journal of Child Neurology, 21,* 719–725.

Kushner, H. I. (1999). *A cursing brain?: The histories of Tourette syndrome.* Cambridge, MA: Harvard University Press.

Leckman, J. F., & Cohen, D. J. (Eds.). (1999). *Tourette's syndrome—tics, obsessions, compulsions: Developmental psychopathology and clinical care.* New York: Wiley.

PART I

Understanding Tourette Syndrome

CHAPTER 2

Characteristics of
Tourette Syndrome

JOHN C. PIACENTINI
AMANDA J. PEARLMAN
TARA S. PERIS

In 1885, Gilles de la Tourette, a 19th-century French neurologist training in the famed Salpêtrière Hospital in Paris, published reports on a small case series of patients suffering from a disorder characterized by rapid involuntary motor movements, hyperexcitability, and unusual vocalizations (Lajonchere, Nortz, & Finger, 1996). From his description of the clinical features and associated characteristics to his speculation about likely genetic underpinnings, childhood onset, and clinical course, his account was remarkably accurate and forms the foundation of the syndrome that today bears his name. For much of the past century, Tourette syndrome (TS) was considered an unusual and exotic condition, a view perpetuated by the fact that only the most severe patients presented for clinical or research study. In the last few decades, however, a swell of neurobiological and psychiatric research has ushered in numerous changes in how the syndrome is conceptualized. Indeed, TS is now recognized as a relatively common neurobehavioral disorder that (1) can be diagnosed reliably, (2) occurs along a continuum of impairment, (3) is sensitive to a variety of environmental factors, and (4) is responsive to a growing array of evidence-based treatment options.

CLINICAL FEATURES

Tics are defined as sudden, repetitive, and stereotyped movements or vo-calizations that draw on one or more muscle groups, typically are expe-rienced as being outside voluntary control, and often mimic the appear-ance of normal movement or behavior (Leckman, King, & Cohen, 1999). Within this classification, they may be further defined as simple or complex tics and as motor or vocal/phonic tics. Simple motor tics in-volve isolated muscle group(s) and manifest in a single anatomical loca-tion. They are characterized by fast, darting, meaningless muscle move-ments. Examples of simple motor tics include excessive eyeblinking, nose twitching, shoulder shrugging, head jerking, or facial grimacing. By con-trast, complex motor tics rely on the coordination of multiple muscle groups, are slower and more protracted in duration, appear more pur-poseful, and include movements such as touching objects or self, squat-ting, jumping, back arching, leg kicking, skipping or hopping, and facial and hand gestures. Simple vocal tics generally are inarticulate single sounds and include vocalizations such as throat clearing, coughing, and grunting or sniffing. Complex vocal tics include intelligible syllables, words, or phrases, including echolalia (repetition of others' words), palilalia (repetition of own words), and coprolalia (swearing). In other cases, they may involve animal noises such as chirping or barking or spontaneous changes in the cadence, volume, or prosody of speech. Un-like simple tics, complex tics can often be mistaken for volitional behav-iors and utterances (Coffey et al., 2000).

Current DSM-IV-TR nosology assigns tic disorders to one of four distinct categories: transient tic disorder, chronic motor or vocal tic dis-order, Tourette's disorder (DSM-IV-TR's term for TS), and tic disorder not otherwise specified (American Psychiatric Association, 2000). Among these conditions, transient tic disorder, characterized by mild tics that are present for at least 4 weeks but not longer than 12 months, is the least severe. Chronic motor or vocal tics and TS reflect more persistent conditions in which frequent tics are present for at least 12 months. In order for a diagnosis of TS to be assigned, there must be a history of multiple motor tics and at least one vocal tic, although these tics need not occur simultaneously. Tic location, type, frequency, and severity may fluctuate over time; however, tics must emerge prior to age 18 to meet criteria for transient tic disorder, chronic motor tics, chronic vocal tics, and TS. Moreover, in order for the TS diagnosis to be assigned, the man-ifestation of tics cannot be attributable to factors such as substance in-toxication, a general medical condition, or a known central nervous sys-tem disease such as Huntington chorea. TS is the most severe form of tic disorder. However, even within this specific subgroup of tic disorders, there is considerable variability, such that clinical presentations can range from those involving infrequent, inconspicuous movements and sounds to explosive, disabling, and painful tic symptoms.

COURSE AND PROGNOSIS

The onset of TS typically occurs between the ages of 6 and 7 and is marked by the emergence of simple tics such as eye blinking, facial, or head/neck tics. Freeman et al. (2000) found that 41% of youths in an international study of TS reported that tics had emerged prior to age 6, and a full 93% reported tic onset prior to age 10. Following initial onset, studies of the clinical course of TS suggest a rostral-to-caudal progression of increasingly complex motor tics over the span of several years (Leckman, Zhang, & Vitale, 1998). Typically, vocal tics appear at age 8 or 9, and complex tics and obsessive–compulsive symptoms (when present) at age 11 or 12. Although vocal tics generally manifest years after the initial motor tics, there are cases where a full register of multiple motor and vocal tics will emerge rapidly over a brief period of a few weeks or more (McCracken, 2000). Children may present in early childhood with signs of disruptive behavioral symptoms such as motoric hyperactivity and inattention, prior to the onset of tics in as many as 50% of cases (Bruun & Budman, 1997). Although tics generally follow a fluctuating course, increasing age is associated with a greater degree of stabilization, and it is not unusual for adolescent and young adult patients to report extended periods during which symptoms diminish or remit altogether. Indeed, longitudinal naturalistic studies of tic disorders suggest that tics may demonstrate persistence over time but that impairment and tic-related dysfunction attenuate as youths age into adults (Coffey et al., 2004). Studies following youngsters with chronic tic disorder longitudinally have found that, for most individuals, tic severity reaches maximum levels in early adolescence, followed by a consistent decrease in symptoms across adolescence. Longitudinal studies indicate that only about 25% of youngsters diagnosed with TS will continue to experience moderate to severe tics into young adulthood (Leckman, Zhang, & Vitale, 1998).

Within an affected individual, tic frequency and severity are also likely to wax and wane over time (Sallee & Spratt, 1999; Spessot & Peterson, 2006). Although exacerbations of tics and tic-related impairment are linked to common psychosocial stressors (e.g., peer and family conflicts, school difficulties, significant change in normal routines) as well as factors such as illnesses, fatigue, and excitement, a degree of random symptom fluctuation is also typical of the condition (Coffey et al., 2000).

EPIDEMIOLOGY

Epidemiological studies aimed at the full spectrum of tic disorders suggest that between 5 and 15% of school-age children may develop transient tics during childhood (Zohar et al., 1992). Using interviews with the parents of school-age children, Lapouse and Monk (1964) estimated the prevalence of all tics, both chronic and transient, at 18% for boys and 11% for girls. However, given the relatively common incidence of transient tics, clinical challenge resides with identifying when transient tics are likely to progress to the more serious and impairing syndrome of TS.

Estimates of the prevalence of TS vary widely across studies, due to differences in study samples, including different age ranges, diagnostic criteria, sample sources, and number of participants. There is consistent evidence, however, suggesting that tic disorders occur more commonly in males than females (5:1) and more frequently in European Americans than African Americans or Latinos (Freeman et al., 2000; Zohar et al., 1999). The overall point prevalence estimates of TS in school-age children range between 3.1 and 4.9/10,000 in teens (male and female, 16- to 17-year-old Israeli army inductees; Apter et al., 1993), and 10.5 to 13/10,000 in children (grades K–8, male–female; Caine et al., 1988; Comings, Himes, & Comings, 1990). The prevalence of TS in community samples ranges from 0.1–1%, increasing to 1–2% when chronic motor or vocal tic disorders are included (Scahill, Sukhodolsky, Williams, & Leckman, 2005). Although studies vary in sampling strategies and diagnostic procedures, the rate of 5–10 per 10,000, derived from population samples, is at least two orders of magnitude higher that estimates from clinical samples (Zohar et al., 1999). The magnitude of this difference underscores the unfortunate reality that a considerable number of individuals who meet criteria for TS may never present for treatment.

PHENOMENOLOGY

Many patients report an urge or sensation that immediately precedes the occurrence of a tic (Banaschewski, Woerner, & Rothenberger, 2003; Leckman, Walker, & Cohen, 1993). Attempts to resist the performance of the tic are described by patients to lead to an intensification of this premonitory urge or sensation. In addition to actively suppressing tics, some individuals endorse voluntarily performing their tics in response to premonitory sensory urges (Sallee & Spratt, 1999). In such instances, tics are performed in an effort to satiate the premonitory sensations (Leckman et al., 1993; Leckman, Cohen, Goetz, & Jankovic, 2001).

Sensory tics such as these generally are focal, localized, or uncomfortable sensations that are relieved by movement of the affected body region. Several studies have documented a high frequency of sensory phenomena immediately preceding tics (Miguel et al., 2000; Spessot & Peterson, 2006; Woods, Piacentini, Himle, & Chang, 2005). However, there are developmental differences in the ability to describe and report on tic behavior, and younger children may be less able to either perceive or articulate sensory or volitional aspects associated with their tic experiences (Banaschewski et al., 2003; Woods et al., 2005). The presence of premonitory sensations distinguishes TS from other movement disorders, such as Parkinson disease, Huntington chorea, and hemiballismus (Scahill, Leckman, & Marek, 1995).

In exploring the link between sensory phenomena and tic expression in TS, some have suggested that the relationship may parallel that observed between obsessions and compulsions in obsessive–compulsive disorder (OCD) (Miguel et al., 2000; Shapiro & Shapiro, 1992). In particular, Miguel et al. (1995) studied intentional repetitive behaviors in both OCD and TS. They found that sensory phenomena (generalized and localized uncontrollable sensations) preceded intentional repetitive behaviors in patients with TS but not in patients with OCD, and that cognitive phenomena (ideas, thoughts, images) and physiological symptoms of anxiety preceded such behaviors in OCD but not in TS. More recent work exploring the distinction between tic-related OCD and OCD alone has supported this distinction, suggesting that bodily sensations and inner tension are linked primarily to TS, whereas "just right" feelings and a need for completeness appear more common in individuals with comorbid OCD and TS (Miguel et al., 2000). The ability of tic expression to alleviate discomfort associated with the premonitory urge suggests that the maintenance, and perhaps even progression, of the disorder during childhood may be related to a negative reinforcement cycle. In this regard, TS is likely similar to OCD wherein compulsive behavior is negatively reinforced by its ability to reduce obsession-triggered distress (Piacentini & Langley, 2004). As will be seen in Chapter 8, this operant model of tic expression and maintenance has significant implications for the nonpharmacological treatment of TS.

COMORBIDITY

More often than not, tics are accompanied by other cognitive and behavioral difficulties, and on average, youths with TS will meet criteria for two additional psychiatric conditions (Freeman et al., 2000). This section presents a brief review of TS comorbidity; the topic is covered more fully in Chapter 4. Chronic tic disorders in childhood have been associated with a wide range of difficulties, including aggression, impulsivity, mood and anxiety disorders, poor social skills, higher levels of family conflict, and obsessive–compulsive behaviors (Leckman et al., 1999; Spessot & Peterson, 2006). However, the conditions that most frequently co-occur with TS are OCD and attention-deficit/hyperactivity disorder (ADHD), with OCD comorbidity generally more common in TS than ADHD (Zohar et al., 1999). The comorbidity of TS and OCD is bidirectional, such that approximately 23% of TS patients meet criteria for OCD and up to 46% demonstrate OCD symptoms in the subclinical range. By contrast, between 7 and 37% of individuals with OCD also meet criteria for TS (Miguel et al., 2001). Notably, Caine et al. (1988) reported that more than half of their sample of individuals with TS displayed extensive comborbid obsessive–compulsive symptomatology, with 7.3% receiving the full diagnosis of OCD and 48% with disproportionate obsessive and compulsive symptoms.

A growing body of literature supports a distinction between individuals comorbid for OCD and TS (i.e., tic-related OCD) and those with only OCD or TS (Miguel, do Rosario-Campos, Shavitt, Hounie, & Mercadante, 2001). For example, Coffey et al. (1998) reported that individuals with both OCD and TS may have higher rates of affective, anxiety, and substance use disorders versus those with either diagnosis in isolation. Individuals with comorbid TS and OCD typically endorse more aggressive obsessions, whereas OCD alone is typified by contamination fears and cleaning compulsions (Sheppard, Bradshaw, Purcell, & Pantelis, 1999). In keeping with findings from the OCD literature, patients with TS often indicate that a sensory–perceptual awareness that something is not "just right" precedes their repetitive behavior (Miguel et al., 1995, 2000, 2001). Indeed, when both disorders are present simultaneously, it can be challenging to differentiate the extent to which a symptom such as repetitive touching or tapping reflects a complex tic or a simple compulsion.

Comorbidity between TS and ADHD is also common (Termine et al., 2006). In clinical samples, 40–60% of children with TS meet criteria for ADHD, indicating possible shared neural circuitry deficits in response inhibition and impulse control (Sheppard et al., 1999; Spessot & Peterson, 2006). Even in mild cases of TS, the incidence of ADHD is seven to eight times that of the general population (Walkup et al., 1999). Similar to comorbid OCD and TS, clinical distinctions have been drawn between TS that co-occurs with ADHD and TS that presents in isolation. Compared to children with TS only, children with TS plus ADHD and those with ADHD alone share a similar profile of comorbid conditions that include depression, anxiety, and disruptive behavior. This finding suggests that the presence of multiple comorbidities in TS is perhaps a function of the comorbid ADHD and not specific to TS itself (Spencer et al., 1998). Family genetic studies have distinguished between ADHD symptoms that appear before tic emergence and those that follow such an event, suggesting that TS and ADHD symptoms are genetically linked when ADHD symptoms follow tic emergence but not when ADHD symptoms precede tic onset (Pauls, Leckman, & Cohen, 1993).

Other common comorbidities include depression, non-OCD anxiety disorders, and learning difficulties primarily in the area of mathematical skills and reading comprehension (Dykens et al., 1990; Freeman et al., 2000; King, Scahill, Findley, & Cohen, 1999). However, assessment of comorbid learning difficulties is often complicated by the distracting effects of the tics themselves on attention, other comorbid psychopathology, and potential demoralization of the child as a result of his or her tic disorder. Notably, Channon, Gunning, Frankl, and Robertson (2006) found that in adults with TS and comorbid psychiatric conditions, cognitive impairments were more related to co-occuring illnesses rather than tic disorder itself. With regard to internalizing disorders, Pitman, Green, Jenike, and Mesulam (1987) found lifetime prevalences of 44% for both generalized anxiety and unipolar depression in patients with TS, a rate that is significantly higher compared to normal controls. In interpreting the high rates of overlap between affective disturbance, anxiety, and TS, many have noted that the chronic, impairing, and potentially stigmatizing nature of tic disorders may account for increased rates of anxiety and depression. Others have posited biological explanations for this phenomenon, indicating that TS maybe associated with increased stress-induced reactivity of the hypothalamic–pituitary–adrenal axis and increased central and peripheral noradrenergic sympathetic activity (Leckman, Walker, Goodman, Pauls, & Cohen, 1994; Lombroso et al., 1995).

CURRENT EXPLANATORY MODELS

Neurobiological

Although Gilles de la Tourette initially hypothesized an organic basis for TS, psychoanalytic theory provided an overarching framework for understanding the etiology of the condition for much of the 20th century (Kushner, 2000). It was only as patients demonstrated favorable responses to pharmacological treatments that perspectives shifted to include biological explanations of TS. Over the past two decades, however, TS has become widely accepted as a neurobehavioral disorder, although understanding of specific causal mechanisms remains incomplete.

As noted in Chapter 5, the hereditary nature of TS is well docu-mented in both family and twin studies of the condition (Kano, Onta, Nagai, Pauls, & Leckman, 2001). Family studies of TS indicate that tics co-occur in both parents and children in 25–41% of families with TS (Hanna, Janjua, Contant, & Jankovic, 1999; Lichter, Dmochowski, Jackson, & Trinidad, 1999). Moreover, twin studies demonstrate that monozygotic twin pairs show much higher concordance rates for TS (53%) compared to dizygotic twins (8%). When examining tic occur-rence more generally, the monozygotic rate is 77% versus 23% for dizygotic twins (Price, Kidd, Cohen, Pauls, & Leckman, 1985).

Findings from twin and family studies of TS have been complemented by a growing base of molecular genetic and imaging research (Abelson et al., 2005; Fredericksen et al., 2002; Peterson et al., 2003; Plessen et al., 2004). Such work has shown that DRD4 and MAO-A genes may contrib-ute to increased risk for TS (Diaz-Anzaldua et al., 2004). It has also isolated rare sequences of Slit and Trk-like 1 (*SLITRK1*) on chromosome 13q31.1 that appear to be associated with TS (Abelson et al., 2005).

In addition to efforts to identify candidate genes, work in this arena also has focused on disordered synaptic neurotransmission resulting in the disinhibition of the cortico–striatal–thalamic–cortical circuitry (Leck-man et al., 2001). Recent functional magnetic resonance imaging studies have shown decreased neuronal activity during periods of suppression in the ventral globus pallidus, putamen, and thalamus, along with in-creased activity in the prefrontal, parietal, temporal, and cingulated cortical areas normally involved in the inhibition of unwanted impulses (Peterson, 2001). In particular, deficits in prefrontal control processes as well as impaired interhemispheric connectivity have been documented in numerous imaging studies (Fredericksen et al., 2002; Peterson et al., 2003; Plessen et al., 2004).

It is worth noting that streptococcal infection may trigger the onset of symptoms in a small subgroup of patients with TS; however, more studies are needed to resolve the relation among group A ß-hemolytic streptococcus, antineuronal antibodies, and TS (Kurlan, 1998).

Environmental

Although ample empirical literature documents that TS is a neurodevel-opmental disorder with salient biological underpinnings (Osmon & Smerz, 2005), there is also evidence that tics may be influenced by envi-ronmental variables (Woods & Himle, 2004; Woods, Watson, Wolfe, Twohig, & Freeman, 2001). Indeed, Woods and Himle (2004) have found compelling evidence that tics may be responsive to reinforcement schedules. In their study, children with TS were either assigned to a condition in which they received a verbal instruction to "do whatever you need to do to keep your tics from happening" or to a condition in which they received both verbal instruction and differential reinforcement of their efforts. They found that differential reinforcement, via a token dispenser, produced significant decreases in tic expression, with a 76% reduction in tics observed in the reinforcement condition versus only 10% in the instruction-only condition. These findings suggest that tics may be responsive to operant schedules and build upon earlier research indicating that vocal tics increased considerably when participants were involved in tic-related conversations compared to discussions of non-tic-related matters (Woods, Watson, Wolfe, Twohig, & Friman, 2001). Although work to date has relied on small sample sizes and, no doubt, bears further replication, Woods and colleagues have provided a basis for further examining environmental variables that may influence tic expression.

In considering these findings, some have argued that externally driven efforts to reduce tics are likely to result in a rebound effect wherein tics return at above-baseline levels after efforts to suppress stop (Bagheri, Kerbeshian, & Burd, 1999). A growing body of evidence is challenging this assertion, however (Himle & Woods, 2005; Meidinger et al., 2005). Meidinger et al. (2005) observed participants at baseline and during periods in which they were asked to suppress their tics while either viewing videotapes, engaging in conversation, or doing nothing. Following the suppression condition, participants were told to stop trying to control the tics and were asked to watch television for another period of time. Suppression—defined as a statistically significantly decrease from baseline—occurred in almost half of the sessions. Although data from individual participants may suggest rebound effects, the study as a whole did not demonstrate a significant amount of increased tic activity in the postsuppression condition, thereby undermining the rebound hypothesis.

Dramatic gains have been made in our understanding of the etiology and clinical phenomenology of TS over the past two decades. Findings from a wide range of neurobiological and genetic investigations (see Chapter 5) have supplanted unproductive psychoanalytic conceptualizations of TS, and more recently, a sophisticated line of behavioral research has led to renewed appreciation of the impact of environmental variables on tic expression and maintenance (e.g., Himle, Woods, Piacentini, & Walkup, 2006; Woods & Himle, 2004). As should be evident throughout the rest of this volume, tic disorders are best understood as a product of the interaction between biology and environment. Perhaps more important is the understanding that effective prevention and treatment require careful consideration of both of these domains (Findley, 2001).

REFERENCES

Abelson, J. F., Kwan, K. Y., O'Roak, B. J., Baek, D. Y., Stillman, A. A., Morgan, T. M., et al. (2005). Sequence variants in SLITRK1 are associated with Tourette's syndrome. *Science, 310,* 317–320.

American Psychiatric Association. (2000). *Diagnostic and statistical manual of mental disorders* (4th ed., text rev.). Washington, DC: Author.

Apter, A., Pauls, D., Bleich, A., Zohar, A., Kron, S., Ratzoni, G., et al. (1993). An epidemiologic study of Gilles de la Tourette's syndrome in Israel. *Archives of General Psychiatry, 50,* 734–738.

Bagheri, M. M., Kerbeshian, J., & Burd, L. (1999). Recognition and management of Tourette's syndrome and tic disorders. *American Family Physician, 59,* 2263–2272.

Banaschewski, T., Woerner, W., & Rothenberger, A. (2003). Premonitory sensory phenomena and suppressibility of tics in Tourette syndrome: Developmental aspects in children and adolescents. *Developmental Medicine and Child Neurology, 45,* 700–703.

Bruun, R., & Budman, C. (1997). The course and prognosis of Tourette syndrome. In J. Jankovic (Ed.), *Neurologic clinics, Vol. 15. Tourette syndrome* (pp. 291–298). Philadelphia: WB Saunders.

Caine, E. D., McBride, M. C., Chiverton, P., Bamford, K. A., Rediess, S., & Shiao, J. (1988). Tourette's syndrome in Monroe County school children. *Neurology, 38*(3), 472–475.

Channon, S., Gunning, A., Frankl, J., & Robertson, M. M. (2006). Tourette's syndrome: Cognitive performance in adults with uncomplicated TS. *Neuropsychology, 20,* 58–65.

Coffey, B. J., Biederman, J., Geller, D., Frazier, J., Spencer, T., Doyle, A., et al. (2004). Reexamining tic persistence and tic-associated impairment in Tourette's disorder: Findings from a naturalistic follow-up study. *Journal of Nervous and Mental Disease, 192,* 776–780.

Coffey, B. J., Biederman, J., Geller, D. A., Spencer, T., Park, K. S., Shapiro, S. J., et al. (2000). The course of Tourette's disorder: A literature review. *Harvard Review of Psychiatry, 8*(4), 192–198.

Coffey, B. J., Miguel, E. C., Biederman, J., Baer, L., Rauch, S. L., & O'Sullivan, R. L., et al. (1998). Tourette's disorder with and without obsessive–compulsive disorder in adults: Are they different? *Journal of Nervous and Mental Disease, 186,* 201–206.

Comings, D. E., Himes, J. A., & Comings, B. G. (1990). An epidemiologic study of Tourette's syndrome in a single school district. *Journal of Clinical Psychiatry, 51*(11), 463–469.

Diaz-Anzaldua, A., Joober, R., Riviere, J. B., Dion, Y., Lesperance, P., Richer, F., et al. (2004). Tourette syndrome and dopaminergic gene: A family-based association study in the French Canadian founder population. *Molecular Psychiatry, 9,* 272–277.

Dykens, E., Leckman, J., Riddle, M., Hardin, M., Schwartz, S., & Cohen, D. (1990). Intellectual, academic, and adaptive functioning of Tourette syndrome children with and without attention deficit disorder. *Journal of Abnormal Child Psychology, 18*(6), 607–615.

Findley, D. (2001). Characteristics of tic disorders. In D. W. Woods & R. E. Miltenberger (Eds.), *Tic disorders, trichotillomania, and other repetitive behavior disorders: Behavioral approaches to analysis and treatment* (pp. 53–71). Norwell, MA: Kluwer Academic.

Fredericksen, K. A., Cutting, L. E., Kates, W. R., Mostofsky, S. H., Singer, H. S., Cooper, K. L., et al. (2002). Disproportionate increases of white matter in right frontal lobe in Tourette syndrome. *Neurology, 58,* 85–89.

Freeman, R. D., Fast, D. K., Burd, L., Kerbeshian, J., Robertson, M. M., & Sandor, P. (2000). An international perspective on Tourette syndrome: Selected findings from 3500 individuals in 22 countries. *Developmental Medicine and Child Neurology, 42,* 436–447.

Hanna, P. A., Janjua, F. N., Contant, C. F., & Jankovic, J. (1999). Bilineal transmission in Tourette syndrome. *Neurology, 53*(4), 813–818.

Himle, M., Woods, D., Piacentini, J., & Walkup, J. (2006). A brief review of habit reversal training for Tourette syndrome. *Journal of Child Neurology, 21,* 719–725.

Kano, Y., Onta, M., Nagai, Y., Pauls, D. L., & Leckman, J. F. (2001). A family study of Tourette syndrome in Japan. *American Journal of Medical Genetics, 105,* 414–421.

King, R. A., Scahill, L., Findley, D., & Cohen, D. J. (1999). Psychosocial and behavioral treatments. In J. F. Leckman & D. J. Cohen (Eds.), *Tourette's syndrome—tics, obsessions, compulsions: Developmental psychopathology and clinical care* (pp. 338–359). New York: Wiley.

Kurlan, R. (1998). Tourette's syndrome and "PANDAS": Will the relation bear out? *Neurology, 50,* 1530–1534.

Kushner, H. I. (2000). A brief history of Tourette syndrome. *Revista Brasiliera de Psiquiatria, 22,* 76–79.

Lajonchere, C., Nortz, M., & Finger, S. (1996). Gilles de la Tourette and the discovery of Tourette syndrome [includes a translation of his 1884 article]. *Archives of Neurology, 53*(6), 567–574.

Lapouse, R., & Monk, M. (1964). Behavior deviations in a representative sample of children: Variation by sex, age, race, class, social class, and family size. *American Journal of Orthopsychiatry, 34,* 436–446.

Leckman, J. F., Cohen, D. J., Goetz, C. G., & Jankovic, J. (2001). Tourette syndrome: Pieces of the puzzle. *Advances in Neurology, 85,* 369–390.

Leckman, J. F., King, R. A., & Cohen, D. J. (1999). Tics and tic disorders. In J. F. Leckman & D. J. Cohen (Eds.), *Tourette's syndrome—tics, obsessions, compulsions: Developmental psychopathology and clinical care* (pp. 23–42). New York: Wiley.

Leckman, J. F., Walker, D. E., & Cohen, D. J. (1993). Premonitory urges in Tourette's syndrome. *American Journal of Psychiatry, 150,* 98–102.

Leckman, J. F., Walker, D. E., Goodman, W. K., Pauls, D. L., & Cohen, D. J. (1994). "Just right" perceptions associated with compulsive behavior in Tourette's syndrome. *American Journal of Psychiatry, 151*(5), 675–680.

Leckman, J. F., Zhang, H., & Vitale, A. (1998). Course of tic severity in Tourette's syndrome: The first two decades. *Pediatrics, 102,* 234–245.

Lichter, D. G., Dmochowski, J., Jackson, L. A., & Trinidad, K. S. (1999). Influence of family history on clinical expression of Tourette's syndrome. *Neurology, 52*(2), 308–316.

Lombroso, P. J., Scahill, L. D., Chappell, P. B., Pauls, D. L., Cohen, D. J., & Leckman, J. F. (1995). Tourette's syndrome: A multigenerational, neuropsychiatric disorder. *Advances in Neurology, 65,* 305–318.

McCracken, J. (2000). Tic disorders. In H. Kaplan & B. Sadock (Eds.), *Comprehensive textbook of psychiatry* (7th ed., pp. 2711–2719). Philadelphia: Lippincott, Williams & Wilkins.

Meidinger, A. L., Miltenberger, R. G., Himle, M., Omvig, M., Trainor, C., & Crosby, R. (2005). An investigation of tic suppression and the rebound effect in Tourette's disorder. *Behavior Modification, 29,* 716–745.

Miguel, E. C., Coffey, B. J., Baer, L., Savage, C. R., Rauch, S. L., & Jenike, M. A. (1995). Phenomenology of intentional repetitive behaviors in obsessive–compulsive disorder and Tourette's disorder. *Journal of Clinical Psychiatry, 56*(6), 246–255.

Miguel, E. C., do Rosario-Campos, M. C., Prado, H. D., Valle, R., Rauch, S. L., Coffey, B. J., et al. (2000). Sensory phenomena in obsessive–compulsive disorder and Tourette's disorder. *Journal of Clinical Psychiatry, 61,* 150–156.

Miguel, E. C., do Rosario-Campos, M. C., Shavitt, R. G., Hounie, A. G., & Mercadante, M. T. (2001). The tic-related obsessive—compulsive disorder phenotype and treatment implications. In D. J. Cohen, J. Jankovic, & C. Goetz (Eds.), *Advances in neurology: Tourette syndrome* (Vol. 85, pp. 43–55). Philadelphia: Lippincott, William & Wilkins.

Osmon, D. C., & Smerz, J. M. (2005). Neuropsychological evaluation in the diagnosis and treatment of Tourette's syndrome. *Behavior Modification, 29,* 746–783.

Pauls, E. L., Leckman, J. F., & Cohen, D. J. (1993). Familial relationship between Gilles de la Tourette syndrome, attention deficit disorder, learning disabilities, speech disorders, and stuttering. *Journal of the American Academy of Child Psychiatry, 32,* 1044–1050.

Peterson, B. S. (2001). Neuroimaging studies of Tourette syndrome: A decade of progress. *Advances in Neurology, 85,* 179–196.

Peterson, B. S., Thomas, P., Kane, M. J., Scahill, L., Zhang, Z., Bronen, R., et al. (2003). Basal ganglia volumes in patients with Gilles de la Tourette syndrome. *Archives of General Psychiatry, 60,* 415–424.

Piacentini, J., & Langley, A. (2004). Cognitive behavior therapy for children with obsessive compulsive disorder. *In Session: Journal of Clinical Psychology, 60,* 1181–1194.

Pitman, R. K., Green, R. C., Jenike, M. A., & Mesulam, M. M. (1987). Clinical comparison of Tourette's disorder and obsessive–compulsive disorder. *American Journal of Psychiatry, 144,* 1166–1171.

Plessen, K. J., Wentzel-Larsen, T., Hugdahl, K., Feineigle, P., Klein, J., Staib, L. H., et al. (2004). Altered interhemispheric connectivity in individuals with Tourette's disorder. *American Journal of Psychiatry, 161,* 2028–2037.

Price, R. A., Kidd, K. K., Cohen, D. L., Pauls, D. L., & Leckman, J. F. (1985). A twin study of Tourette syndrome. *Archives of General Psychiatry, 42,* 815–820.

Sallee, F. R., & Spratt, E. G. (1999). Tic disorders. In R. T. Ammerman, M. Hersen, & C. G. Last (Eds.), *Prescriptive treatments for children and adolescents* (2nd ed., pp. 261–276). New York: Wiley.

Scahill, L. D., Leckman, J. F., & Marek, K. L. (1995). Sensory phenomena in Tourette's syndrome. In W. J. Weiner & A. E. Lang (Eds.), *Advances in neurology: Vol. 65. Behavioral neurology of movement disorders.* New York: Raven Press.

Scahill, L. D., Sukhodolsky, D., Williams, S., & Leckman, J. (2005). Public health significance of tic disorders in children and adolescents. *Advances in Neurology, 96,* 240–248.

Shapiro, A. K., & Shapiro, E. (1992). Evaluation of the reported association of obsessive–compulsive symptoms or disorder with Tourette's disorder. *Comprehensive Psychiatry, 33*(3), 152–165.

Sheppard, D. M., Bradshaw, J. L., Purcell, R., & Pantelis, C. (1999). Tourette's and comorbid syndromes: Obsessive compulsive and attention deficit hyperactivity disorder—A common etiology? *Clinical Psychology Review, 19*(5), 531–552.

Spencer, T., Biederman, J., Harding, M., O'Donnell, D., Wilens, T., Faraone, S., et al. (1998). Disentangling the overlap between Tourette's disorder and ADHD. *Journal of Child Psychology and Psychiatry, 39*(7), 1037–1044.

Spessot, A. L., & Peterson, B. S. (2006). Tourette's syndrome: A multifactorial, developmental psychopathology. In D. Cicchetti & D. J. Cohen (Eds.), *Developmental psychopathology: Vol 3. Risk, disorder, and adaptation* (2nd ed., pp. 436–469). Hoboken, NJ: Wiley.

Termine, C., Balottin, U., Rossi, G., Maisano, F., Salini, S., Di Nardo, R., et al. (2006). Psychopathology in children and adolescents with Tourette's syndrome: A controlled study. *Brain and Development, 28,* 69–75.

Walkup, J. T., Khan, S., Schuerholz, L., Paik, Y., Leckman, J. F., & Schultz, R. (1999). Phenomenology and natural history of tic-related ADHD and learning disabilities. In J. F. Leckman & D. J. Cohen (Eds.), *Tourette's syndrome—tics, obsessions, compulsions: Developmental pathology and clinical care* (pp. 63–79). New York: Wiley.

Woods, D. W., & Himle, M. B. (2004). Creating tic suppression: Comparing the effects of verbal instruction to differential reinforcement. *Journal of Applied Behavior Analysis, 37,* 417–420.

Woods, D., Piacentini, J., Himle, M., & Chang, S. (2005). Initial development and psycho-
    metric properties of the Premonitory Urge for Tics Scale (PUTS) in children with
    Tourette syndrome. *Journal of Developmental and Behavioral Pediatrics, 26,* 1–7.
Woods, D. W., Watson, T. S., Wolfe, E., Twohig, M. P., & Friman, P. C. (2001). Analyzing the
    influence of tic-related talk on vocal and motor tics in children with Tourette's syn-
    drome. *Journal of Applied Behavior Analysis, 34,* 353–356.
Zohar, A. H., Apter, A., King, R. A., Pauls, D. L., Jeckman, J. F., & Cohen, D. J. (1999). Epi-
    demiological studies. In J. F. Leckman & D. J. Cohen (Eds.), *Tourette's syndrome—tics,
    obsessions, compulsions: Developmental pathology and clinical care* (pp. 177–193).
    New York: Wiley.
Zohar, A. H., Ratzoni, G., Pauls, D. L., Apter, A., Bleich, A., Kron, S., et al. (1992). An epide-
    miological study of obsessive–compulsive disorder and related disorders in Israeli ado-
    lescents. *Journal of the American Academy of Child and Adolescent Psychiatry, 31*(6),
    1057–1061.

CHAPTER 3

Assessment of Tic Disorders

Douglas W. Woods
John C. Piacentini
Michael B. Himle

Tourette syndrome (TS) is generally considered to be the most severe on a spectrum of tic disorders that includes chronic tic disorder (CTD) and transient tic disorder (TTD; American Psychiatric Association, 2000). A comprehensive assessment of tic disorders should involve four major areas. The first three—diagnosis/differential diagnosis, assessment of tic symptoms, and description of the functional impact produced by tics—are discussed in this chapter. The fourth, assessment of comorbid conditions, is considered in Chapter 4.

STEP 1: DIAGNOSIS/DIFFERENTIAL DIAGNOSIS

Because there is no specific medical test for tics, clinicians must rely on interviews and observations to establish a diagnosis. Using the diagnostic criteria described in Chapter 2, it is relatively easy to distinguish between the different tic disorders (e.g., transient, chronic motor, chronic vocal, TS). However, it is more difficult to determine whether a specific movement is a symptom of tic disorder or a result of some other condition. A positive family history for tic disorder provides strong support for a tic disorder diagnosis, but other conditions could be confused with a tic disorder, ranging from other movement disorders to allergies or psychiatric disturbances in which repetitive movements are common.

Movement disorders that may appear similar to tics include myoclonus, dystonia, Sydenham or Huntington chorea, and restless legs syndrome. Given that many mental health practitioners are unfamiliar with the various movement disorders, it is recommended that individuals with a questionable tic disorder presentation initially be referred to a neurologist or psychiatrist specializing in these disorders. There are no clear-cut guidelines for what makes a tic presentation "questionable," but generally, the absence of facial tics either currently or historically, tics that do not wax and wane or fail to change in bodily location, late onset (after the age of 18) with no prior history of tics, and the presence of complex tics with no history of simple tics all serve as possible indicators that another movement disorder could be present.

A medical evaluation may also be helpful in ruling out other possible explanations for behaviors appearing as tics. For example, throat clearing or sniffing may be related to allergies, and eye squinting/blinking may be related to one of several eye problems (e.g., poor vision, eye infection). Likewise a medical evaluation could be used to rule out seizure activity or joint or vertebrae alignment problems that produce a continual discomfort, which is corrected with a repetitive movement.

Another common differential diagnostic concern involves distinguishing tic disorders from stereotypic movement disorder, and complex tics from compulsions associated with obsessive–compulsive disorder (OCD). There is considerable gray area in these differential diagnoses, but the following strategies are commonly used to distinguish tics from these other psychiatric conditions.

The difference between repetitive behaviors associated with stereotypic movement disorders and those suggestive of tic disorders can generally be determined by three factors. First, if a patient has a developmental disability, it is more likely that a repetitive behavior (especially a more complex one such as hand flapping or body rocking) is a symptom of a stereotypic movement disorder rather than a tic disorder. This is not to say that tic disorders do not occur in those with a developmental disability. Rather, it is the case that stereotypic movement disorder is more common than tic disorders in this population (Berkson & Davenport, 1962; Long, Miltenberger, & Rapp, 1998). Second, if the patient presents with a single stereotypic movement that does not vary in anatomical location and does not wax and wane in severity, it is more likely a symptom of a stereotypic movement disorder. Finally, if the patient has a single complex movement in the absence of a reported or observed history of more simple head tics, it would suggest the presence of a stereotypic movement disorder.

Given the comorbid overlap between tic disorders and OCD, clinicians are often presented with the diagnostic dilemma of determining whether a particular behavior is a complex tic or an OCD-related compulsion. Again, no clear-cut strategy exists for distinguishing between the two, but a few heuristics may apply. First, if a client fails to report physical anxiety or specific cognitive content (e.g., "If I don't do this, something bad will happen") prior to the repetitive behavior, especially when simple tics are also present, then the behavior is likely to be a complex tic rather than a manifestation of OCD. Second, complex tics are more likely to be preceded by a vague urge or tension than are compulsions associated with OCD (Miguel et al., 1995). Finally, complex tics may be less ego-dystonic than compulsive behaviors.

STEP 2: ASSESSMENT OF TIC SYMPTOMS

After a tic disorder diagnosis is established, an assessment of symptoms and associated phenomena must be conducted. Tic symptoms should be assessed in three domains: physical characteristics and severity, premonitory phenomena, and environmental influences on tic expression.

Assessing the Physical Characteristics and Severity of Tics

Assessment of tic symptom severity should include multiple dimensions of expression: tic topography, number, frequency, complexity, noticability, intensity, degree of interference experienced, subjective distress, and temporal stability (i.e., waxing and waning). Assessing all domains allows the clinician to consider how each contributes to an individual's disorder. For example, a patient with a single, infrequent, and physically painful tic who has been socially excluded may report much more distress than an individual with several facial and bodily tics that occur frequently but with less intensity and noticability. A thorough assessment of tics should be conducted using the following assessment modalities.

Clinical Interviews

One of the most useful strategies for assessing tic disorders is a clinical interview with the patient and other relevant parties (e.g., spouse, parent, teachers, family). The first step in the interview process is to gather information about the onset and course of symptoms and family history of tic disorder. It is useful to know the age of onset as well as descriptive information regarding the topography, frequency, intensity, and stability of initial tics. As noted earlier, tics commonly develop in a head-down pattern, and simple tics (e.g., eye blinking) usually appear before complex tics (if complex tics are present). In addition, it is not uncommon for initial tics to be transient, with prolonged periods during which the tics are absent or not noticed. Indeed, even later in the disorder, tics tend to wax and wane in frequency and intensity across both short (i.e., minutes and hours) and long (i.e., days, weeks, and months) time periods (Leckman, King, & Cohen, 1999).

Semistructured clinical interviews are also used to provide symptom information and quantification of severity. Perhaps the most widely used instrument is the Yale Global Tic Severity Scale (YGTSS; Leckman et al., 1989), which is a clinician-administered, semistructured interview that can be conducted relatively quickly (approximately 15–30 minutes) and has been shown to have adequate psychometric properties. Throughout the interview, the examiner gathers information separately for motor and phonic tics. The YGTSS consists of three main components: a symptom checklist, tic severity ratings, and an assessment of impairment. The checklist segment of the YGTSS includes an extensive list of tic topographies most commonly endorsed by individuals with tics. As the examiner reads through the checklist, the respondent provides yes/no responses regarding current or past presence of the symptom and elaboration on the nature of the symptom (e.g., specific topography, intensity) when relevant. The tic severity ratings of the YGTSS are composed of assessments in various dimensions, including the number, frequency, intensity or noticability, complexity or purposefulness, and degree to which tics interrupt or interfere with intended actions. Each dimension is rated on a 0- to 5-point scale, and motor and phonic tics are rated separately. A total tic severity score ranging from 0- to 50 is calculated by summing the five, 5-point scales across motor and vocal tics. Higher scores indicate more severe tic symptoms. Data from clinical samples have shown a mean total tic severity score of 21.9 for mixed adult/child samples (SD = 8.7; Leckman et al., 1989), and 25.9 for child samples (SD = 10.1; Woods, Piacentini, Himle, & Chang, 2005).

In addition to the total tic score, the YGTSS provides an overall rating of impairment, ranging from 0 (no impairment) to 50 (severe impairment causing severe disability and distress). Ratings are anchored by qualitative categorizations (minimal, mild, moderate, marked, severe) and descriptions to aid the examiner in his or her rating.

Self-Report Inventories

Several tic self-report inventories exist are available that are easy to administer and may be especially useful in providing brief snapshots of tic number and frequency over repeated administrations. The two most frequently studied are the Yale Tourette Syndrome Symptom List—Revised (TSSL-R; Cohen, Detlor, Young, & Shaywitz, 1980) and the Motor tic, Obsessions and compulsions, Vocal tic Evaluation Survey (MOVES; Gaffney, Sieg, & Hellings, 1994). The TSSL lists multiple motor and vocal tics (divided into simple and complex), which the client rates as either present or absent during each day of the previous week. For each tic that did occur, the client is asked to provide a 0–5 severity rating for each day. The TSSL can be a useful adjunct to the interview procedures described above, but it should be interpreted cautiously because the scale's psychometric properties have not been adequately evaluated (Kompoliti & Goetz, 1997).

The MOVES (Gaffney et al., 1994) requires the individual to rate how often he or she has experienced the 20 symptoms described on the inventory. Items on the MOVES include inquiries about motor tics, vocal tics, obsessions, and compulsions. Ratings are made on a 4-point ordinal scale (corresponding to *never, sometimes, often,* and *always*). The MOVES appears to correlate adequately with the YGTSS, but rigorous psychometric studies have not been conducted (Gaffney et al., 1994).

The Hopkins Motor/Vocal Tic Scale (Walkup, Rosenberg, Brown, & Singer, 1992) requires a respondent to rate, using a 5-point (1 = none, 2 = mild, 3 = moderate, 4 = moderately severe, 5 = severe) scale, the severity of each tic present over the previous week. The scale should be completed independently by the patient (or parent) and the examiner. The final item on the scale is a single rating of the current severity across symptoms, ranging from "worst ever" to "no symptoms." The Hopkins scale correlates highly with the total motor and vocal tic scales of the YGTSS, but more rigorous psychometric studies have not been conducted (Walkup et al., 1992). Although the TSSL, MOVES, and Hopkins scales are easy to administer and provide useful information, they may provide little insight into the duration, impairment, or interference that result from the symptoms.

In a recent collaborative study, our labs developed a self-report measure for children. The Parent Tic Questionnaire (PTQ; see Appendix 3.1) is a brief self-report measure that instructs parents to rate the presence/absence of 14 motor and 14 vocal tics along with their frequency, intensity, and controllability. The PTQ is scored by computing and summing weighted scores for each of the items (i.e., tics). Weighted scores are derived by multiplying the presence/absence of each tic (1 = present, 0 = absent) by the frequency rating (constantly = 4, hourly = 3, daily = 2, weekly = 1) and intensity rating of each tic (0–8). Using this scoring system, each tic receives a weighted score ranging from 0 (absent) to 32 (maximum frequency and intensity). Motor and vocal tic subscale scores are computed by summing the weighted scores for motor and vocal tics, respectively. An overall score is computed by summing the motor and vocal tic subscale scores. Initial psychometrics for the instrument showed excellent test–retest reliability over 1 and 2 weeks (correlations ranging from .71 to .89). Concurrent validity was also generally good, with strong correlations between the PTQ and the YGTSS subscales (correlations ranging from .59 to .83 for tic presence/absence, from .30 to .58 for tic frequency, and from .58 to .79 for tic intensity; Piacentini, Woods, Chang, & Himle, 2007).

Direct Observation

Clinical interviews and self-reports provide a wealth of information about an individual's symptoms. However, it is often useful to include a measure that is not reliant on patient report. Direct observation procedures allow the examiner to obtain an objective measure of tic expression. Because recent research suggests that brief (e.g., 5-minute) clinic-based observations can be temporally stable and as informative as more extended home-based observations (Himle et al., 2006), it may be useful and practical for clinicians to obtain such observations as part of routine clinical assessment.

Direct observation typically involves video recordings of the patient while he or she is sitting in an observation or therapy room. Observations can be conducted with recording equipment concealed or in plain view. After the observation is complete, the assessor must score the recordings. The first step in scoring is to define each tic. Next, the recordings should be scored using frequency count (Chappell et al., 1994) or partial interval methods (e.g., Woods, Miltenberger, & Lumley, 1996). Frequency count scoring requires the rater to count the tics as they occur, which may be useful for low-frequency tics. Partial-interval (PI) scoring requires the examiner to break the 5-minute observation period into thirty 10-second intervals and then note whether tics were present or absent during each of the 10-second intervals. The percent of intervals with tics is then calculated as the tic score. An example of a PI scoring sheet is provided in Appendix 3.2. The PI scoring method is more useful for high-frequency tic presentations. The use of both frequency count and PI methods have been found to be temporally stable, sensitive to change, and contributing unique information above self- or clinician report (Harrop & Daniels, 1986; Himle et al., 2006; Repp, Roberts, Slack, Repp, & Berkler, 1976).

If the examiner is interested in obtaining more than just tic occurrence from direct observation data, the Rush Videotape-Based Tic Rating Scale (Goetz, Tanner, Wilson, & Shannon, 1987) and the Modified Rush Videotape-Based Tic Rating Scale (Goetz, Pappert, Louis, Raman,

& Leurgans, 1999) may be useful. The original Rush-based scoring system is a videotape protocol in which the patient is overtly recorded while sitting alone in an examination room. During the observation segments, the patient is videotaped from two different perspectives: a full body (i.e., "far") view and a head/shoulders (i.e., "near"). The videotape is later scored for tic distribution (motor tics only), frequency, and severity. To score the distribution of motor tics, the examiner indicates those areas of the body affected (11 are listed in the protocol: eyes, nose, mouth, neck, shoulders, arms, hands, trunk, pelvis, legs, and feet). Frequency is measured via discrete trial recording, and severity is determined via a 0–5 ordinal rating scale for motor tics, vocal tics, and the most severe tic. Descriptively, the motor tic severity scale ranges from "absent" to "extreme," with descriptions that include the subjective normality, topography, and complexity of the movement. The vocal tic severity scale also ranges from "absent" to "extreme," with similar descriptions.

To use the modified system, the patient's tics (obtained using the same observation protocol) are rated (on a 0–4 ordinal scale) on five domains: location, frequency, severity of motor tics, and frequency and severity of vocal tics. The examiner then sums these ratings and derives a composite (or global) severity score. Both of the Rush scoring systems have been shown to have adequate psychometric properties (Goetz et al., 1987, 1999). According to the authors, the advantages of the modified scoring system is that it allows internal comparisons among domains and provides an overall composite score, allowing the scale to be used as a primary outcome measure (Goetz et al., 1999). The primary advantage of the Rush systems is that they assess multiple dimensions of symptom severity (i.e., frequency, topography, severity), and the observation includes recording from two camera perspectives, near and far, allowing the examiner to detect both subtle and gross movements.

As a caveat, we must point out that direct observation should be considered as a supplement, not a sufficient alternative, to the traditional clinical methods such as the interviews discussed above. Tics are believed to be temporarily suppressible, and, as noted earlier, tics are often reactive to environmental influences. The contrived nature of the clinician's office (or more generally, the assessment situation) may not represent patients' typical living arrangements, and it is plausible that their symptom presentation during assessment may not represent what they experience on a daily basis. In our experience, it is not uncommon for parents of children with tics to tell us that the child's presentation at our clinic is much more severe (or much more benign) than what they experience at home. Furthermore, not all tics can be observed practically. For example, tics involving the torso are likely to be unobservable unless clothing is removed (which is often not practical or appropriate), and some tics (such as compulsive touching and echolalia) will not be observed if the individual is alone. Even readily observable tics that are very subtle may not be detected by video recording equipment. Although direct observation provides unique and useful information, the examiner should be aware of these limitations.

Assessing Premonitory Sensations

In addition to the obvious symptoms of tics, many with TS report unpleasant and distressing somatosensory events prior to performing a tic (traditionally referred to as "premonitory urges"). These private events are often reported with either specificity ("It feels like energy [or tension, a tickle, an itch]") or vagueness ("It feels like something just isn't right"). Most often, premonitory urges are temporarily lessened upon the performance of the tic and can occur at the specific site of the tic or globally throughout large regions of the body. Assessment of pre-tic phenomena is important for a few reasons. First, these sensations may be uncomfortable and disturbing to the patient. Second, awareness of pre-tic thoughts or sensations may be important for treatment planning and may become an actual target of treatment. Third, as mentioned earlier, complex tics that are preceded by vague urges or tensions that are often difficult to differentiate from symptoms of OCD. A detailed assessment of these private antecedents will help the examiner to ensure an appropriate diagnosis.

Assessment of premonitory phenomena is usually accomplished during the clinical interview. In our experience, older patients and individuals who have suffered from the disorder for longer periods of time are usually quite adept at describing their pre-tic sensations. Younger and less experienced individuals, however, can often benefit from the use of standardized scales.

The Premonitory Urge for Tics Scale (PUTS; Appendix 3.3) assesses premonitory urge severity (Woods et al., 2005). This nine-item self-report measure asks individuals to rate several premonitory urge descriptions on a 0–4 point ordinal scale anchored by "not at all true" and "very true." The instrument is scored by simply summing the nine items. In a clinic sample, the mean score of the PUTS was 18.5 (SD = 7.3). The PUTS appears to be internally consistent (a = .81) and temporally stable at 1 (r = .79) and 2 (r = .86) weeks (Woods et al., 2005). In addition, the PUTS total score is correlated with overall tic severity as measured by the YGTSS (r = .31), along with the number (r = .35), complexity (r =

.49), and interference ($r = .36$) subscales of the YGTSS. The scale seems most appropriate for those 10 years of age and older (Woods et al., 2005).

It may also be useful to obtain information about the location and intensity of premonitory urges. Leckman, Walker, and Cohen (1993) asked participants to indicate the location of pre-tic sensations using full-page depictions of human figures that included both dorsal and ventral views and were separated into 87 separate surface regions. Although these ratings were used experimentally, clinical examiners may find them useful when assessing the location of premonitory urges. In addition, they can easily be modified to allow the patient to indicate the relative intensity or severity of urges if multiple phenomena are reported.

Assessing the Effects of Environmental Events on Tic Suppression/Expression

Because tics are susceptible to environmental or contextual influences, it is important to consider such events and how they may influence tic expression. Contextual events can occur before (antecedent) or after (consequence) tics and can increase (facilitate) or decrease (inhibit) tics (Piacentini et al., 2006; Woods, Watson, Wolfe, Twohig, & Friman, 2001). At a minimum, common antecedent events, including cognitions, premonitory urges, mood states, physical settings, social interaction, and activities, should be discussed to determine if such events influence tic expression.

A thorough assessment of the social consequences of tics will often provide a wealth of useful information. Although it is rare that tics are caused or maintained exclusively by social factors, it is not uncommon for an individual to experience a variety of social reactions to the symptoms of his or her disorder. Such events may influence the patient in a variety of ways. For example, social consequences may worsen tics by inadvertently reinforcing them through welcomed attention or escape from tasks or demands. Social consequences (e.g., ridicule, staring, teasing, questioning) may also result in avoidance of events or settings, may provide motivation for the individual to attempt to suppress his or her tics (i.e., inhibition), or may exacerbate tics through a variety of indirect mechanisms (e.g., increasing anxiety).

Perhaps the most efficient and comprehensive method for assessing the effects of contextual variables on tics is the use of a functional assessment interview. By conducting a thorough functional assessment interview, the examiner will be better able to tailor treatment to the individual patient. In conducting such an assessment, the examiner asks the patient (or parent) to identify settings and events that predict exacerbations or reductions in tics. For each of these antecedent variables, various conse- quences are explored for tic occurrence in that setting and for the poten- tial of the setting to make the tics more or less likely. Based on the patient's responses, function-based treatment recommendations can be developed and implemented. For example, if a parent states that his or her child's vocal tic typically occurs in undesirable public places (e.g., after-school events) and that the tic frequently results in the child leaving or being removed from that public place (e.g., going home to play videogames), it is possible that the child is being reinforced for having that tic in public (because doing so allows the child to go home and en- gage in a desirable activity). In this scenario, a function-based treatment recommendation might include having the child stay in the public place for increasing periods of time.

STEP 3: ASSESSMENT OF CURRENT FUNCTIONING

In addition to tic symptoms, it is important to assess how well a patient is functioning with his or her disorder. In addition to a global assessment of functioning, the examiner should inquire about current and past sub- stance use and/or abuse, level of interpersonal, familial, educational, and occupational functioning, and overall quality of life. Research has shown that individuals with TS often experience significant psychiatric comorbidity (see Scahill et al., Chapter 4, this volume), are viewed as less acceptable than their peers (Boudjouk, Woods, Miltenberger, & Long, 2000), experience greater levels of unemployment (Shady, Broder, Staley, Furer, & Papadopolos, 1995), and experience decreased overall quality of life (Elstner, Selai, Trimle, & Robertson, 2001). In addition, many individuals with TS are likely to be on medication, many of which have potential side effect profiles that range from mild annoyances to severe and irreversible symptoms (for reviews, see Peterson & Azrin, 1993; Sandor, 2003). In addition to information gathered from the clini- cal interview, an examiner may find it useful to assess adaptive function- ing and quality of life. A variety of instruments are available to aid the examiner in assessing these domains.

SUMMARY

The assessment of tic disorders should include four basic domains. After establishing a diagnosis and differentiating tics from a host of movement disorders, other medical conditions, and psychiatric conditions, clini- cians must assess various dimensions of the tics. These dimensions include the physical features of tics (e.g., topography, number, frequency, severity, intensity), the premonitory phenomena, and how various environmental antecedents and consequences may impact tic expression. The third domain of assessment should involve a detailed account of how tics may impact academic, social, and occupational functioning. The final area of assessment, evaluation for comorbid conditions, is the topic described in Chapter 4.

REFERENCES

American Psychiatric Association. (2000). *Diagnostic and statistical manual of mental disorders* (4th ed., text rev.). Washington, DC: Author.

Berkson, G., & Davenport, R. K. (1962). Stereotyped movements in mental defectives: I. Initial survey. *American Journal of Mental Deficiency, 66,* 849–852.

Boudjouk, P., Woods, D. W., Miltenberger, R. G., & Long, E. S. (2000). Negative peer evaluation in adolescents: Effects of tic disorders and trichotillomania. *Child and Family Behavior Therapy, 22,* 17–28.

Chappell, P. B., McSwiggan-Hardin, M. T., Scahill, L., Rubenstein, M., Walker, D. E., Cohen, D. J., et al. (1994). Videotape tic counts in the assessment of Tourette's syndrome: Stability, reliability, and validity. *Journal of the American Academy of Child and Adolescent Psychiatry, 33,* 386–393.

Cohen, D. J., Detlor, J., Young, J. G., & Shaywitz, B. A. (1980). Clonidine ameliorates Gilles de la Tourette syndrome. *Archives of General Psychiatry, 37,* 1350–1357.

Elstner, K., Selai, C. E., Trimble, M. R., & Robertson, M. M. (2001). Quality of life (QOL) of patients with Gilles de la Tourette syndrome. *Acta Psychiatrica Scandinavica, 103,* 52–59.

Gaffney, G. R., Sieg, K., & Hellings, J. (1994). The MOVES: A self-rating scale for Tourette's syndrome. *Journal of Child and Adolescent Psychopharmacology, 4,* 269–280.

Goetz, C. G., Pappert, E. J., Louis, E. D., Raman, R., & Leurgans, S. (1999). Advantages of a modified scoring method for the Rush video-based tic rating scale. *Movement Disorders, 14,* 502–506.

Goetz, C. G., Tanner, C. M., Wilson, R. S., & Shannon, K. M. (1987). A rating scale for Gilles de la Tourette's syndrome: Description, reliability, and validity data. *Neurology, 37,* 1542–1544.

Harrop, A., & Daniels, M. (1986). Methods of time sampling: A reappraisal of momentary time sampling and partial interval recording. *Journal of Applied Behavior Analysis, 19,* 73–77.

Himle, M. B., Chang, S., Woods, D. W., Pearlman, A., Buzzella, B., Bunaciu, L., et al. (2006). Direct observation of tics in children with chronic tic disorders: Reliability, validity, and feasibility. *Journal of Applied Behavior Analysis, 39,* 429–440.

Kompoliti, K., & Goetz, C. G. (1997). Clinical rating and quantitative assessment of tics. *Neurologic Clinics, 15,* 239–254.

Leckman, J. F., King, R. A., & Cohen, D. J. (1999). Tics and tic disorders. In J. F. Leckman & D. J. Cohen (Eds.), *Tourette's syndrome—tics, obsessions, compulsions: developmental psychopathology and clinical care* (pp. 23–42). New York: Wiley.

Leckman, J. F., Riddle, M. A., Hardin, M. T., Ort, S. I., Swartz, K. L., Stevenson, J., et al. (1989). The Yale Global Tic Severity Scale: Initial testing of a clinician-rated scale of tic severity. *Journal of the American Academy of Child and Adolescent Psychiatry, 28*, 566–573.

Leckman, J. F., Walker, D. E., & Cohen, D. J. (1993). Premonitory urges in Tourette's syndrome. *American Journal of Psychiatry, 150*, 98–102.

Long, E. S., Miltenberger, R. G., & Rapp, J. T. (1998). A survey of habit behaviors exhibited by individuals with mental retardation. *Behavioral Interventions, 13*, 79–89.

Miguel, E. C., Coffey, B. J., Baer, L., Savage, C. R., Rauch, S. L., & Jenike, M. A. (1995). Phenomenology of intentional repetitive behaviors in obsessive compulsive disorder and Tourette's disorder. *Journal of Clinical Psychiatry, 56*, 246–255.

Peterson, A. L., & Azrin, N. H. (1993). Behavioral and pharmacological treatments for TS: A review. *Applied and Preventative Psychology, 24*, 231–242.

Piacentini, J. C., Himle, M. B., Chang, S., Baruch, D. E., Pearlman, A., Buzzella, B., et al. (2006). Reactivity of tic observation procedures to situation and setting: A multisite study. *Journal of Abnormal Child Psychology, 34*, 647–656.

Piacentini, J. C., Woods, D. W., Chang, S., & Himle, M. B. (2007). *Parent Tic Questionnaire.* Manuscript in preparation.

Repp, A. C., Roberts, D. M., Slack, D. J., Repp, C. F., & Berkler, M. S. (1976). A comparison of frequency, interval, and time-sampling methods of data collection. *Journal of Applied Behavior Analysis, 9*, 501–508.

Sandor, P. (2003). Pharmacological management of tics in patients with Tourette syndrome. *Journal of Psychosomatic Research, 55*, 41–48.

Shady, G., Broder, R., Staley, D., Furer, P., & Papadopolos, R. B. (1995). Tourette syndrome and employment: Descriptors, predictors, and problems. *Psychiatric Rehabilitation Journal, 19*, 35–42.

Walkup, J., Rosenberg, L. A., Brown, J., & Singer, H. S. (1992). The validity of instruments measuring the severity in Tourette syndrome. *Journal of the American Academy of Child and Adolescent Psychiatry, 31*, 472–477.

Woods, D. W., Miltenberger, R. G., & Lumley, V. A. (1996). Sequential application of major habit-reversal components to treat motor tics in children. *Journal of Applied Behavior Analysis, 29*, 483–493.

Woods, D. W., Piacentini, J. C., Himle, M. B., & Chang, S. (2005). Premonitory Urge for Tics Scale (PUTS): Initial psychometric results and examination of the premonitory urge phenomenon in children with tic disorders. *Journal of Developmental and Behavioral Pediatrics, 26*, 397–403.

Woods, D. W., Watson, T. S., Wolfe, E., Twohig, M. P., & Friman, P. C. (2001). Analyzing the influence of tic-related talk on vocal and motor tics in children with Tourette's syndrome. *Journal of Applied Behavior Analysis, 34*, 353–356.

APPENDIX 3.1. Parent Tic Questionnaire (PTQ)

For each of the tics listed below, please mark "yes" or "no" as to whether your child has had the tic in the <u>past week.</u> For each tic you mark as "yes," please mark how FREQUENTLY the tic occurred this week, according to the following:

> <u>C</u>onstantly, almost all the time during the day
> <u>H</u>ourly, at least once per hour
> <u>D</u>aily, at least several times per day
> <u>W</u>eekly, just a few times

Under INTENSITY, rate how intense you believe the tic felt to your child over the past week. For example, if it was very mild, like a weak twitch, that would be a "1" or "2." A much more forceful tic that would be very noticeable to others and may even be painful would be rated as a "6" or even higher. Any tic that would be obviously noticeable to others should be rated as at least a "4."

Finally, under CONTROL, please rate how much control you think your child had over the tic this past week; that is, to what extent do you think your child could resist the urge for this tic. A rating of "0" indicates absolutely no control at all, whereas an "8" means complete control and the ability to resist or stop the tic immediately without any problem.

MOTOR TICS	Present Yes No	Frequency C H D W	Intensity (0–8)	Control (0–8)
Eye blinking	☐ ☐	C H D W	_____	_____
Eye rolling/darting	☐ ☐	C H D W	_____	_____
Head jerk	☐ ☐	C H D W	_____	_____
Facial grimace	☐ ☐	C H D W	_____	_____
Mouth/tongue movements	☐ ☐	C H D W	_____	_____
Shoulder shrugs	☐ ☐	C H D W	_____	_____
Chest/stomach tightening	☐ ☐	C H D W	_____	_____
Pelvic tensing movements	☐ ☐	C H D W	_____	_____
Leg/feet movements	☐ ☐	C H D W	_____	_____
Arm/hand movements	☐ ☐	C H D W	_____	_____

(*continued on next page*)

MOTOR TICS (*continued*)

	Present Yes No	Frequency C H D W	Intensity (0–8)	Control (0–8)
Echopraxia (copying another's gestures)	☐ ☐	C H D W	_____	_____
Copropraxia (obscene gestures)	☐ ☐	C H D W	_____	_____
Other motor tics _____	☐ ☐	C H D W	_____	_____
Complex motor combinations (multiple tics at once)	☐ ☐	C H D W	_____	_____

VOCAL TICS

	Present Yes No	Frequency C H D W	Intensity (0–8)	Control (0–8)
Grunting	☐ ☐	C H D W	_____	_____
Sniffing	☐ ☐	C H D W	_____	_____
Snorting	☐ ☐	C H D W	_____	_____
Coughing	☐ ☐	C H D W	_____	_____
Animal noises	☐ ☐	C H D W	_____	_____
Syllables	☐ ☐	C H D W	_____	_____
Words	☐ ☐	C H D W	_____	_____
Phrases	☐ ☐	C H D W	_____	_____
Echolalia (repeating vocalizations of others)	☐ ☐	C H D W	_____	_____

APPENDIX 3.2. Partial Interval 10-Second Scoring Sheet (PI-10)

10-Minute Interval

Participant _____   Visit _____

Directions: For each 10-second block, note whether or not a tic occurs. For tics occurring continuously across both blocks, mark both boxes. Score the observation segment by dividing the number of marked boxes by the total number of boxes and multiply by 100.

1	00	10	20	30	40	50
2	00	10	20	30	40	50
3	00	10	20	30	40	50
4	00	10	20	30	40	50
5	00	10	20	30	40	50
6	00	10	20	30	40	50
7	00	10	20	30	40	50
8	00	10	20	30	40	50
9	00	10	20	30	40	50
10	00	10	20	30	40	50

APPENDIX 3.3. Premonitory Urge for Tics Scale (PUTS)

Please answer the following questions. Try to be very honest when you answer them. Circle the number that best describes how you feel.

	Not at all true	A little true	Pretty much true	Very much true
1. Right before I do a tic, I feel like my insides are itchy.	1	2	3	4
2. Right before I do a tic, I feel pressure inside my brain or body.	1	2	3	4
3. Right before I do a tic, I feel "wound up" or tense inside.	1	2	3	4
4. Right before I do a tic, I feel like something is not "just right."	1	2	3	4
5. Right before I do a tic, I feel like something isn't complete.	1	2	3	4
6. Right before I do a tic, I feel like there is energy in my body that needs to get out.	1	2	3	4
7. I have these feelings almost all the time before I do a tic.	1	2	3	4
8. These feelings happen for every tic I have.	1	2	3	4
9. After I do the tic, the itchiness, energy, pressure, tense feelings, or feelings that something isn't "just right" or complete go away, at least for a little while.	1	2	3	4

From Douglas W. Woods, John C. Piacentini, and Michael B. Himle, "Assessment of Tic Disorders." In *Treating Tourette Syndrome and Tic Disorders: A Guide for Practitioners*, edited by Douglas W. Woods, John C. Piacentini, and John T. Walkup. Copyright 2007 by The Guilford Press. Permission to photocopy this appendix is granted to purchasers of this book for personal use only (see copyright page for details).

CHAPTER 4

Assessment of Co-Occurring Psychiatric Conditions in Tic Disorders

LAWRENCE SCAHILL
DENIS G. SUKHODOLSKY
ROBERT A. KING

Tourette syndrome (TS) is frequently associated with obsessive–compulsive symptoms, hyperactivity, impulsive behavior, and inattention (Jankovic, 2001; Leckman, 2002). The identification of co-occurring conditions is an important first step in the appropriate treatment for patients with TS. In addition to the closely associated conditions of obsessive–compulsive disorder (OCD) and attention-deficit/hyperactivity disorder (ADHD), children and adolescents with TS are subject to other psychiatric disorders such as other anxiety disorders and depression as well as developmental disorders such as autism. Assessment of potentially co-occurring disorders such as depression, anxiety, or autism is essential because the presence of one of these conditions may be more pressing than the tics, may directly or indirectly influence the severity of tics, and may add to the child's overall disability. Thus, comprehensive clinical assessment also includes screening, followed by closer diagnostic inquiry of these disorders when screening information is positive. This chapter reviews the contemporary approach to assessment of OCD,

ADHD, and other psychiatric disorders (e.g., pervasive developmental disorders, other anxiety disorders and depression) that may co-occur in children with TS. Selected assessment tools to aid in the evaluation are briefly described in each section

ASSESSMENT OF OCD

OCD is defined by the presence of recurrent, unwanted worries, thoughts, images or impulses (obsessions) that are difficult to dislodge and/or the presence of repetitive behavior that the person feels driven to perform (compulsions). Attempts to resist these repetitive behaviors typically increase anxiety and the urge to perform the compulsion. To meet the diagnostic criteria, the obsessions or compulsions must waste time (at least an hour per day) and interfere with daily living (American Psychiatric Association, 2000). Most adolescent and adult patients readily agree that their obsessive worries and repetitive habits are excessive, but this realization may not be present in younger children.

The lifetime prevalence of OCD is estimated to be 2–3% in adults (Karno, Golding, Sorenson, & Burnam, 1988). Similar estimates have been observed in adolescent samples (Flament et al., 1988; Valleni-Basile et al., 1995; Zohar et al., 1992), but the prevalence appears to be lower in pre-adolescents. For example, Costello et al. (1996) estimated a prevalence of 2 per 1,000 in children below the age of 13 years. In addition, there were no cases of OCD in the longitudinal study of a birth cohort when the sample was evaluated at 11 years of age (McGee, Feehan, Williams, & Anderson, 1992). When the same cohort was assessed at 18 years of age, however, the investigators observed an OCD prevalence of 4% (Douglass, Moffitt, Dar, McGee, & Silva, 1995). The reasons for this pattern of age-specific prevalence for OCD are unclear.

The initial evaluation should include a detailed review of the onset and course of obsessive–compulsive symptoms. Adolescents should be interviewed separately (to give the parent and the adolescent the opportunity to speak as freely as possible) and conjointly with their parents. Common obsessions in children and adolescents include worry about contamination, fear of harm coming to self or family members, worry about acting on unwanted aggressive impulses, and concern about order and symmetry (Scahill et al., 2003). Many children and adolescents describe the obsessions as occurring "out of the blue"—but careful discussion (perhaps over multiple interviews) shows that the obsessive worries are likely to be triggered by specific events and situations. Common compulsions include hand washing, cleaning rituals, repetitive requests for reassurance, arranging objects in patterns, touching habits, checking, counting, and repeating routine activities (e.g., setting down a glass or flipping a light switch over and over again) to achieve a sense of completion. In many cases, there is a close relationship between the obsessive worry and the compulsive ritual, such as with contamination and hand washing. Similarly, another child may report that the purpose of a touching ritual is to prevent harm to the self or to a family member. By contrast, other patients state that the ritual is done to achieve a sense of completion. In either case, the performance of the compulsion often results in a decrease (albeit, brief) in anxiety or discomfort, which reinforces the compulsive habit.

Studies in children (Scahill et al., 2003) and adults (Leckman, 2002) suggest that the OCD symptoms in children with TS differ in fundamental ways from patients with OCD without tics. The OCD patients with TS tend to describe repetition of behaviors to achieve a sense of completion. By contrast, children with OCD without tics typically report that the repetitive behavior is performed to reduce a recurring worry about harm or contamination. Thus, the first step in differentiating the compulsions in TS versus OCD is to ask about the purpose of the behavior. Children with compulsive behavior and tics are less likely to endorse a cognition as the trigger for the behavior and more likely to describe a need for symmetry and a drive to achieve a sense of completion.

Assessment Tools

Several quantitative ratings are available for assessment of OCD in children with TS, including clinician ratings, self-reports, and parent reports. The most commonly used clinician rating in children and adolescents is the Children's Yale–Brown Obsessive–Compulsive Scales (CYBOCS; Scahill et al., 1997). The CYBOCS, which was derived from the original YBOCS developed for use in adults (Goodman, Price, Rasmussen, Mazure, Delgado, et al., 1989; Goodman, Price, Rasmussen, Mazure, Fleischmann, et al., 1989), rates time spent, degree of interference, degree of distress, level of resistance, and degree of control over the obsessions and compulsions. Detailed self-report versions of the YBOCS have also been introduced for evaluating the presence and severity of obsessive–compulsive symptoms and may be useful (Rosenfeld, Dar, Anderson, Kobak, & Greist, 1992; Steketee, Frost, & Bogart, 1996).

ASSESSMENT OF SEPARATION ANXIETY DISORDER AND GENERALIZED ANXIETY DISORDER

The most common anxiety disorder in prepubertal children is separation anxiety disorder (SAD), which affects as many as 3.5% of children in this age group (Costello et al., 1996). Girls are at greater risk for SAD than boys. SAD is characterized by a recurring pattern of acute distress upon separation from the primary caretaker—typically, the mother. Because of this distress, the child is reluctant, or may even refuse, to separate from the primary caretaker. In the school setting, SAD may give rise to dramatic scenes in which a child clings desperately to a bewildered mother at the entrance to the school. The child may protest when the parents plan a night out and usually will not tolerate staying overnight away from home. Children with SAD typically express worry about the safety of the primary caregiver; others may express worry about their own safety when separated from the primary caretaker.

Generalized anxiety disorder (GAD) is defined by the presence of excessive worry about everyday life. The term *excessive* indicates that the degree of worry is exaggerated and is a source of impairment. For example, many children may express worry about upcoming events such as returning to school, joining the Girl Scouts, going to camp, going to the dentist, or facing school examinations. The child with GAD dwells on the worry and may express fundamental doubt about competence and acceptance by others. As the event draws nearer, the distress tends to mount and may lead to avoidance. GAD is more common in girls and has an estimated prevalence in children of 1–2% (Costello et al., 1996). The differential diagnosis of GAD, SAD, and OCD may be difficult in some cases. In OCD, the expressed worries are usually thematically connected, though not tightly linked to everyday life. For example, in OCD worries about harm coming to the self or a family member need not be prompted by separation or minor injury. By contrast, worries for the child with SAD are more narrowly focused and triggered by, separation. For the child with GAD, the worries may seem ever changing because they are connected to everyday life events. Children with any anxiety disorder may seek reassurance, express feeling tense, and have recurrent somatic complaints of headaches and stomachaches. Here again, looking for themes may assist with differential diagnosis. For example, somatic complaints in a child with OCD may follow contact with a perceived form of contamination. Somatic complaints in a child with GAD may be coincident with expressed worries about competence. Some children may have more than one anxiety disorder, which may further complicate differential diagnosis.

Assessment Tools for Non-OCD Anxiety Disorders

Data from clinical samples suggest that anxiety disorders are more common in children with TS than the general population (Coffey, Biederman, Smoller, et al., 2000). Although not necessarily borne out by controlled studies, there is general agreement that the presence of anxiety

can increases tics (Coffey, Biederman, Geller, et al., 2000; King &
Scahill, 2001). Thus, the clinical interview should include screening
questions about GAD and SAD. Screening for anxiety disorders may be
aided through the use of parent and child ratings. The Mood and Feelings Questionnaire (MFQ) is a 32-item scale that can be completed by a
parent; there is also a child self-report version for children 11 years of
age and older (Costello & Angold, 1988). Both versions are simple to
administer, score, and interpret. Although not diagnostic, interpretation
of the MFQ is aided by thresholds derived from community-based studies (Costello & Angold, 1988). Another child-self report instrument for
collecting data on anxiety symptoms is the Multidimensional Anxiety
Scale for Children (MASC; March, Sullivan, Stallings, Conners, &
Parker, 1997). It can be used in children as a young as 8, and, like the
MFQ, there are normative data upon which to base interpretation. An
advantage of the MASC is that is parallels DSM symptoms more closely
than the MFQ. Disadvantages include the length (37 items) and its
slightly more complicated scoring.

ASSESSMENT OF ADHD

ADHD is characterized by the early onset of an enduring pattern of inattention and/or hyperactivity and impulsive behavior (American Psychiatrist Association, 2000). To establish the diagnosis of ADHD and to
measure the symptom severity in children and adolescents requires information from multiple informants, including parents, teachers, and the
child. The use of multiple informants helps determine whether the behavioral pattern is consistent across settings and the impact of ADHD
symptoms on family life, peer interaction, and academic progress. Clinical observation is also important but may be deceiving, because some
children may not show the behavioral manifestations of ADHD during a
clinic visit. ADHD affects 2–10% of school-age children, depending on
the definition and sampling methods used (Scahill & Schwab-Stone,
2000). The symptoms of ADHD—impulsiveness, overactivity, disruptiveness, poor concentration—are among the most common reasons for
seeking mental health treatment in the pediatric population.

Assessment Tools

The most cost-efficient way to collect information from multiple informants across settings and to measure change with treatment is through
the use of parent and teacher rating scales. Conners Parent and Teacher
Rating Scales (Conners, 1997; Goyette, Conners, & Ulrich, 1978); the

ADHD Rating Scale (DuPaul, Power, Anastopoulos, & Reid, 1998), and the SNAP-IV (Swanson et al., 2001) are examples of reliable and valid behavior scales. Each of the items on the scales is scored from 0 (symptom not present) to 3 (severe). The ADHD Rating Scale and the SNAP-IV have a one-to-one correspondence with DSM-IV symptoms of ADHD. Based on clinical and population data, an average per item score of 2.0 on either the SNAP-IV or the ADHD Rating Scale is highly predictive of ADHD. Both scales have also been shown to be sensitive to change with treatment. For example, in the Multimodal Treatment Study of ADHD (MTA Cooperative Group, 1999), children with ADHD treated with medication (primarily methylphenidate) in the research centers showed 50–60% improvement on the teacher-rated SNAP-IV. The ADHD Rating Scale has also been used to measure change (Michelson et al., 2001; Scahill et al., 2001).

As useful as these ADHD rating scales can be, there are potential limitations. First, scores may be influenced by the parent's reading ability or cultural background. Second, teacher ratings may be inflated by the child's disruptive behavior. Thus, although scales such as the SNAP-IV and ADHD Rating Scale are valuable for the clinical evaluation of ADHD in children with TS, they cannot be relied upon as the only means of making the diagnosis.

Tics and Stimulants

Stimulants are the first-line agents for the treatment of ADHD (Greenhill et al., 1996; MTA Cooperative Group, 1999). In the MTA study (1999) involving a total of 579 children, the children who were treated in the research centers achieved an average of 50–60% improvement on teacher-rated ADHD symptoms. Of the roughly 280 children who started the trial on methylphenidate in the research centers, three-fourths remained on methylphenidate for the entire 14-month study. However, stimulants fail in 10–20% of children with ADHD (Elia, Borcherding, Rapoport, & Keysor, 1991). Treatment may fail due to lack of efficacy or adverse effects. The de novo emergence or increase in preexisting tics has been reported in case studies over the past three decades (Erenberg, Cruse, & Rothner, 1985; Golden, 1974; Lipkin, Goldstein, & Adesman, 1994; Lowe, Cohen, Detlor, Kremenitzer, & Shaywitz, 1982; Riddle et al., 1995; Varley, Vincent, Varley, & Calderon, 2001). Two placebo-controlled trials that *excluded* subjects with tic disorders (Barkley, McMurray, Edelbrock, & Robbins, 1990; Borcherding, Keysor, Rapoport, Elia, & Amass, 1990) also reported the emergence of tics in children treated with stimulants.

Despite this body of evidence from clinical trials and case reports, three short-term, placebo-controlled studies in children with ADHD and tic disorders reported no increase in tics attributable to stimulant medication (Castellanos et al., 1997; Gadow, Sverd, Sprafkin, Nolan, & Ezor, 1995; Tourette's Syndrome Study Group, 2002). Two naturalistic studies also provide information on the longer-term effects of stimulants in children with TS (Gadow, Sverd, Sprafkin, Nolan, & Grossman, 1999; Law & Schachar, 1999). Although most children in these longer-term studies did not show an increase in tics, acute exacerbations did occur in a few children, resulting in discontinuation of the stimulant. Taken together, these findings suggest that the assessment of children with ADHD and tics requires a review of tics and ADHD symptoms and may involve an on–off stimulant trial.

ASSESSMENT OF DISRUPTIVE BEHAVIOR DISORDERS

In DSM-IV-TR (American Psychiatric Association, 2000) the disruptive behavior disorders include conduct disorder (CD) and oppositional defiant disorder (ODD). ODD is defined by persistent noncompliance with rules and expectations, arguing with adult authority figures, low frustration tolerance, angry outbursts, and a tendency to blame others for interpersonal conflicts. This pattern of behavior begins early in life—even as early as preschool age (Lavigne et al., 2001). In children with TS, therefore, ODD may precede the onset of tics by several years. The prevalence of ODD is estimated at 5–10% in school-age children (Costello et al., 1996). It is distinguishable from CD, which is characterized by more serious antisocial behavior and direct violations of the rights of others, such as truancy, running away from home, stealing, vandalism, and aggression toward others. Children with TS appear to be at high risk for the explosive behavior, argumentativeness, and noncompliance that define ODD; however, they do not appear to be at increased risk for conduct disorder (see Sukhodolsky & Scahill, Chapter 10, this volume).

Assessment Tools

As with ADHD, the assessment of ODD relies on data collection from multiple informants—especially parents and teachers. The SNAP-IV and the ADHD Rating Scale have companion checklists for ODD (DuPaul et al., 1998; Swanson et al., 2001). These measures, which are based on DSM-IV symptoms for ODD, are also rated on a 0–3 scale, with higher scores corresponding to greater symptom severity. For both scales, an average per item score of 1.5 should alert the clinician to the likelihood that symptoms in this domain may be clinically meaningful and worthy of further inquiry (DuPaul et al., 1998; Swanson et al., 2001).

ASSESSMENT OF PERVASIVE DEVELOPMENTAL DISORDERS

The pervasive developmental disorders (PDDs) are a group of disorders characterized by severe impairments across multiple domains of development (American Psychiatric Association, 2000). Although it is not a defining feature of PDDs, a high percentage of these children are cognitively delayed as well. The most common forms of PDD include autistic disorder (autism), Asperger syndrome, and pervasive developmental disorder not otherwise specified (PDDNOS). These disorders share several common features, including delayed socialization, stereotypies (e.g., rocking and hand flapping), and overfocus on narrow interests (e.g., playing the same videotape over and over, peculiar preoccupations such as trains, electric fans, or air conditioners). Another common feature, which is essential for the diagnosis of autism, is language delay. Children with PDD tend to be rigid and insistent on following routines. An estimated at 20–30% of children with PDD have serious behavioral problems characterized by tantrums, aggression, and self-injury (RUPP Autism Network, 2002).

Differential Diagnosis of PDD

Autism is characterized by the early onset of impairments in all three PDD domains: socialization, communication, and repetitive behavior (stereotypies and restricted interests) (Volkmar & Pauls, 2003; Woodbury-Smith, Klin, & Volkmar, 2005). Many children with autism have little or no functional speech. Even for those children who develop language, the history is remarkable for language that is both delayed and deviant (echoing, neologisms, pronoun reversals). By contrast, children with Asperger syndrome do not have prominent language delay, and their intellectual functioning is likely to be normal or near normal. Their speech is often described as pedantic, and there is a general failure to recognize social cues—but language delay is not part of the patient's history. The most prominent feature in Asperger syndrome is the preoccupation with a narrow field of interest, such as an unusual degree of interest in a common topic—for example, horses or dinosaurs. Alternatively, the child may become immersed in a more esoteric interest such as the makes and models of air conditioners or succession of British royalty. The child's interest in this topic may intrude on any conversation. For example, when introduced to someone new, the child may immediately ask if the person has an air conditioner at home and then ask about the make and model. Children with Asperger syndrome may not notice that their interest on a specific topic is not shared by the listener. They may go on with their discourse, despite the lack of interest on the part of their listener. This persistence manifests both an inability to read social cues as well as the overfocus on the restricted interest. Children with TS may also perseverate on topic. Parents may report that the child "can't let go . . . " The difference is that in TS, the topic may swift from one week to the next and based on current events rather than an overencompassing topic that endures over time.

PDDNOS is the residual category for children who have social delay but may have milder forms of communication disability than children with autism. Affected children with PDDNOS may exhibit stereotypy or other repetitive behavior, they do not show the all-encompassing restricted interest as the child with Asperger syndrome.

Several recent epidemiological surveys indicate that the PDDs are more common than previously believed (Fombonne, 2003). The prevalence of autism is estimated at 10 to 20 per 10,000 in children, which is 2–10 times greater than previous estimates. This apparent increase in the detected prevalence probably reflects improved classification of children with developmental disorders rather than a true increase in prevalence. For example, a study of the special education registry in California showed a threefold increase in children classified with autism from the late 1980s to the mid-1990s. During this same period, there was also a substantial decrease in the number of children classified with mental retardation only. Another apparent source of the increase in the number of cases with autism came from children in the normal range of intelligence (Croen, Grether, Hoogstrate, & Selvin, 2002).

The prevalence of Asperger syndrome is presumed to be less common than autism and in the range of 2–5 per 10,000 in children. Although Asperger syndrome was first described over 50 years ago, it did not enter the official PDD nomenclature until 1994, and prevalence has not been well studied. Given the few community surveys that have focused on prevalence of Asperger syndrome, the level of confidence in the current estimate is not strong. The prevalence of PDDNOS is estimated to be in the range of 20–40 per 10,000 children (Fombonne, 2003).

The co-occurrence of PDD and TS in community samples is difficult to estimate, as few studies have been large enough to provide reliable estimates. Indeed, most reports on the co-occurrence of PDD and TS have come from clinical samples. In cases for whom the diagnosis of PDD (autism, Asperger's, or PDDNOS) is already established, parents may hope that the identification of TS will offer new directions for the treatment of PDD. Although understandable, this hope is unlikely to be realized except in cases of untreated tics. On the other hand, a new diagnosis of PDD in a child with TS could have a large impact on treatment planning, especially in the school setting.

Assessment Tools

The diagnosis of PDD is based on developmental history to establish the age of onset of delays in socialization, communication, and repetitive behavior. This review of development is followed by a careful examination of current functioning to determine whether impairments have persisted across these same domains. As noted above, the differential diagnosis of autism and Asperger syndrome turns on the history of delayed and deviant language in autism. By contrast, Asperger syndrome is not characterized by language delay. In addition to the core features of PDD, assessment should also consider intellectual capacity, adaptive functioning, and behavioral profiles.

The diagnosis of PDD can be aided by structured interview, such as the Autism Diagnostic Interview—Revised (ADI-R; Lord, Rutter, & Le Couteur, 1994). This interview covers the patient's current and past language functioning, social interactions, as well as restricted interests and stereotyped behaviors. The ADI-R is widely used in research settings but is not yet commonplace in clinical practice. Responses on the ADI-R can be scored, and thresholds have been established for the diagnosis of autism. Cutoff scores have not been established for Asperger syndrome or for PDDNOS. One drawback of the ADI-R is that it takes about 2 hours to complete.

One instrument that may be more commonly used in clinical practice to assist with diagnosis is the Childhood Autism Rating Scale (CARS; Schopler, Reichler, DeVellis, & Daly, 1980). The CARS is a 15-item scale that is rated by an experienced clinician following an interview with the parent and child. It permits the clinician to consider information gathered during the interview as well as from existing records and clinical observation. The 15-item scale is also able to distinguish mild to moderate autism from severe autism. Scores range from 15 to 60; a score of 30 is often used as the cutoff for autistic disorder. As with the ADI-R, there are no established thresholds for Asperger syndrome disorder or for PDDNOS. The diagnosis of PDD in a child with TS proceeds in much the same way as a child with PDD who does not have TS. An area of potential confusion in the assessment of a child with developmental delays and tics is stereotypies. In PDD, this term refers to abnormal movements such as hand flapping, rocking, waving fingers, or pacing. Hand flapping and rocking are unlikely to be mistaken for tics— but other repetitive behaviors in children with PDD may be more difficult to differentiate from tics. For example, rather than body rocking, a child with PDD may exhibit a variation of shifting weight from one foot to the other in a more tic-like fashion. The assessment principles of frequency, intensity, and interference still apply. Stereotypies and tics may respond to the same medications (RUPP Autism Network, 2002).

ASSESSMENT OF DEPRESSION

Depression is defined by symptoms of sadness, sleep and appetite disturbance, demoralization, change in activity level (usually decline), and loss of interest in usual activities—some or all of which persist for 2 weeks or more. The patient may also describe feeling worthless or hopeless, may ruminate on morbid themes, and may express suicidal ideation (American Psychiatric Association, 2000). The co-occurrence of depression in TS has been a matter of debate over the past two decades for the following reasons (Comings & Comings, 1987; King & Scahill, 2001; Pauls, Leckman, & Cohen, 1994). First, TS is a chronic condition, and the burden of chronic disease is often cited as a risk factor for depression (Burg & Abrams, 2001; Culpepper, 2002); however, reports from clinical case series do not show a dramatic increase in the frequency of depression in children and adolescents with TS alone, compared to the general population (Sukhodolsky et al., 2003). Second, it has been reported that depression recurs at a higher than expected rate in the families of children with TS. Comings and Comings (1987) argue that the burden of chronic disease is not a sufficient explanation. This finding was not replicated in a subsequent study (Pauls et al., 1994).

Third, the co-occurrence of OCD and depression is high (Flament et al., 1990). This observation, plus the effectiveness of selective serotonin reuptake inhibitors (SSRIs) for the treatment of depression and OCD, has led to speculation about possible shared neurobiology for these two disorders (Fitzgerald, MacMaster, Paulson, & Rosenberg, 1999). Indeed, children and adolescents with TS and OCD appear to be at higher risk for depression than those with TS alone. For example, in a clinically ascertained sample of children with TS, OCD, ADHD, (some with two or more of these conditions), Sukhodolsky and colleagues observed a prevalence of depression of 14% in children with TS only (Sukhodolsky et al., 2003). By contrast, children with OCD, alone or in combination with ADHD, had a much higher rate of depression (28% and 58%, respectively; Sukhodolsky et al., 2005). Taken together, these findings suggest that clinical samples of children and adolescents with TS alone may be at slightly increased risk of depression; those with OCD or OCD plus ADHD are at higher risk.

Assessment Tools

Based on these observations, children with TS should be screened for depressive symptoms, and greater attention to depression is warranted in children with TS in combination with OCD or ADHD. The clinical interview can review the child's interests and friendships as a way of identifying any recent decline in interests or involvements. Similarly, conversation about current activity level, sleep, and appetite can help to establish a change in these activities of daily living. If answers to these initial inquiries are positive, the clinician can follow with more specific questions about the presence of sadness, hopelessness, and suicidal ideation and plan.

Assessment tools that may be useful in the screening and diagnosis of depression include the parent-rated Child Behavior Checklist, which provides information about internalizing symptoms, relevant to depression (Achenbach, 1991). DSM-IV-based parent questionnaires such as the Child and Adolescent Symptom Inventory may provide more diagnosis-specific information (Gadow & Sprafkin, 1998). However, the assessment cannot rely completely on parent measures. Self-reports, such as the Children's Depression Inventory (CDI), although not diagnostic, permit the child to endorse depressive symptoms without having to verbalize issues that may be difficult to discuss. Structured interviews such as the Diagnostic Interview Schedule for Children (Shaffer, Fisher, Lucas, Dulcan, & Schwab-Stone, 2000) and the Anxiety Interview Schedule (Silverman & Nelles, 1988) provide a more systematic method of establishing the diagnosis of depression in pediatric patients.

ASSESSMENT OF BIPOLAR DISORDER

DSM-IV identifies two broad types of bipolar disorder: I and II. Bipolar I is characterized by the occurrence of a manic episode in the absence of depression. In contrast, bipolar II disorder is marked by a history of major depression and hypomanic episodes. A manic episode is defined by the presence of elevated or irritable mood, decreased need for sleep, racing thoughts, pressured speech, and increased goal-directed activity. Whether discrete manic episodes occur in children is a matter of considerable controversy (Findling, Kowatch, & Post, 2003), and questions remain about the validity of diagnosing bipolar illness in children. Available data suggest that bipolar disorder resembling the adult form of the illness is rare in prepubertal children, with gradual increase in prevalence during adolescence (Costello et al., 1996; Lewinsohn, Klein, & Seeley, 1995). If an expanded phenotype were accepted, however, the disorder would be more common. For example, Lewinsohn and colleagues (1995) surveyed nearly 2,000 adolescents from a single community and identified a prevalence of 1% for bipolar I and II combined. Another 5% showed core features of bipolar disorder, such as mood swings, irritability, sleep disturbance, and grandiosity. Although the youngsters with core features did not meet the criteria for bipolar illness, a high percentage did show evidence of functional impairment. These same investigators conducted a follow-up study of these adolescents 4–5 years later. The adolescents who showed core features without meeting criteria for bipolar illness were no more likely to develop bipolar upon follow-up than those in the general population. In fact, these adolescents with subthreshold bipolar symptoms in the first study were more likely to exhibit depression or anxiety disorders than bipolar illness at follow-up. Taken together, these findings indicate that subthreshold variants of bipolar illness are common—but these variants may not be part of a bipolar *spectrum*. Until the matter of threshold is resolved, the identification of bipolar illness in children will continue to be uncertain and controversial.

Given this uncertainty, treatment implications are also unclear. For example, it is unclear whether children and adolescents with TS and *core features* of bipolar illness should be treated with mood-stabilizing medications such as divalproex or lithium. This clinical question has not been evaluated in TS populations and only minimally studied in adolescent samples without TS (Donovan et al., 2000). The argument that treatment with a mood stabilizer could slow the progress from core symptoms to bipolar illness is not supported by the follow-up study conducted by Lewinsohn, Seeley, Buckley, and Klein (2002). Therefore, the usefulness of pharmacotherapy in children and adolescents with TS, accompanied by core bipolar symptoms who do not meet criteria for a bipolar illness, awaits further study.

Assessment Tools

Screening for bipolar disorder begins with observation in the clinical interview. During the interview, the clinician takes note of the tone, tempo, volume, and content of speech. Pressured speech and discourse that moves rapidly from one topic to another are cardinal signs of mania or hypomania. Grandiose ideas, such as implausible plans to make money or poorly thought-out plans to take trips to faraway places, may also be expressed in the open-ended clinical interview. Questions about recent activities and sleep may reveal little or no sleep for several days and increased pursuit of specific activities, perhaps involving sexual promiscuity or even productive activities such as painting or writing. In some cases of mania or hypomania, irritability is more prominent than elated mood. The difference between hypomania and mania is a matter of degree and duration. By definition, mania is characterized by marked impairment lasting for at least a week; in hypomania the impairment is of a lesser degree and the duration is at least 4 days.

Current guidelines clearly point out the difficulty of applying adult criteria to children and adolescents with bipolar disorder (Kowatch et al., 2005). In addition, conditions such as ADHD, ODD, anxiety, and depression have features such as hyperactivity, distractibility, garrulousness, mood instability, or irritability that are commonly observed in bipolar disorder. Even more confusing is the problem that ADHD or ODD may co-occur in youths with bipolar disorder. Thus, current guidelines recommend careful focus on the frequency, intensity, number, and duration of bipolar symptoms. Techniques such as charting the time line of mood symptoms is often useful. In clear cases, the episodic nature of the symptoms as well as the associated impairment will be easily identified. Instruments such as Schedule for Affective Disorders and Schizophrenia for School-Age Children (K-SADS) or Children's Interview for Psychiatric Symptoms (ChIPs) may be useful for organizing symptom elicitation and diagnosis (Kowatch et al., 2005).

ASSESSMENT OF AGGRESSIVE AND EXPLOSIVE BEHAVIOR

The frequency of aggression in patients with TS varies from 26 to 75% depending on the sample (Bliss, 1980; Moldofsky, Tullis, & Lamon, 1974; Stefl, 1984). When present, aggression and explosive behavior in children and adolescents with TS is multidetermined and often causes significant impairment in social and family functioning (Sukhodolsky et al., 2003). Therefore, aggression and explosive behavior may become a focus of treatment and require separate evaluation.

Assessment Tools

Clinical evaluation of aggressive and explosive behavior may include psychiatric interviews, parent ratings, and child reports (Collett, Ohan, & Myers, 2003). The choice and interpretation of these assessment instruments are related to the purpose of the given instrument. For example, questions about aggressive behavior in a semistructured psychiatric interview such as K-SADS (Kaufman et al., 1997) occur in the module on CD. Dimensional ratings scales, such as Aggression subscale of the Child Behavior Checklist (Achenbach, 1991), offer the capacity to quantify aggressiveness in an individual child (or group) in relation to standard scores. Self-reports, such as the Children's Inventory of Anger (Nelson &

Finch, 2000), may also be compared to population norms, but may have the drawback of underreporting.

There is no agreed-upon taxonomy for aggressive behaviors to guide evaluations. Some helpful classifications distinguish between overt and covert antisocial acts and verbal, physical, and object-directed aggression (Connor, 2002). Information about possible patient, family, and environment risk factors for aggression as well as the situations preceding aggressive acts is essential in clinical assessment. Situations and events that trigger and the consequences that follow aggressive behavior are fundamental to understanding the function of the behavior. Individual characteristics, such as style of emotional regulation and social-cognition, are particularly relevant to clinical case formulation. Finally, clinicians also need to evaluate frequency and seriousness of aggressive acts, possible association of aggression with co-occurring psychiatric conditions, and the impact of aggression on adaptive functioning.

CONCLUSION

TS is defined by the presence of motor and phonic tics. In addition to tics, there are several other potential sources of morbidity, including ADHD, OCD, anxiety and depression, disruptive behavior and aggression, and pervasive developmental disorders. For many children with TS, one or more of these co-occurring features may be the source of greater impairment than the tics. Indeed, data from clinical and community samples indicate that children with TS and ADHD are more impaired than children with TS only (Scahill et al., 2005; Sukhodolsky et al., 2003; see also Sukhodolsky & Scahill, Chapter 10, this volume). Although the evidence base is inadequate, emerging data from several studies offer guidance to clinicians on the management of tics, ADHD, and OCD in children with TS. In the absence of any specific information on co-occurring anxiety, depression, or pervasive developmental disorder, the assessment and treatment of these conditions in children with TS should follow best practice for children affected with those disorders who do not have TS. More study is needed to guide clinical practice on the treatment of disruptive behavior and aggression in children with TS.

REFERENCES

Achenbach, T. M. (1991). *Manual for the Child Behavior Checklist/4–18 and 1991 Profile.* Burlington, VT: University of Vermont Press.
American Psychiatric Association. (2000). *Diagnostic and statistical manual of mental disorders* (4th ed., text rev.). Washington, DC: Author.

Barkley, R. A., McMurray, M. B., Edelbrock, C. S., & Robbins, K. (1990). Side effects of methylphenidate in children with attention deficit hyperactivity disorder: A systemic, placebo-controlled evaluation. *Pediatrics, 86*(2), 184–192.

Bliss, J. (1980). Sensory experiences of Gilles de la Tourette syndrome. *Archives of General Psychiatry, 37*(12), 1343–1347.

Borcherding, B. G., Keysor, C. S., Rapoport, J. L., Elia, J., & Amass, J. (1990). Motor/vocal tics and compulsive behaviors on stimulant drugs: Is there a common vulnerability? *Psychiatry Research, 33*(1), 83–94.

Burg, M. M., & Abrams, D. (2001). Depression in chronic medical illness: The case of coronary heart disease. *Journal of Clinical Psychology, 57*(11), 1323–1337.

Castellanos, F., Giedd, J. N., Elia, J., Marsh, W. L., Rithie, G. F., Hamburger, S. D., et al. (1997). Controlled stimulant treatment of ADHD and comorbid Tourette's syndrome: Effects of stimulant and dose. *Journal of the American Academy of Child and Adolescent Psychiatry, 36*(5), 589–596.

Coffey, B. J., Biederman, J., Geller, D. A., Spencer, T. J., Kim, G. S., Bellordre, C. A., et al. (2000). Distinguishing illness severity from tic severity in children and adolescents with Tourette's disorder. *Journal of the American Academy of Child and Adolescent Psychiatry, 39*(5), 556–561.

Coffey, B. J., Biederman, J., Smoller, J. W., Geller, D. A., Sarin, P., Schwartz, S., et al. (2000). Anxiety disorders and tic severity in juveniles with Tourette's disorder. *Journal of the American Academy of Child and Adolescent Psychiatry, 39*(5), 562–568.

Collett, B. R., Ohan, J. L., & Myers, K. M. (2003). Ten-year review of rating scales: VI. Scales assessing externalizing behaviors. *Journal of the American Academy of Child and Adolescent Psychiatry, 42*(10), 1143–1170.

Comings, D. E., & Comings, B. G. (1987). A controlled study of Tourette syndrome: I. Attention-deficit disorder, learning disorders, and school problems. *American Journal of Human Genetics, 41*(5), 701–741.

Conners, C. K. (1997). *Conners' Rating Scales—Revised.* North Tonawanda, NY: Multi-Health Systems.

Connor, D. F. (2002). *Aggression and antisocial behavior in children and adolescents.* New York: Guilford Press.

Costello, E. J., & Angold, A. (1988). Scales to assess child and adolescent depression: Checklists, screens, and nets. *Journal of the American Academy of Child and Adolescent Psychiatry, 27*(6), 726–737.

Costello, E. J., Angold, A., Burns, B. J., Stangl, D. K., Tweed, D. L., Erkanli, A., et al. (1996). The Great Smoky Mountains Study of youth: Goals, design, methods, and the prevalence of DSM-III-R disorders. *Archives of General Psychiatry, 53*(12), 1129–1136.

Croen, L. A., Grether, J. K., Hoogstrate, J., & Selvin, S. (2002). The changing prevalence of autism in California. *Journal of Autism and Developmental Disorders, 32*(3), 207–215.

Culpepper, L. (2002). Depression and chronic medical illness: Diabetes as a model. *Psychiatric Annals, 32*(9), 528–534.

Donovan, S. J., Stewart, J. W., Nunes, E. V., Quitkin, F. M., Parides, M., Daniel, W., et al. (2000). Divalproex treatment for youth with explosive temper and mood lability: A double-blind, placebo-controlled crossover design. *American Journal of Psychiatry, 157*(5), 818–820.

Douglass, H. M., Moffitt, T. E., Dar, R., McGee, R., & Silva, P. (1995). Obsessive–compulsive disorder in a birth cohort of 18-year-olds: Prevalence and predictors. *Journal of the American Academy of Child and Adolescent Psychiatry, 34*(11), 1424–1431.

DuPaul, G. J., Power, T. J., Anastopoulos, A. D., & Reid, R. (1998). *ADHD Rating Scale-IV.* New York: Guilford Press.

Elia, J., Borcherding, B. G., Rapoport, J. L., & Keysor, C. S. (1991). Methylphenidate and dextroamphetamine treatments of hyperactivity: Are there true nonresponders? *Psychiatry Research, 36*(2), 141–155.

Erenberg, G., Cruse, R. P., & Rothner, A. D. (1985). Gilles de la Tourette's syndrome: Effects of stimulant drugs. *Neurology, 35*(9), 1346–1348.

Findling, R. L., Kowatch, R. A., & Post, R. M. (2003). *Pediatric bipolar disorder: A handbook for clinicians.* London: Murtin Dunitz.

Fitzgerald, K. D., MacMaster, F. P., Paulson, L. D., & Rosenberg, D. R. (1999). Neurobiology of childhood obsessive–compulsive disorder. *Child and Adolescent Psychiatric Clinics of North America, 8*(3), 533–575.

Flament, M. F., Koby, E., Rapoport, J. L., Berg, C. J., Zahn, T., Cox, C., et al. (1990). Childhood obsessive–compulsive disorder: A prospective follow-up study. *Journal of Child Psychology and Psychiatry and Allied Disciplines, 31*(3), 363–380.

Flament, M. F., Whitaker, A., Rapoport, J. L., Davies, M., Zaremba Berg, C., Kalikow, K., et al. (1988). Obsessive–compulsive disorder in adolescence: An epidemiological study. *Journal of the American Academy of Child and Adolescent Psychiatry, 27*(6), 764–771.

Fombonne, E. (2003). Epidemiological surveys of autism and other pervasive developmental disorders: An update. *Journal of Autism and Developmental Disorders, 33*(4), 365–382.

Gadow, K. D., & Sprafkin, J. (1998). *Child Symptom Inventory–4.* Stony Brook, NY: Checkmate Plus.

Gadow, K. D., Sverd, J., Sprafkin, J., Nolan, E. E., & Ezor, S. N. (1995). Efficacy of methylphenidate for attention-deficit hyperactivity disorder in children with tic disorder. *Archives of General Psychiatry, 52*(6), 444–455.

Gadow, K. D., Sverd, J., Sprafkin, J., Nolan, E. E., & Grossman, S. (1999). Long-term methylphenidate therapy in children with comorbid attention-deficit hyperactivity disorder and chronic multiple tic disorder. *Archives of General Psychiatry, 56*(4), 330–336.

Golden, G. S. (1974). Gilles de la Tourette's syndrome following methylphenidate administration. *Developmental Medicine and Child Neurology, 16*(1), 76–78.

Goodman, W. K., Price, L. H., Rasmussen, S. A., Mazure, C., Delgado, P., Heninger, G. R., et al. (1989). The Yale–Brown Obsessive Compulsive Scale: II. Validity. *Archives of General Psychiatry, 46*(11), 1012–1016.

Goodman, W. K., Price, L. H., Rasmussen, S. A., Mazure, C., Fleischmann, R. L., Hill, C. L., et al. (1989). The Yale–Brown Obsessive Compulsive Scale: I. Development, use, and reliability. *Archives of General Psychiatry, 46*(11), 1006–1011.

Goyette, C. H., Conners, C. K., & Ulrich, R. F. (1978). Normative data on revised Conners Parent and Teacher Rating Scales. *Journal of Abnormal Child Psychology, 6*(2), 221–236.

Greenhill, L. L., Abikoff, H. B., Arnold, L. E., Cantwell, D. P., Conners, C. K., Elliott, G., et al. (1996). Medication treatment strategies in the MTA study: Relevance to clinicians and researchers. *Journal of the American Academy of Child and Adolescent Psychiatry, 35*(10), 1304–1313.

Jankovic, J. (2001). Tourette's syndrome. *New England Journal of Medicine, 345*(16), 1184–1192.

Karno, M., Golding, J. M., Sorenson, S. B., & Burnam, M. A. (1988). The epidemiology of obsessive–compulsive disorder in five U.S. communities. *Archives of General Psychiatry, 45*(12), 1094–1099.

Kaufman, J., Birmaher, B., Brent, D., Rao, U., Flynn, C., Moreci, P., et al. (1997). Schedule for Affective Disorders and Schizophrenia for School-Age Children—Present and Lifetime Version (K-SADS-PL): Initial reliability and validity data. *Journal of the American Academy of Child and Adolescent Psychiatry, 36*(7), 980–988.

King, R. A., & Scahill, L. (2001). Emotional and behavioral difficulties associated with Tourette syndrome. *Advances in Neurology, 85*, 79–88.

Kowatch, R. A. Fristad, M., Birmaher, B., Wagner, K. D., Findling, R. L. Hellander, M.. & Child Psychiatric Workgroup on Bipolar Disorder. (2005). Treatment guidelines for children and adolescents with bipolar disorder. *Journal of the American Academy of Child and Adolescent Psychiatry, 44*(3), 213–235.

Lavigne, J. V., Cicchetti, C., Gibbons, R. D., Binns, H. J., Larsen, L., & Devito, C. (2001). Oppositional defiant disorder with onset in preschool years: Longitudinal stability and pathways to other disorders. *Journal of the American Academy of Child and Adolescent Psychiatry, 40*(12), 1393–1400.

Law, S. F., & Schachar, R. J. (1999). Do typical clinical doses of methylphenidate cause tics in children treated for attention-deficit hyperactivity disorder? *Journal of the American Academy of Child and Adolescent Psychiatry, 38*(8), 944–951.

Leckman, J. F. (2002). Tourette's syndrome. *Lancet, 360*(9345), 1577–1586.

Lewinsohn, P. M., Klein, D. N., & Seeley, J. R. (1995). Bipolar disorders in a community sample of older adolescents: Prevalence, phenomenology, comorbidity, and course. *Journal of the American Academy of Child and Adolescent Psychiatry, 34*(4), 454–463.

Lewinsohn, P. M., Seeley, J. R., Buckley, M. E., & Klein, D. N. (2002). Bipolar disorder in adolescence and young adulthood. *Child and Adolescent Psychiatric Clinics of North America, 11*(3), 461–475.

Lipkin, P. H., Goldstein, I. J., & Adesman, A. R. (1994). Tics and dyskinesias associated with stimulant treatment in attention-deficit hyperactivity disorder. *Archives of Pediatrics and Adolescent Medicine, 148*(8), 859–861.

Lord, C., Rutter, M., & Le Couteur, A. (1994). Autism Diagnostic Interview—Revised: A revised version of a diagnostic interview for caregivers of individuals with possible pervasive developmental disorders. *Journal of Autism and Developmental Disorders, 24*(5), 659–685.

Lowe, T. L., Cohen, D. J., Detlor, J., Kremenitzer, M. W., & Shaywitz, B. A. (1982). Stimulant medications precipitate Tourette's syndrome. *Journal of the American Medical Association, 247*(12), 1729–1731.

March, J. S., Sullivan, K., Stallings, P., Conners, C. K., & Parker, J. D. A. (1997). The Multidimensional Anxiety Scale for Children (MASC): Factor structure, reliability, and validity. *Journal of the American Academy of Child and Adolescent Psychiatry, 36*(4), 554–565.

McGee, R., Feehan, M., Williams, S., & Anderson, J. (1992). DSM-III disorders from age 11 to age 15 years. *Journal of the American Academy of Child and Adolescent Psychiatry, 31*(1), 50–59.

Michelson, D., Faries, D., Wernicke, J., Kelsey, D., Kendrick, K., Sallee, F. R., et al. (2001). Atomoxetine in the treatment of children and adolescents with attention-deficit/hyperactivity disorder: A randomized, placebo-controlled, dose–response study. *Pediatrics, 108*(5), E83.

Moldofsky, H., Tullis, C., & Lamon, R. (1974). Multiple tic syndrome (Gilles de la Tourette's syndrome). *Journal of Nervous and Mental Disease, 159*(4), 282–292.

MTA Cooperative Group. (1999). A 14-month randomized clinical trial of treatment strategies for attention-deficit/hyperactivity disorder: Multimodal treatment study of children with ADHD. *Archives of General Psychiatry, 56*(12), 1073–1086.

Nelson, W. M., & Finch, A. J. (2000). *Children's Inventory of Anger.* Los Angeles: Western Psychological Services.

Pauls, D. L., Leckman, J. F., & Cohen, D. J. (1994). Evidence against a genetic relationship between Tourette's syndrome and anxiety, depression, panic and phobic disorders. *British Journal of Psychiatry, 164*(2), 215–221.

Riddle, M. A., Lynch, K. A., Scahill, L., deVries, A., Cohen, D. J., & Leckman, J. F. (1995). Methylphenidate discontinuation and reinitiation during long-term treatment of children with Tourette's disorder and attention-deficit hyperactivity disorder: A pilot study. *Journal of Child and Adolescent Psychopharmacology, 5*(3), 205–214.

Rosenfeld, R., Dar, R., Anderson, D., Kobak, K. A., & Greist, J. H. (1992). A computer-administered version of the Yale–Brown Obsessive Compulsive Scale. *Psychological Assessment, 4,* 329–332.

RUPP Autism Network. (2002). Risperidone in children with autism and serious behavioral problems. *New England Journal of Medicine, 347*(5), 314–321.

Scahill, L., Chappell, P. B., Kim, Y. S., Schultz, R. T., Katsovich, L., Shepherd, E., et al. (2001). A placebo-controlled study of guanfacine in the treatment of children with tic disorders and attention deficit hyperactivity disorder. *American Journal of Psychiatry, 158*(7), 1067–1074.

Scahill, L., King, R. A., Carlson, A., do Rosario-Campos, M. C., Leckman, J. F., Kano, Y., et al. (2003). Influence of age and tic disorders on obsessive–compulsive disorder in a pediatric sample. *Journal of Child and Adolescent Psychopharmacology, 13*(Suppl. 1), 7–8.

Scahill, L., Riddle, M. A., McSwiggin-Hardin, M., Goodman, W. K., Ort, S. I., King, R. A., et al. (1997). Children's Yale–Brown Obsessive Compulsive Scale: Reliability and validity. *Journal of the American Academy of Child and Adolescent Psychiatry, 36*(6), 844–852.

Scahill, L., & Schwab-Stone, M. (2000). Epidemiology of ADHD in school-age children. *Child and Adolescent Psychiatric Clinics of North America, 9*(3), 541–555.

Scahill, L., Williams, S. K., Schwab-Stone, M., Applegate, J., & Leckman, J. F. (2006). Disruptive behavior problems in a community sample of children with tic disorders. *Advances in Neurology, 99,* 184–190.

Schopler, E., Reichler, R. J., DeVellis, R. F., & Daly, K. (1980). Toward objective classification of childhood autism: Childhood Autism Rating Scale (CARS). *Journal of Autism and Developmental Disorders, 10*(1), 91–103.

Shaffer, D., Fisher, P., Lucas, C. P., Dulcan, M. K., & Schwab-Stone, M. E. (2000). NIMH Diagnostic Interview Schedule for Children—Version IV (NIMH DISC-IV): Description, differences from previous versions, and reliability of some common diagnoses. *Journal of the American Academy of Child and Adolescent Psychiatry, 39*(1), 28–38.

Silverman, W. K., & Nelles, W. B. (1988). The anxiety disorders interview schedule for children. *Journal of the American Academy of Child and Adolescent Psychiatry, 27*(6), 772–778.

Stefl, M. E. (1984). Mental health needs associated with Tourette syndrome. *American Journal of Public Health, 74*(12), 1310–1313.

Steketee, G., Frost, R., & Bogart, K. (1996). The Yale–Brown Obsessive Compulsive Scale: Interview versus self-report. *Behaviour Research and Therapy, 34*(8), 675–684.

Sukhodolsky, D. G., do Rosario-Campos, M. C., Scahill, L., Katsovich, L., Pauls, D. L., Peterson, B. S., et al. (2005). Adaptive, emotional, and family functioning of children with obsessive–compulsive disorder and comorbid attention deficit hyperactivity disorder. *American Journal of Psychiatry, 162*(6), 1125–1132.

Sukhodolsky, D. G., Scahill, L., Zhang, H., Peterson, B. S., King, R. A., Lombroso, P. J., et al. (2003). Disruptive behavior in children with Tourette's syndrome: Association with ADHD comorbidity, tic severity, and functional impairment. *Journal of the American Academy of Child and Adolescent Psychiatry, 42*(1), 98–105.

Swanson, J. M., Kraemer, H. C., Hinshaw, S. P., Arnold, L. E., Conners, C. K., Abikoff, H. B., et al. (2001). Clinical relevance of the primary findings of the MTA: Success rates based on severity of ADHD and ODD symptoms at the end of treatment. *Journal of the American Academy of Child and Adolescent Psychiatry, 40*(2), 168–179.

Tourette's Syndrome Study Group. (2002). Treatment of ADHD in children with tics: A randomized controlled trial. *Neurology, 58*(4), 527–536.

Valleni-Basile, L. A., Garrison, C. Z., Jackson, K. L., Waller, J. L., McKeown, R. E., Addy, C. L., et al. (1995). Family and psychosocial predictors of obsessive compulsive disorder in a community sample of young adolescents. *Journal of Child and Family Studies, 4,* 193–206.

Varley, C. K., Vincent, J., Varley, P., & Calderon, R. (2001). Emergence of tics in children with attention deficit hyperactivity disorder treated with stimulant medications. *Comprehensive Psychiatry, 42*(3), 228–233.

Volkmar, F. R., & Pauls, D. (2003). Autism. *Lancet, 362*(9390), 1133–1141.

Woodbury-Smith, M., Klin, A., & Volkmar, F. (2005). Asperger's syndrome: A comparison of clinical diagnoses and those made according to the ICD-10 and DSM-IV. *Journal of Autism and Developmental Disorders, 35*(2), 235–240.

Zohar, A. H., Ratzoni, G., Pauls, D. L., Apter, A., Bleich, A., Kron, S., et al. (1992). An epidemiological study of obsessive–compulsive disorder and related disorders in Israeli adolescents. *Journal of the American Academy of Child and Adolescent Psychiatry, 31*(6), 1057–1061.

CHAPTER 5

Genetic and Neurobiological Bases for Tourette Syndrome

JANA LEARY
TYLER REIMSCHISEL
HARVEY S. SINGER

Demonstration that a complex disorder such as Tourette syndrome (TS) has a genetic origin with neurobiological underpinnings requires a sequential process of scientific study. For example, steps used to identify the genetic basis of a disease often include (1) clinical observation of familial clustering, (2) utilization of twin studies to distinguish genetic contribution from environmental contribution, (3) determination of the mode of transmission, and (4) discovery of causative genes. Similarly, confirmation of a neurobiological basis for a disorder requires (1) determination of the anatomical localization of the biological lesion, (2) identification of potentially causative neurophysiological abnormalities, and (3) discovery of precise neurochemical disturbances that may be contributing to the pathophysiology. The goal of this chapter is to use the aforementioned categories to outline the scientific advances for both the genetics and neurobiology of TS.

GENETICS OF TS

Beginning with Georges Gilles de la Tourette's initial description of the syndrome that carries his name, clinicians have identified the increased rates of tic disorders in family members. Family studies have repeatedly demonstrated an increased risk of TS in relatives of affected individuals as compared to the incidence in the general population (Hebebrand, Nothen, Ziegler, et al., 1997; Pauls, Raymond, Stevenson, & Leckman, 1991; Kano, Ohta, Nagai, Pauls, & Leckman, 2001). Twins studies, which provide the most powerful evidence for a genetic basis in TS, have documented an increased concordance rate in identical (77–94%) versus nonidentical twins (23%) (Hyde, Aaronson, Randolph, Rickler, & Weinberger, 1992; Price, Kidd, Cohen, Pauls, & Leckman, 1985; Shapiro, Shapiro, Bruun, & Sweet, 1978). Hence, both twin and family studies have strongly suggested that one or more genes contribute to the pathogenesis of TS. Several approaches, including complex segregation analysis, linkage analysis, candidate gene evaluation, studies of molecular polymorphisms, association studies, and investigations of cytogenetic abnormalities, have been used to identify the causative gene(s). The aim of the genetics portion of this chapter is to review each of these techniques and to discuss the results pertaining to TS.

Segregation Analysis

The statistical approach most commonly used to identify the mode of inheritance is segregation analysis. To complete a segregation analysis, multiple families containing at least one person with TS are evaluated for tic symptoms and co-occurring disorders. The data are processed by a computer program that analyzes the pedigree information by following different algorithms for each potential mode of inheritance. These complex mathematical programs then determine the maximum likelihood of each mode of inheritance with the highest likelihood score suggestive of the true mode of transmission in the population studied.

Results in Families with TS

Results of segregation analyses have been inconsistent. The earliest studies suggested an autosomal dominant (AD) mode of inheritance (Eapen, Pauls, & Robertson, 1993; Walkup et al., 1996; Pauls & Leckman, 1986; Comings & Comings, 1984), that was not confirmed by other studies. For example, two large linkage studies, which together scanned the entire genome, found no DNA regions linked to the TS phenotype using an AD model (Barr et al., 1999; Pakstis et al., 1991). Furthermore, other investigators have determined that the most suitable model for their observed pedigrees was a mixed model, that is, one major gene with contributing minor genes and environmental factors (Walkup et al., 1996; Comings, Comings, Devor, & Cloniger, 1984). Seuchter et al.

(2000) reported the mode of transmission to be non-Mendelian but consistent with an unrestricted model rather than the mixed model previously described (Seuchter et al., 2000). In sum, segregation analyses using larger samples suggest a more complex non-Mendelian inheritance pattern for TS. Unfortunately, this change in our understanding of the complex nature of TS genetics has not been adequately conveyed to patients, families, and the popular media, who continue to consider TS a simple AD condition.

Complicating Factors

A number of reasons have been postulated—including phenotypic heterogeneity, polygenicity, and epigenetic factors—to explain the lack of a clear finding in family studies.

Phenotypic Heterogeneity

Due to the established yet still ill-defined relationship between chronic tic disorders (CT) and obsessive–compulsive disorder (OCD) (Paul, Towbin, Leckman, Zahner, & Cohen, 1986; Pitman, Green, Jenike, & Mesulam, 1987; Grad, Pelcovitz, Olson, Matthews, & Grad, 1987), TS should be considered a phenotypically heterogeneous disorder in which the same genetic perturbation(s) may manifest differently among individuals. This understanding requires each investigator to define his or her own affected phenotype before collecting data for segregation analysis. As might be predicted, many groups have selected different definitions. Comings et al. (1984) defined their phenotype as TS or multiple tics, whereas Seuchter et al. (2000) defined the affected as TS, CT, tic disorder not otherwise specified (TDNOS), or OCD. Thus, if these disorders are less genetically related than assumed—that is, if each has a separate mode of inheritance—then different definitions of the affected phenotype could lead to nonconvergent results.

Polygenicity

The phenotype of a polygenic disorder is determined by mutations in multiple genes, of which no single gene is pathogenic alone. These multiple genes, in turn, contribute to different systems or pathways that eventually converge to cause the underlying pathophysiology. Polygenicity results in a complex trait—a disease caused by multiple DNA alterations and environmental influences. If TS is, in fact, a polygenic complex trait, then each family analyzed in the segregation analyses could have different combinations of genes contributing to the TS phenotype, and nonconvergent results would be understandable, if not to be expected.

Epigenetic Factors

Epigenetic factors—factors that alter the expression of a gene rather than its sequence—could also be the cause of inconsistent results from segregation analyses. Examples of these factors are discussed in detail later in the chapter. In brief, statistical methods used in segregation analyses do not have the capacity to define epigenetic parameters; this incapacity may thereby overlook possible contributors to inaccurate analyses.

Linkage Analysis

Linkage analysis is an approach commonly used to find causative genes by attempting to identify a DNA marker of known location that is inherited significantly more often in affected family members than in unaffected members. If such a DNA segment is found, it is then inferred that a pathogenic gene, which is at least partially responsible for the pathogenesis of a disorder, lies near that marker.

Understanding linkage analysis requires knowledge of the process of recombination, which can occur during cell division. Figure 5.1 illustrates recombination between two chromosomes containing a hypothetical allele T (contributing to the TS phenotype) and DNA marker S. Four genotypes result upon completion of meiosis: nonrecombinant TS and ts (identical to the original parental combinations) and recombinant Ts and tS (crossing over occurred between the two loci). If these loci are on different chromosomes or on separate arms of one chromosome, independent assortment will result in equal proportions of each type of offspring. However, if the loci are present on the same chromosome (and usually physically close in space), they could be linked, assorting together during meiosis, resulting in a lower frequency of recombination.

In these analyses, because of the size and complexity of each family's pedigree, investigators use computer programs to analyze possible linkage. Results are reported as log of odds (LOD) score—essentially the ratio of the likelihood that two loci are linked divided by the likelihood that they are not linked. An LOD score greater than 3 at a particular marker site is said to be statistically significant for linkage—suggesting that a causative gene or regulatory element is located near that marker. An LOD score greater than 2 is not considered strong evidence of linkage, but may be pursued with other genetic techniques such as "fine mapping." The latter is a process that looks more closely at the area uti-

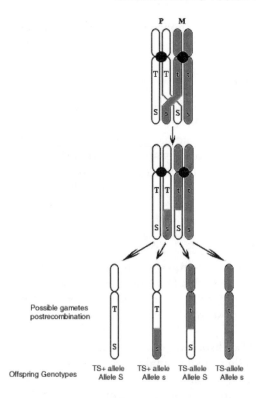

FIGURE 5.1. A single crossover between two homologous chromosomes in meiosis results in two nonrecombinant genotypes in offspring (TS and ts) and two recombinant genotypes (Ts and tS). Frequencies of the nonrecombinant and recombinant genotypes are utilized to calculate LOD scores and demonstrate linkage.

lizing multiple markers to define a narrower segment of DNA that could be linked to the TS phenotype.

Results in TS

Linkage studies have identified multiple different chromosomal segments linked to the TS phenotype, rather than only one or a few unifying DNA regions. A Tourette Syndrome International Consortium for Genetics, identifying alleles shared more often by two affected siblings than expected by chance alone, found two regions of interest on chromosomes 4q and 8p (TSAICG, 1999). In further analyses by this same group, linkage analysis in 238 affected sib-pair families and 18 multigenerational families identified significant evidence for linkage to a marker on chromosome 2p32.2 (TSAICG, 2007). This latter investigation also identified other chromosomal regions, including 3p, 3q, and 14q, with LOD scores greater than 2.5 in sib-pair samples but not in multigenerational pedigrees. Verkerk et al. (2006), using multipoint analysis, found a single linkage peak (LOD score 2.55) with marker D3S1311 on chromosome 3q. Simonic et al. (2001) identified significant evidence for linkage on chromosomes 2p, 8q, and 11q. Linkage to the DNA segment on chromosome 11q in their TS patients was similar to that reported by Merette et al. (2000). McMahon et al. (1996) found regions on chromosomes 17q and 8q that were suggestive of linkage, although they did not reach statistically significant LOD scores. Barr et al. (1999) identified regions on chromosomes 19p and 5p suggestive of linkage (did not reach statistical significance) in more than one family. Although their analyses also identified regions on chromosomes 5, 7, 11, 13, 14, 16, and 19 with significant LOD scores, the program used in the analysis is known to have high false-positive rates. Adding to the diversity of findings, Curtis et al. (2004) has reported evidence of linkage on chromosomes 5, 10, and 13. In summary, results continue to suggest a complex inheritance model with locus heterogeneity and a gene of major effect. A potential region on chromosome 2p32.2 is of particular interest because it has been identified in both sib-pair and large families. Additionally, the chromosomal region 11q23–24, identified in patients with TS by two independent groups, warrants further investigation.

Complicating Factors

Multiple variables may account for the lack of consistent findings in linkage analyses. First, some methods require the investigator to define the mode of inheritance. As seen in the previous section, the mode of transmission for TS is not yet definitively understood. Secondly, if TS is truly a complex genetic disorder, as suggested by the segregation analyses, it is possible that linkage studies may merely be reflecting that complexity. For example, if multiple genes at different sites can contribute to the TS phenotype, clearly many different chromosomal regions would be identified by linkage studies. Thirdly, although the scientific process is very rigorous, errors can occur in the assessment of the individual subjects and in the determination of individual genotypes. Finally, it is possible that current genetic approaches are inadequate to detect the abnormality. In this regard, although the use of 300 markers throughout the genome is thought to provide sufficient density to demonstrate a statistically significant linkage for an AD disease, it is possible that even more markers are necessary to demonstrate linkage for a more complex disorder such as TS. Genetic methods, especially the technology of gene finding, are expanding rapidly and offer the hope that the gene(s) for TS will soon be identified.

Candidate Gene Studies

Another approach is to combine linkage analysis with our expanding knowledge of the neurobiology of TS; that is, to determine if specific genes are involved in TS. For example, cortical–striatal–thalamic–cortical (CSTC) circuit abnormalities have long been established in TS, making all genes that encode neurotransmitters and synaptic proteins in these circuits' excellent candidate genes. In many instances, as a result of the Human Genome Project, the locations of these genes are already known. Hence, investigators have attempted to establish whether there is linkage between known specific genes and TS.

Results in Patients with TS

Despite the promise of candidate gene approaches, studies completed to date have had mostly negative or unconfirmed findings. For example, even though the dopaminergic system has been proposed to play a part in TS pathogenesis (Bruggeman et al., 2001), no consistent linkage or association could be demonstrated between patients with TS and the dopamine D2–D5 receptor alleles (Hebebrand et al., 1997; Diaz-Anzaldua et al., 2004; Devor, Dill-Devor, & Magee, 1998; Barr, Wigg, Zivko, Sandor, & Tsui, 1997) or mutations in the D1 receptor (Thompson, Comings, Feder, George, & O'Dowd, 1998) or dopamine ß-hydroxylase gene (Ozbay et al., 2006). Association studies or mutation screenings also yielded negative results for the dopamine and norepinephrine transporters (Diaz-Anzaldua et al., 2004; Stober et al., 1999). Linkage was also not demonstrated between TS and the glycine, GABA, glutamate, α- and ß-adrenergic, or glucocorticoid receptor alleles (Barr et al., 1999; Brett, Curtis, Robertson, & Gurling, 1997), or between TS and a functional polymorphism in the catechol-O-methyltransferase gene (Barr, Wigg, & Sandor, 1999).

Complicating Factors

Methodological issues, as described above for segregation analyses and linkage studies, may again explain the lack of candidate gene findings. In addition, if TS is more of a polygenic condition, then negative candidate gene results would be expected. If multiple loci can contribute to the TS phenotype, it is also possible that each study simply did not recruit adequate families with a phenotype contribution from the particular susceptibility gene being scrutinized. Additionally, it is possible that investigators are simply not studying the correct candidate genes. For example, a microarray analysis that identified genes with abnormal expression in the putamen of deceased TS patients suggested that the VAMP-2 and glutamate receptor metabotropic 3 genes had abnormal expression and concentrations of product (Hong et al., 2004). Therefore, utilizing our expanding knowledge of TS neurobiology, we recognize that many more candidate genes remain to be studied, including those implicated by microarray analyses and those involved with neurotransmitter release and second messenger pathways.

Association Studies of Polymorphisms Using a Candidate Gene Approach

The failure of family and candidate gene studies to identify a precise linkage to TS has led investigators to examine polymorphism (changes in DNA sequence) associations. Using known polymorphisms located on candidate genes, investigators have attempted to determine whether specific polymorphisms are more commonly seen in TS individuals and families than in control populations. Association studies, unlike candidate gene studies, make no assumptions about a marker's possible genetic contribution to TS. By using polymorphisms, these studies attempt to demonstrate an association between a marker and the TS phenotype. Unfortunately, this approach cannot prove causation, only a potential association. False positives are relatively common and often occur due to use of inappropriate control groups, such as subjects with ethnic backgrounds that differ from the affected subjects.

Results in Patients with TS

In a study performed in the Singer laboratory (Yoon et al., in press), DNA was obtained from 266 individuals with TS ± attention-deficit/hyperactivity disorder (ADHD) and 236 controls that were matched for ethnicity. Polymorphisms investigated included the dopamine transporter (DAT1 *Dde*I and DAT1 VNTR), dopamine receptor (D4 Upstream Repeat and D4 VNTR), dopamine converting enzyme (dopamine ß-hydroxylase), and the acid phosphatase locus 1 (ACP1) gene. A significant association, using a genotype-based association analysis, was identified for the TS-total and TS-only versus control groups for the DAT1 *Dde*I polymorphism (nucleotides AG vs. AA, $p = .004$ and $p = .01$, respectively). A statistical reevaluation of DAT1 *Dde*I polymorphism following population stratification confirmed the association for the TS-total and TS-only groups, but the degree of significance was reduced. This study has thus identified a significant association between the presence of TS and a DAT polymorphism. Because abnormalities of the dopamine transporter have been hypothesized in the pathophysiology of TS, the possibility that a susceptibility factor or functional allele affects the expression of the phenotype cannot be excluded.

Associations have also been reported between the dopamine receptor D4 (DRD4) 7 repeat allele and the TS phenotype (Grice et al., 1996; Abelson et al., 2005; Cruz et al., 1997). However, other investigators reported no greater frequency of the 7 repeat allele in TS patients than was observed in control groups (Hebebrand et al., 1997; Huang et al., 2002). This controversy has yet to be resolved. All other polymorphisms investigated in candidate genes returned negative results. The a-2A and a-1C adrenergic receptors (located near markers linked to TS by sib-pair studies) and the central cannabinoid receptor gene (*CNR1*), implicated in TS pathogenesis because of the positive effects of marijuana on frequency of tic symptoms, all failed to demonstrate any polymorphisms significantly associated with the TS phenotype (Xu et al., 2003; Gadzicki et al., 2004). Similarly, the ACP1*A allele of a protein tyrosine phosphatase gene, thought to contribute to TS by regulating serotoninergic and dopaminergic systems, revealed no association with TS (Bottini et al., 2002).

Complicating Factors

Limitations of polymorphism studies are numerous and include inaccurate definition of the phenotype; failure to eliminate the possibility that a specific polymorphism could be linked to other coexisting neuropsychiatric issues such as ADHD, OCD, anxiety, or depression; and the inclusion of control populations that are insufficient in size, unmatched for age and gender, and not screened for population stratification. Lastly, there is the possibility that association screening studies evaluating multiple polymorphisms can be influenced by a multiple testing effect. Hence, additional association studies in larger numbers of well-characterized TS patients and their parents will be necessary to clarify the clinical association between TS and the DAT1 *DdeI* locus.

Chromosomal Abnormalities

Investigation of chromosomal abnormalities has become an alternative method of identifying candidate genes. If a chromosomal abnormality is observed in a patient with TS, it is possible that the abnormality is coincidental and has no contribution to the pathogenesis of TS. However, if a gene is disrupted by the chromosomal abnormality, this gene could potentially be causative and should therefore be investigated as a candidate gene. This is especially true if the pedigree data suggest that family members with a tic disorder also share a higher frequency of the chromosomal abnormality.

Results in Patients with TS with Chromosomal Translocations

CHROMOSOME 13Q

Based on the presence of a de novo chromosomal inversion at 13q31.1 in a child with TS, Abelson and colleagues (2005) evaluated proximal candidate genes, leading to a possible association with *SLITRK1*. *SLITRK1* is a gene with an associated protein that binds to extracellular signaling molecules and affects the growth and shape of neurons during development (Aruga & Mikoshiba, 2003). This gene derives its name from its similarity to *Slit*, a well-known gene in growing neurons during brain development, and Trk, a family of tyrosine protein kinase receptors. *SLITRK1* is expressed in specific regions of the brain that are known to be affected in TS. Because the abnormality was identified in a single family and results have not been confirmed in additional TS populations, *SLITRK1* is not considered "the" gene for TS (Deng, Le, Xie, & Jankovic, 2006). This finding is, however, an important early step in understanding how genetic abnormalities may ultimately result in TS symptoms (Selling, 1929).

CHROMOSOME 18Q

An 18q22.3 breakpoint was identified in multiple TS patients having balanced t(7;18) translocations (Boghosian-Sell, Comings, & Overhauser, 1996), and similarly, State et al. (2003) observed an 18q22.1–q22.2 inversion in a TS patient. Unfortunately, the DNA regions flanking these breakpoints demonstrated no linkage with TS (Heutink et al., 1990).

CHROMOSOME 7Q

Two studies have suggested regions on chromosome 7q to be of interest. Kroisel et al. (2001) identified a de novo duplication of the 7q22.1–33.1 region, and Verkerk et al. (2003) identified a complex insertion/translocation involving chromosome 2 and 7q35–36 in a TS-affected family. Upon further investigation, Verkerk et al. identified the *CNTNAP2* gene, encoding a neurexin located in the nodes of Ranvier, near the breakpoint. However, mutation screens or linkage studies have yet to be performed to confirm the contribution of this gene to the TS phenotype.

CHROMOSOME 8Q

In the study of a TS patient with a balanced t(3;8) chromosomal translocation, Brett, Curtis, Robertson, Dahlitz, and Gurling (1996) discovered breakpoints at 3p21.3 and 8q24.1. More recently, a TS-affected family with a balanced t(1;8) translocation revealed breakpoints at 1q22.1 and 8q22.1, near regions previously linked to TS by Simonic et al. (2001) and Matsumoto et al. (2000). Further study revealed the *CBFA2T1* gene (encoding a transcription factor) just distal to the 8q breakpoint, but unrelated TS patients displayed no mutations in this gene. Similarly, two TS families with balanced t(6;8) translocations displayed breakpoints in the 8q13 region (Crawford et al., 2003). The 8q13 region is of particular interest because the breakpoint occurred in the same 250-kb region in both unrelated families, and this segment also lies between two regions linked to TS by Simonic et al. (2001) and Taylor et al. (1991). Further candidate gene studies are necessary in this DNA segment.

CHROMOSOME 9P

Chromosomal deletions involving chromosome 9p have been described in two studies of individuals with TS (Taylor et al., 1991; Singh, Howe, Jordan, & Hara, 1982). A search for genes in the deleted regions has yet to be performed.

Complicating Factors

The results of these studies are somewhat more consistent than the others in that we have seen some replication of findings. As mentioned, certain DNA regions identified are in need of further research to determine candidate genes in those segments. As for investigative groups that took the extra step and searched for candidate genes, to no avail, one must keep in mind that their breakpoint could be disrupting the promoter or enhancer of an important contributing gene. More research is necessary to confirm this possibility.

Epigenetic and Environmental Factors

Epigenetic factors could be another explanation for why it has been so challenging to identify the gene(s) for TS. Epigenetic factors, unlike genetic factors, are not related to the sequence of DNA but instead impact a gene's regulation and thus its expression. Investigators are now exploring whether epigenetic factors such as *imprinting* (effect of the transmitting parent on gene expression in an offspring), or environmental factors such as maternal stress, poor prenatal care, low birth weight, and others, could alter the expression of a gene involved in TS pathogenesis. Burd, Severud, Klug, and Kerbeshian (1999) in a retrospective review, has identified an association between poor prenatal care and frequency of TS in children. A study of imprinting in families with TS reported that maternal transmission of the disorder resulted in a more complex pattern of motor tics (Lichter, Jackson, & Schacter, 1995). Further replication asynchrony (which can occur upon imprinting) has been demonstrated in a TS patient with a chromosomal inversion (State et al., 2003).

NEUROBIOLOGY OF TS

Advances in the neurobiology of TS can be divided into three major areas: neuroanatomy, neurophysiology, and neurochemistry (Table 5.1).

Where Is the Neuroanatomical Lesion in TS?

CSTC circuitry has long been suspected in TS pathogenesis. Five parallel CSTC circuits, identified in primates, could correlate with clinical symptomology in TS: (1) a motor pathway contributing to motor tic pathogenesis; (2) an oculomotor pathway causing generation of ocular

---

TABLE 5.1. Three Neurobiological Questions and Hypotheses Proposed to Answer Each

1. Proposed sites for the primary neuroanatomical lesion
   a. Frontal cortex
   b. Striatum
   c. Thalamus
   d. Midbrain
2. Potential neurophysiological abnormality
   a. Excess striatal excitation
   b. Altered interstriatal circuitry
   c. Altered striatal output
   d. Excess thalamic–cortical excitation
   e. Altered thalamic–striatal excitation
   f. Impaired cortical inhibition
3. Possible neurochemical bases for TS pathogenesis
   a. Dopamine
      1. Abnormal tonic/phasic DA release system
      2. Dopamine hyperinnervation
      3. Supersensitive dopamine receptors
      4. Excess presynaptic DA synthesis
   b. Glutamate
   c. GABA
   d. Serotonin
   e. Acetylcholine
   f. Neuropeptides

tics; (3) a dorsolateral prefrontal pathway contributing to attention deficits; (4) a lateral orbitofrontal pathway involved in OCD pathogenesis, and, finally; (5) the anterior cingulate pathway, causing behavioral problems and OCD (Alexander, DeLong, & Strick, 1986; Cummings, 1993; see Figure 5.2).

Although most investigators do not dispute CSTC involvement in TS pathogenesis, the precise location of the neuroanatomical lesion within these circuits is unknown. Several approaches have been used to determine the neuroanatomical localization, including neurological and psychological examinations, brain imaging, and neuropathological studies. Results have suggested involvement of both cortical and subcortical (striatal) regions in TS. Recognizing that these regions are integrated by circuits, it is possible that a disruptive lesion in either site could cause common symptoms.

Studies Suggestive of a Cortical Lesion in TS

Executive functioning is thought to depend on an intact and properly functioning prefrontal cortex. Psychological examinations in children with TS, regardless of ADHD status, have reproducibly revealed abnormalities in executive functioning such as planning, organization, inhibition of behavior, and sequenced behavior (Harris et al., 1995; Schuerholz, Baumgardner, Singer, Reiss, & Denckla, 1996; Mahone,

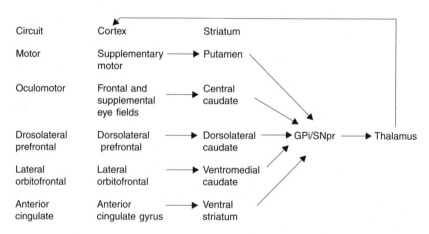

FIGURE 5.2. Five parallel CSTC circuits. Cortical areas project to various striatal areas, proceeding through the GPi/SNpr to the thalamus, and finally returning to the cortex, completing the circuit. GPi, globus pallidus interna; SNpr, substantia nigra pars reticulata.

Koth, Cutting, Singer, & Denckla, 2001; Muller et al., 2003). Motor evaluations in TS patients have identified deficits in sequence motor task performance further suggesting prefrontal and frontal cortical dysfunction (Sheppard, Bradshaw, Georgiou, Bradshaw, & Lee, 2000). Lastly tasks assessing a precision grip coupled with functional MRI studies, documented a decreased activation of secondary cortical motor areas, suggesting a dysfunction of secondary motor cortices (Serrien et al., 2002).

A variety of radiographic studies, including simple magnetic resonance imaging (MRI), positron emission tomography (PET), and single photon emission computerized tomography (SPECT) studies, volumetric MRI, and functional MRI, have identified cortical abnormalities in TS patients. Although the majority of routine computerized tomographies (CTs) and MRIs have failed to identify any abnormalities that could convincingly be associated with TS pathogenesis, several case reports have shown frontal lesions that could be associated with TS symptomatology (McAbee, Ward, & Manning, 1999; Yochelson & David, 2000). Although such findings do not prove causation, they do suggest the potential for some contribution of frontal cortical abnormalities to TS pathogenesis. In contrast, volumetric MRI and functional MRI have consistently identified cortical abnormalities in TS. Volumetric MRI has identified larger dorsolateral prefrontal regions in TS children relative to TS adults and controls (Peterson et al., 2001), which were inversely proportional to tic severity (Gerard & Peterson, 2003). Such volumetric changes are not well understood and could be associated with an adaptive rather than pathogenic process in TS (Gerard & Peterson, 2003). Volumetric change in frontal white matter has been noted in two TS studies: (1) Frederickson et al. (2002) reported a volumetric increase of white matter in the right frontal lobe, whereas (2) studies by Kates et al. (2002) revealed decreased cortical white matter in deep left frontal areas. In addition, the size of the corpus callosum, a brain structure involved in interhemispheric communication, has been shown to have both increased and decreased size in individuals with TS (Baumgardner et al., 1996; Peterson et al., 1994). Functional MRI studies of TS patients have suggested cortical abnormalities in the sensory–motor and supplemental motor cortices (Biswal et al., 1998) and proposed that prefrontal cortical functioning was involved in tic suppression (Peterson et al., 1998). PET studies have shown decreased metabolic activity within the frontal, cingulate, and insular cortices (Baxter, 1990; Baxter, Schwartz, Guze, Bergman, & Szuba, 1990; Stoetter et al., 1992). Similarly, SPECT studies have reported decreased blood flow bilaterally in cingular and dorsolateral prefrontal cortices (Diler, Reyhanli, Toros, Kibar, & Auci, 2002). Transcranial magnetic stimulation studies suggest that tics originate from impaired inhibition at the level of the motor cortex (Moll et al., 1999).

Studies Suggestive of a Basal Ganglia Lesion in TS

Many of the same study approaches that were used to investigate cortical abnormalities have also identified changes within the basal ganglia (BG) patients with TS but the same caveats: that is, abnormalities in individual patients are only suggestive. Studies comparing patients with TS to controls may identify either a pathological state or an adaptation to such as state.

Bilateral globus pallidus (GP) lesions have been identified by MRI in a 17-year-old with ADHD, OCD, stuttering, and gait abnormalities (Demirkol, Erdem, Inan, & Guney, 1999). Volumetric MRI studies have reproducibly identified decreased size or asymmetry of the caudate nucleus, putamen, or lenticular nuclei (GP/putamen) in children and adults with TS (Peterson et al., 1993; Hyde et al., 1995; Singer et al., 1993; Moriarity et al., 1997). Functional MRI has identified signal intensity changes in the BG and thalamus during the expression of tics (Peterson et al., 1998). Similar to results in the cortex, a greater magnitude of signal change correlated with less severe tic expression, suggesting that tic suppression involves both the prefrontal cortex and caudate. PET studies have reported bilaterally increased or decreased glucose utilization within the BG of individuals with TS (Baxter, 1990; Baxter et al., 1990), and SPECT studies have identified decreased blood flow to the BG in some patients with TS (Hall, Costa, & Shields, 1991). Several investigators have also emphasized involvement of the ventral striatum in TS. In studies assessing functional coupling of regional cerebral metabolic rates for glucose, connectivity of the ventral striatum differentiated subjects with TS from control subjects (Jeffries et al., 2002). The ventral striatum is also involved with the formation of habit memories and is a regulator of stereotyped behaviors.

Several comprehensive neuropathological studies have reported contradictory results: (1) a histological examination of the striatum from a 42-year-old patient with TS showed increased density of neurons, a finding often seen in very young children, suggesting an "arrested development" of the caudate/putamen (Balthasar, 1957); (2) tissue samples from an 18-year-old individual with TS failed to identify any abnormalities within the cerebellum, red nucleus, olivary nucleus, cortex, BG, or cervical spinal cord (DeWult & van Bogaret, 1941); and (3) a quantitative postmortem study of the BG in patients with TS showed a profound imbalance in the number of parvalbumin-positive neurons—that is, increased in the GPi and decreased in the striatum as compared to controls (Kalanithi et al., 2005).

What Is the Neurophysiological Abnormality in TS?

Recognition that the CSTC circuit is composed of a variety of excitatory/inhibitory signals, it has been proposed that a physiological disturbance within the cortex or striatum, particularly signals causing increased stimulation or decreased inhibition, could contribute to TS (see Figure 5.3). Excess excitation of cortical neurons (potentially leading to tic formation) can occur via increased thalamic input or decreased inhibition via cortical interneurons; hence, two common pathophysiological hypotheses for TS have emerged: (1) excess thalamic excitation and (2) impaired cortical inhibition. *Excess thalamic excitation* can be caused by two striatal abnormalities: decreased activity or effect of striatal neurons contributing to the indirect path, or excessive activity or effect of striatal neurons contributing to the direct path. *Impaired cortical inhibition* could be caused by de-

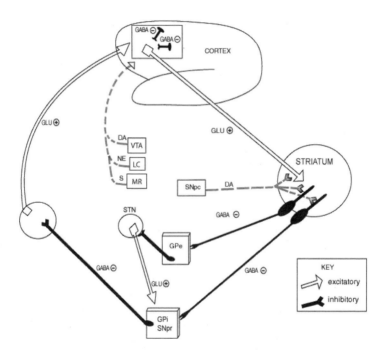

FIGURE 5.3. Pathophysiology of TS. This figure illustrates the cortical–striatal–thalamic–cortical pathway and ascending cortical inputs. Hypothesized abnormalities have included disorders of excess excitation or diminished inhibition, disruptions in the frontal cortex and striatum, and abnormalities of various synaptic neurotransmitters. *DA*, dopamine; *GABA*, gamma-aminobutyric acid; *GLU*, glutamate; *GPe*, globus pallidus externa; *GPi*, globus pallidus interna; *LC*, locus coeruleus; *MR*, median raphe; *NE*, norepinephrine; *S*, serotonin; *SNpc*, substantia nigra pans compacta; *SNpr*, substantia nigra pans reticulata; *STN*, subthalamic nucleus; *VTA*, ventral tegmental area.

creased activity or effect of cortical interneurons or alterations of input from brainstem neurotransmitter systems. To date, transcranial stimulation studies (Moll et al., 1999; Zieman, Paulus, & Rothenberger, 1997; Moll et al., 2001) and event-related (brain) potential (ERP) studies (Johannes, Kube, Wieringa, Matzke, & Munte, 1997; Johannes et al., 2001, 2002; Oades, Dittman-Balcar, Schepker, Eggers, & Zerbin, 1996; van Woerkom, Roos, & van Dijk, 1994) suggest that impaired cortical inhibition may contribute specifically to TS pathophysiology. Additional potential sites for neurophysiological abnormalities are listed in Table 5.1.

What Is the Neurochemical Basis for TS Pathogenesis?

Neurochemical hypotheses tend to be based on extrapolations from clinical responses to specific classes of medications; from cerebrospinal fluid (CSF), blood, and urine studies in relatively small numbers of patients; from neurochemical assays on a few postmortem brain tissues; and from PET/SPECT studies (Singer & Minzer, 2003; Harris & Singer, 2006).

Dopaminergic System

The dopaminergic system continues to receive much interest due to its significant involvement in CSTC circuitry and the demonstrated therapeutic benefit of neuroleptics in patients with TS. In CSTC circuits, dopaminergic neurons from the substantia nigra project to the striatum and affect all frontal–subcortical functions, though the specific inhibitory and excitatory effects of dopamine (DA) are dependent on the type of receptors with which it interacts postsynaptically. Dopaminergic input from the substantia nigra pars compacta (SNpc) influences striatal activity via several mechanisms, including (1) postsynaptic activating D1 receptors present on direct pathway medium-sized striatal neurons (MSSNs), and postsynaptic inhibitory D2 receptors on indirect pathway MSSNs; (2) postsynaptic DA receptors on striatal cholinergic interneurons; and (3) presynaptic DA receptors on presynaptic glutamatergic cortical–striatal terminals. Dopaminergic neurons arising from the ventral tegmental area also innervate prefrontal regions, and DA receptors are present on both pyramidal neurons (activating) and interneurons (inhibiting) in the prefrontal cortex.

Based on the aforementioned dopaminergic innervations, there are two possible mechanisms whereby DA involvement could lead to the genesis of tics: (1) excess DA activity causing hyperexcitation of thalamic nuclei and resulting in hyperstimulation of the cortex, and/or (2) excess DA activity via the ventral tegmental area, causing increased activation of frontal cortical neurons (or decreased inhibition of interneurons). Investigators have suggested that such an enhanced dopaminergic activity could result from (1) supersensitive postsynaptic striatal receptors; (2) striatal DA hyperinnervation; (3) increased striatal presynaptic production of DA, leading to increased release; (4) elevated DA release upon stimulation without abnormal presynaptic synthesis; or (5) cortical DA abnormalities.

SUPERSENSITIVE STRIATAL DA RECEPTORS

Three studies document increased D2 receptor binding (1) in the caudate (Wolf et al., 1996); (2) in postmortem brain (Singer, Hahn, & Moran, 1991); and (3) in a PET study (Wong et al., 1997).

STRIATAL DOPAMINE HYPERINNERVATION

Postmortem brain and SPECT studies have demonstrated increased binding to the DA transporter (DAT) consistent with hyperinnervation in patients with TS (Singer et al., 1991; Malison et al., 1995; Muller-Vahl et al., 2000). However, other DAT studies could not confirm these findings (Wong et al., 1998; Stamen Kovic et al., 2001; Meyer et al., 1999), and PET studies using vesicular monoamine transporter binding have shown excess binding limited to the ventral striatum (Albin et al., 2003).

INCREASED STRIATAL PRESYNAPTIC PRODUCTION OF DA LEADING TO INCREASED RELEASE

A single PET study has shown higher concentrations of [^{18}F]fluorodopa in the caudate of patients with TS compared to controls, suggestive of higher dopa decarboxylase activity in these individuals (Ernst et al., 1999). Although an interesting finding, it needs to be confirmed by other studies.

ELEVATED DA RELEASE UPON STIMULATION WITHOUT ABNORMAL PRESYNAPTIC SYNTHESIS

Administration of amphetamine, a stimulant that induces release and inhibits reuptake of DA, caused significantly greater DA release in the putamen of patients with TS relative to controls (Singer et al., 2002). One hypothesis that may explain this phenomenon, without invoking increased presynaptic synthesis, is increased stimulus-dependent dopamine release (Grace, 1993). If there were excess DAT activity in TS patients, then DA would be taken up from the synaptic cleft, resulting in a higher presynaptic DA concentration. This dysfunctional transporter system could, in turn, explain the higher stimulus-dependent phasic DA release displayed in patients with TS upon amphetamine challenge.

CORTICAL DA ABNORMALITIES

Recent postmortem studies have identified increased densities of D2 and DAT receptor protein in the prefrontal cortex of patients with TS (Minzer, Lee, Hong, & Singer, 2004; Yoon, Gause, Leckman, & Singer, 2006). Because dopaminergic fibers arise from the ventral tegmental area and form synapses on both frontal pyramidal neurons (activating) and interneurons (inhibiting), a prefrontal dopaminergic abnormality has been hypothesized, which leads to excess striatal glutamatergic stimulation and tic genesis.

Glutamate, GABA, and Serotonin

Although many other neurotransmitter systems contribute to CSTC circuitry, evidence for disturbances in other neurotransmitter systems is currently very limited. For example, the functional significance of reduced glutamate in postmortem GP tissue samples has yet to be elucidated (Anderson et al., 1992). Glutamate decarboxylase activity and gamma-aminobutyric acid (GABA) levels have been normal in various TS tissue samples from both cortical and subcortical regions (Anderson et al., 1992a, 1992b; Singer, Hahn, Krowiak, Nelson, & Moran, 1990; van Woerkom, Rosenbaum, & Enna, 1982).

Several studies have suggested a possible serotoninergic disturbance in TS, including (1) CSF studies showing abnormally low levels of 5-HIAA (the principal serotonin metabolite) in some individuals with TS (Singer, Tune, Butler, Zaczek, & Coyle, 1982; Butler, Koslow, Seifert, Caprioli, & Singer, 1979; Cohen, Shaywitz, Caparulo, Young, & Bowers, 1978); (2) postmortem studies reporting decreased concentrations of 5-HIAA and tryptophan (a serotonin precursor) in the BG of patients with TS (Anderson et al., 1992a, 1992b); (3) whole blood, plasma analysis, and urinalysis showing low levels of serotonin and tryptophan in blood and decreased excretion of serotonin in individuals with TS (Leckman et al., 1995; Comings, 1990); and (4) microarray analyses (Hong et al., 2004). Heinz and colleagues (Heinz et al., 1998) reported a negative correlation between vocal tics and [^{123}I]beta-CIT binding in the midbrain and thalamus, indicating that serotoninergic neurotransmission in the midbrain and serotoninergic or noradrenergic neurotransmission in the thalamus may be important factors in the expression of TS. Use of [^{123}I]beta-CIT and SPECT to investigate serotonin transporter binding capacity in patients with TS also found impaired serotoninergic function that appeared to be associated with OCD (Muller-Vahl et al., 2005). Lastly, in view of the importance of cortical dopaminergic changes in TS, there is growing interest in the modulatory influence of serotonergic pathways on DA release.

SUMMARY

TS Genetics

Although genetic involvement in TS pathogenesis is well established, finding the gene(s) for TS is proving to be a very difficult endeavor. If one believes that the pathogenesis of TS is occurring at the level of the gene, TS should be considered a complex trait. In complex traits, the disease phenotype may become apparent only when particular combinations of susceptibility genes have been acquired. This concept may be especially applicable to TS, wherein the inheritance of different combinations of alleles could modify the phenotype expression and perhaps explain variations of tic patterns/severity or the presence of comorbidities in different individuals with TS. Alternatively, if one considers the perturbation responsible for TS pathogenesis to be slightly removed from the DNA sequence, than one might conclude that the nonconvergent results presented in this chapter could simply be caused by a failure to include the possible contribution of epigenetic factors in each analytical model. Although investigators are now taking interest in potential epigenetic influences in TS, evidence of their contribution is currently very limited, meriting further research.

TS Neurobiology

Much progress has been made in understanding the neurobiology of TS, although no concrete conclusions are available. Expanding evidence supports the concept of a CSTC circuit abnormality, but whether the primary defect resides in the cortex or striatum is unclear. Recent findings of increased dopaminergic abnormalities in prefrontal postmortem tissue suggest that further focus should be directed toward cortical abnormalities in TS. Physiological hypotheses vary between excess cortical excitation and impaired cortical inhibition. Neurochemical studies have emphasized a role for DA, with a phasic model of DA release being a unifying hypothesis, but other neurotransmitters may also be involved. Clearly, additional research efforts are necessary before we have a comprehensive understanding of the pathophysiology of this complex disorder.

REFERENCES

Abelson, J. F., Kwan, K. Y., O'Roak, B. J., et al. (2005). Sequence variants in SLITRK1 are associated with Tourette's syndrome. *Science*, *310*, 317–320.

Albin, R. L., Koeppe, R. A., Bohnen, N. I., et al. (2003). Increased ventral striatal monoaminergic innervation in Tourette syndrome. *Neurology*, *61*, 310–315.

Alexander, G. E., DeLong, M. R., & Strick, P. L. (1986). Parallel organization of functionally segregated circuits linking basal ganglia and cortex. *Annual Review of Neuroscience*, *9*, 357–381.

Anderson, G. M., Pollak, E. S., Chatterjee, D., Leckman, J. F., Riddle, M. A., & Cohen, D. J. (1992a). Postmortem analysis of subcortical monoamines and amino acids in Tourette syndrome. *Advances in Neurology*, *58*, 123–133.

Anderson, G. M., Pollak, E. S., Chatterjee, D., Leckman, J. F., Riddle, M. A., & Cohen, D. J. (1992b). Brain monoamines and amino acids in Gilles de la Tourette's syndrome: A preliminary study of subcortical regions. *Archives of General Psychiatry*, *49*, 584–586.

Aruga, J., & Mikoshiba, K. (2003). Identification and characterization of SLITRK, a novel neuronal transmembrane protein family controlling neurite outgrowth. *Molecular and Cellular Neuroscience*, *24*, 117–129.

Balthasar, K. (1957). Über das anatomische Substrat der generalisierten Tic-Krankheit: Entwicklungshemmung des corpus striatum. *Archives of Psychiatry Berlin*, *195*, 531–549.

Barr, C. L., Wigg, K. G., Pakstis, A. J., et al. (1999). Genome scan for linkage to Gilles de la Tourette syndrome. *American Journal of Medical Genetics*, *88*, 437–445.

Barr, C. L., Wigg, K. G., & Sandor, P. (1999). Catechol-O-methyltransferase and Gilles de la Tourette syndrome. *Molecular Psychiatry*, *4*, 492–495.

Barr, C. L., Wigg, K. G., Zovko, E., Sandor, P., & Tsui, L. C. (1997). Linkage study of the dopamine D5 receptor gene and Gilles de la Tourette syndrome. *American Journal of Medical Genetics*, *74*, 58–61.

Baumgardner, T. L., Singer, H. S., Denckla, M. B., et al. (1996). Corpus callosum morphology in children with Tourette syndrome and attention deficit hyperactivity disorder. *Neurology*, *47*, 477–482.

Baxter, L. R. (1990). Brain imaging as a tool in establishing a theory of brain pathology in obsessive compulsive disorder. *Journal of Clinical Psychiatry 51*(Suppl.), 22–25; discussion 26.

Baxter, L. R., Jr., Schwartz, J. M., Guze, B. H., Bergman, K., & Szuba, M. P. (1990). PET imaging in obsessive compulsive disorder with and without depression. *Journal of Clinical Psychiatry*, *51*(Suppl.), 61–69; discussion 70.

Biswal, B., Ulmer, J. L., Krippendorf, R. L., et al. (1998). Abnormal cerebral activation associated with a motor task in Tourette syndrome. *American Journal of Neuroradiology*, *19*, 1509–1512.

Boghosian-Sell, L., Comings, D. E., & Overhauser, J. (1996). Tourette syndrome in a pedigree with a 7;18 translocation: Identification of a YAC spanning the translocation breakpoint at 18q22.3. *American Journal of Human Genetics*, *59*, 999–1005.

Bottini, N., MacMurray, J., Rostamkani, M., McGue, M., Iacono, W. G., & Comings, D. E. (2002). Association between the low molecular weight cytosolic acid phosphatase gene ACP1*A and comorbid features of Tourette syndrome. *Neuroscience Letters*, *330*, 198–200.

Brett, P. M., Curtis, D., Robertson, M. M., Dahlitz, M., Gurling, H. M. (1996). Linkage analysis and exclusion of regions of chromosomes 3 and 8 in Gilles de la Tourette syndrome following the identification of a balanced reciprocal translocation 46 XY, t(3:8)(p21.3 q24.1) in a case of Tourette syndrome. *Psychiatric Genetics*, *6*, 99–105.

Brett, P. M., Curtis, D., Robertson, M. M., & Gurling, H. M. (1997). Neuroreceptor subunit genes and the genetic susceptibility to Gilles de la Tourette syndrome. *Biological Psychiatry, 42,* 941–947.

Bruggeman, R., van der Linden, C., Buitelaar, J. K., Gericke, G. S., Hawkridge, S. M., & Temlett, J. A. (2001). Risperidone versus pimozide in Tourette's disorder: A comparative double-blind parallel-group study. *Journal of Clinical Psychiatry, 62,* 50–56.

Burd, L., Severud, R., Klug, M. G., & Kerbeshian, J. (1999). Prenatal and perinatal risk factors for Tourette disorder. *Journal of Perinatal Medicine, 27,* 295–302.

Butler, I. J., Koslow, S. H., Seifert, W. E., Jr., Caprioli, R. M., & Singer, H. S. (1979). Biogenic amine metabolism in Tourette syndrome. *Annals of Neurology, 6,* 37–39.

Cohen, D. J., Shaywitz, B. A., Caparulo, B., Young, J. G., & Bowers, M. B., Jr. (1978). Chronic, multiple tics of Gilles de la Tourette's disease: CSF acid monoamine metabolites after probenecid administration. *Archives of General Psychiatry, 35,* 245–250.

Comings, D. E. (1990). Blood serotonin and tryptophan in Tourette syndrome. *American Journal of Medical Genetics, 36,* 418–430.

Comings, D. E., & Comings, B. G. (1984). Tourette's syndrome and attention deficit disorder with hyperactivity: Are they genetically related? *Journal of the American Academy of Child Psychiatry, 23,* 138–146.

Comings, D. E., Comings, B. G., Devor, E. J., & Cloninger, C. R. (1984). Detection of major gene for Gilles de la Tourette syndrome. *American Journal of Human Genetics, 36,* 586–600.

Crawford, F. C., Ait-Ghezala, G., Morris, M., et al. (2003). Translocation breakpoint in two unrelated Tourette syndrome cases, within a region previously linked to the disorder. *Human Genetics, 113,* 154–161.

Cruz, C., Camarena, B., King, N., et al. (1997). Increased prevalence of the seven-repeat variant of the dopamine D4 receptor gene in patients with obsessive–compulsive disorder with tics. *Neuroscience Letters, 231,* 1–4.

Cummings, J. L. (1993). Frontal–subcortical circuits and human behavior. *Archives of Neurology, 50,* 873–880.

Curtis, D., Brett, P., Dearlove, A. M., et al. (2004). Genome scan of Tourette syndrome in a single large pedigree shows some support for linkage to regions of chromosomes 5, 10 and 13. *Psychiatric Genetics, 14,* 83–87.

Demirkol, A., Erdem, H., Inan, L., Yigit, A., & Guney, M. (1999). Bilateral globus pallidus lesions in a patient with Tourette syndrome and related disorders. *Biological Psychiatry, 46,* 863–867.

Deng, H., Le, W. D., Xie, W. J., & Jankovic, J. (2006). Examination of the SLITRK1 gene in Caucasian patients with Tourette syndrome. *Acta Neurologica Scandinavica, 114,* 400–402.

Devor, E. J., Dill-Devor, R. M., & Magee, H. J. (1998). The Bal I and Msp I polymorphisms in the dopamine D3 receptor gene display: Linkage disequilibrium with each other but no association with Tourette syndrome. *Psychiatric Genetics, 8,* 49–52.

Dewult, A., & van Bogaret, L. (1941). Études anatomocliniques de syndrôme hypercinétiques complexes. *Monatsschrift fur Psychiatrie und Neurologie, 104,* 53–61.

Diaz-Anzaldua, A., Joober, R., Riviere, J. B., et al. (2004). Tourette syndrome and dopaminergic genes: A family-based association study in the French Canadian founder population. *Molecular Psychiatry, 9,* 272–277.

Diler, R. S., Reyhanli, M., Toros, F., Kibar, M., & Avci, A. (2002). Tc-99m-ECD SPECT brain imaging in children with Tourette's syndrome. *Yonsei Medical Journal, 43,* 403–410.

Eapen, V., Pauls, D. L., & Robertson, M. M. (1993). Evidence for autosomal dominant transmission in Tourette's syndrome: United Kingdom cohort study. *British Journal of Psychiatry, 162,* 593–596.

Ernst, M., Zametkin, A. J., Jons, P. H., Matochik, J. A., Pascualvaca, D., Cohen, R. M. (1999). High presynaptic dopaminergic activity in children with Tourette's disorder. *Journal of the American Academy of Child and Adolescent Psychiatry, 38,* 86–94.

Fredericksen, K. A., Cutting, L. E., Kates, W. R., et al. (2002). Disproportionate increases of white matter in right frontal lobe in Tourette syndrome. *Neurology, 58,* 85–89.

Gadzicki, D., Muller-Vahl, K. R., Heller, D., et al. (2004). Tourette syndrome is not caused by mutations in the central cannabinoid receptor (CNR1) gene. *American Journal of Medical Genetics, 127B,* 97–103.

Gerard, E, & Peterson, B. S. (2003). Developmental processes and brain imaging studies in Tourette syndrome. *Journal of Psychosomatic Research, 55,* 13–22.

Grace, A. A. (1993). Cortical regulation of subcortical dopamine systems and its possible relevance to schizophrenia. *Journal of Neural Transmission General Section, 91,* 111–134.

Grad, L. R., Pelcovitz, D., Olson, M., Matthews, M., & Grad, G. J. (1987). Obsessive-compulsive symptomatology in children with Tourette's syndrome. *Journal of the American Academy of Child and Adolescent Psychiatry, 26,* 69–73.

Grice, D. E., Leckman, J. F., Pauls, D. L., et al. (1996). Linkage disequilibrium between an allele at the dopamine D4 receptor locus and Tourette syndrome, by the transmission-disequilibrium test. *American Journal of Human Genetics, 59,* 644–652.

Hall, M., Costa, D. C., Shields, J. (1991). Brain perfusion patterns with ^{99}Tc^{m}: HMPAO/SPECT in patients with Gilles de la Tourette syndrome—short report. In H. A. E. Schmidt (Ed.), *Nuclear medicine: The state of the art of nuclear medicine in Europe* (pp. 243–245). Stuttgart: Schattauer.

Harris, E. L., Schuerholz, L. J., Singer, H. S., et al. (1995). Executive function in children with Tourette syndrome and/or attention deficit hyperactivity disorder. *Journal of International Neuropsychological Society, 1,* 511–516.

Harris, K., & Singer, H. S. (2006). Tic disorders: Neural circuits, neurochemistry, and neuroimmunology. *Journal of Child Neurologyogy, 21,* 678–689.

Hebebrand, J., Nothen, M. M., Ziegler, A., et al. (1997). Nonreplication of linkage disequilibrium between the dopamine D4 receptor locus and Tourette syndrome. *American Journal of Human Genetics, 61,* 238–239.

Heinz, A., Knable, M. B., Wolf, S. S., et al. (1998). Tourette's syndrome: [I^{123}]-beta-CIT SPECT correlates of vocal tic severity. *Neurology, 51,* 1069–1074.

Heutink, P., van de Wetering, B. J., Breedveld, G. J., et al. (1990). No evidence for genetic linkage of Gilles de la Tourette syndrome on chromosomes 7 and 18. *Journal of Medical Genetics, 27,* 433–436.

Hong, J. J., Loiselle, C. R., Yoon, D. Y., Lee, O., Becker, K. G., & Singer, H. S. (2004). Microarray analysis in Tourette syndrome postmortem putamen. *Journal of the Neurological Sciences, 225,* 57–64.

Huang, Y., Liu, X., Li, T., et al. (2002). [Transmission disequilibrium test of DRD4 exon III 48bp variant number tandem repeat polymorphism and tic disorder]. *Zhonghua Yi Xue Yi Chuan Xue Za Zhi, 19,* 100–103.

Hyde, T. M., Aaronson, B. A., Randolph, C., Rickler, K. C., & Weinberger, D. R. (1992). Relationship of birth weight to the phenotypic expression of Gilles de la Tourette's syndrome in monozygotic twins. *Neurology, 42,* 652–658.

Hyde, T. M., Stacey, M. E., Coppola, R., Handel, S. F., Rickler, K. C., Weinberger, D. R. (1995). Cerebral morphometric abnormalities in Tourette's syndrome: A quantitative MRI study of monozygotic twins. *Neurology, 45,* 1176–1182.

Jeffries, K. J., Schooler, C., Schoenbach, C., Herscovitch, P., Chase, T. N., & Braun, A. R. (2002). The functional neuroanatomy of Tourette's syndrome: An FDG PET study. III. Functional coupling of regional cerebral metabolic rates. *Neuropsychopharmacology, 27,* 92–104.

Johannes, S., Kube, C., Wieringa, B. M., Matzke, M., & Munte, T. F. (1997). Brain potentials and time estimation in humans. *Neuroscience Letters, 231,* 63–66.

Johannes, S., Wieringa, B. M., Nager, W., Muller-Vahl, K. R., Dengler, R., & Munte, T. F. (2001). Electrophysiological measures and dual-task performance in Tourette syndrome indicate deficient divided attention mechanisms. *European Journal of Neurology, 8,* 253–260.

Johannes, S., Wieringa, B. M., Nager, W., Muller-Vahl, K. R., Dengler, R., & Munte, T. F. (2002). Excessive action monitoring in Tourette syndrome. *Journal of Neurology, 249,* 961–966.

Kalanithi, P. S., Zheng, W., Kataoka, Y., et al. (2005). Altered parvalbumin-positive neuron distribution in basal ganglia of individuals with Tourette syndrome. *Proceedings of the National Academy of Sciences USA, 102,* 13307–13312.

Kano, Y., Ohta, M., Nagai, Y., Pauls, D. L., & Leckman, J. F. (2001). A family study of Tourette syndrome in Japan. *American Journal of Medical Genetics, 105,* 414–421.

Kates, W. R., Frederiksen, M., Mostofsky, S. H., et al. (2002). MRI parcellation of the frontal lobe in boys with attention deficit hyperactivity disorder or Tourette syndrome. *Psychiatry Research, 116,* 63–81.

Kroisel, P. M., Petek, E., Emberger, W., Windpassinger, C., Wladika, W., & Wagner, K. (2001). Candidate region for Gilles de la Tourette syndrome at 7q31. *American Journal of Medical Genetics, 101,* 259–261.

Leckman, J. F., Goodman, W. K., Anderson, G. M., et al. (1995). Cerebrospinal fluid biogenic amines in obsessive compulsive disorder, Tourette's syndrome, and healthy controls. *Neuropsychopharmacology, 12,* 73–86.

Lichter, D. G., Jackson, L. A., & Schachter, M. (1995). Clinical evidence of genomic imprinting in Tourette's syndrome. *Neurology, 45,* 924–928.

Mahone, E. M., Koth, C. W., Cutting, L., Singer, H. S., & Denckla, M. B. (2001). Executive function in fluency and recall measures among children with Tourette syndrome or ADHD. *Journal of the International Neuropsychological Society, 7,* 102–111.

Malison, R. T., McDougle, C. J., van Dyck, C. H., et al. (1995). [^{123}I]-beta-CIT SPECT imaging of striatal dopamine transporter binding in Tourette's disorder. *American Journal of Psychiatry, 152,* 1359–1361.

Matsumoto, N., David, D. E., Johnson, E. W., et al. (2000). Breakpoint sequences of an 1;8 translocation in a family with Gilles de la Tourette syndrome. *European Journal of Human Genetics, 8,* 875–883.

McAbee, G. N., Wark, J. E., & Manning, A. (1999). Tourette syndrome associated with unilateral cystic changes in the gyrus rectus. *Pediatric Neurology, 20,* 322–324.

McMahon, W. M., van de Wetering, B. J., Filloux, F., Betit, K., Coon, H., & Leppert, M. (1996). Bilineal transmission and phenotypic variation of Tourette's disorder in a large pedigree. *Journal of the American Academy of Child and Adolescent Psychiatry, 35,* 672–680.

Merette, C., Brassard, A., Potvin, A., et al. (2000). Significant linkage for Tourette syndrome in a large French Canadian family. *American Journal of Human Genetics, 67,* 1008–1013.

Meyer, P., Bohnen, N. I., Minoshima, S., et al. (1999). Striatal presynaptic monoaminergic vesicles are not increased in Tourette's syndrome. *Neurology, 53,* 371–374.

Minzer, K., Lee, O., Hong, J. J., & Singer, H. S. (2004). Increased prefrontal D2 protein in Tourette syndrome: A postmortem analysis of frontal cortex and striatum. *Journal of the Neurological Sciences, 219,* 55–61.

Moll, G. H., Heinrich, H., Trott, G. E., Wirth, S., Bock, N., & Rothenberger, A. (2001). Children with comorbid attention-deficit-hyperactivity disorder and tic disorder: Evidence for additive inhibitory deficits within the motor system. *Annals of Neurology, 49,* 393–396.

Moll, G. H., Wischer, S., Heinrich, H., Tergau, F., Paulus, W., & Rothenberger, A. (1999). Deficient motor control in children with tic disorder: Evidence from transcranial magnetic stimulation. *Neuroscience Letters*, *272*, 37–40.

Moriarty, J., Varma, A. R., Stevens, J., Fish, M., Trimble, M. R., Robertson, M. M. (1997). A volumetric MRI study of Gilles de la Tourette's syndrome. *Neurology*, *49*, 410–415.

Muller, S. V., Johannes, S., Wieringa, B., et al. (2003). Disturbed monitoring and response inhibition in patients with Gilles de la Tourette syndrome and co-morbid obsessive compulsive disorder. *Behavioural Neurology*, *14*, 29–37.

Muller-Vahl, K. R., Berding, G., Brucke, T., et al. (2000). Dopamine transporter binding in Gilles de la Tourette syndrome. *Journal of Neurology*, *247*, 514–520.

Muller-Vahl, K. R., Meyer, G. J., Knapp, W. H., et al. (2005). Serotonin transporter binding in Tourette syndrome. *Neuroscience Letters*, *385*, 120–125.

Oades, R. D., Dittmann-Balcar, A., Schepker, R., Eggers, C., & Zerbin, D. Auditory event-related potentials (ERPs) and mismatch negativity (MMN) in healthy children and those with attention-deficit or Tourette/tic symptoms. *Biological Psychology*, *43*, 163–185.

Ozbay, F., Wigg, K. G., Turanli, E. T., et al. (2006). Analysis of the dopamine beta hydroxylase gene in Gilles de la Tourette syndrome. *American Journal of Medical Genetics B: Neuropsychiatric Genetics*, *141*, 673–677.

Pakstis, A. J., Heutink, P., Pauls, D. L., et al. (1991). Progress in the search for genetic linkage with Tourette syndrome: An exclusion map covering more than 50% of the autosomal genome. *American Journal of Human Genetics*, *48*, 281–294.

Pauls, D. L., & Leckman, J. F. (1986). The inheritance of Gilles de la Tourette's syndrome and associated behaviors: Evidence for autosomal dominant transmission. *New England Journal of Medicine*, *315*, 993–997.

Pauls, D. L., Raymond, C. L., Stevenson, J. M., & Leckman, J. F. (1991). A family study of Gilles de la Tourette syndrome. *American Journal of Human Genetics*, *48*, 154–163.

Pauls, D. L., Towbin, K. E., Leckman, J. F., Zahner, G. E., & Cohen, D. J. (1986). Gilles de la Tourette's syndrome and obsessive–compulsive disorder: Evidence supporting a genetic relationship. *Archives of General Psychiatry*, *43*, 1180–1182.

Peterson, B., Riddle, M. A., Cohen, D. J., et al. (1993). Reduced basal ganglia volumes in Tourette's syndrome using three-dimensional reconstruction techniques from magnetic resonance images. *Neurology*, *43*, 941–949.

Peterson, B. S., Leckman, J. F., Duncan, J. S., et al. (1994). Corpus callosum morphology from magnetic resonance images in Tourette's syndrome. *Psychiatry Research*, *55*, 85–99.

Peterson, B. S., Skudlarski, P., Anderson, A. W., et al. (1998). A functional magnetic resonance imaging study of tic suppression in Tourette syndrome. *Archives of General Psychiatry*, *55*, 326–333.

Peterson, B. S., Staib, L., Scahill, L., et al. (2001). Regional brain and ventricular volumes in Tourette syndrome. *Archives of General Psychiatry*, *58*, 427–440.

Peterson, B. S., Thomas, P., Kane, M. J., et al. (2003). Basal ganglia volumes in patients with Gilles de la Tourette syndrome. *Archives of General Psychiatry*, *60*, 415–424.

Pitman, R. K., Green, R. C., Jenike, M. A., & Mesulam, M. M. (1987). Clinical comparison of Tourette's disorder and obsessive–compulsive disorder. *American Journal of Psychiatry*, *144*, 1166–1171.

Price, R. A., Kidd, K. K., Cohen, D. J., Pauls, D. L., & Leckman, J. F. (1985). A twin study of Tourette syndrome. *Archives of General Psychiatry*, *42*, 815–820.

Schuerholz, L. J., Baumgardner, T. L., Singer, H. S., Reiss, A. L., & Denckla, M. B. (1996). Neuropsychological status of children with Tourette's syndrome with and without attention deficit hyperactivity disorder. *Neurology*, *46*, 958–965.

Selling, L. (1929). The role of infection in the etiology of tics. *Archives of Neurology and Psychiatry*, *22*, 1163–1171.

Serrien, D. J., Nirkko, A. C., Loher, T. J., Lovblad, K. O., Burgunder, J. M., & Wiesendanger, M. (2002). Movement control of manipulative tasks in patients with Gilles de la Tourette syndrome. *Brain, 125,* 290–300.

Seuchter, S. A., Hebebrand, J., Klug, B., et al. (2000). Complex segregation analysis of families ascertained through Gilles de la Tourette syndrome. *Genetic Epidemiology, 18,* 33–47.

Shapiro, A. K., Shapiro, E. S., Bruun, R. D., & Sweet, R. D. (1978). *Gilles de la Tourette syndrome.* New York: Raven Press.

Sheppard, D. M., Bradshaw, J. L., Georgiou, N., Bradshaw, J. A., & Lee, P. (2000). Movement sequencing in children with Tourette's syndrome and attention deficit hyperactivity disorder. *Movement Disorders, 15,* 1184–1193.

Simonic, I., Nyholt, D. R., Gericke, G, S., et al. (2001). Further evidence for linkage of Gilles de la Tourette syndrome (GTS) susceptibility loci on chromosomes 2p11, 8q22 and 11q23–24 in South African Afrikaners. *American Journal of Medical Genetics, 105,* 163–167.

Singer, H. S., Hahn, I. H., Krowiak, E., Nelson, E., & Moran, T. (1990). Tourette's syndrome: A neurochemical analysis of postmortem cortical brain tissue. *Annals of Neurology, 27,* 443–446.

Singer, H. S., Hahn, I. H., & Moran, T. H. (1991). Abnormal dopamine uptake sites in postmortem striatum from patients with Tourette's syndrome. *Annals of Neurology, 30,* 558–562.

Singer, H. S., & Minzer, K. (2003). Neurobiology of Tourette syndrome: Concepts of neuroanatomical localization and neurochemical abnormalities. *Brain and Development, 25*(Suppl.), S70–S84.

Singer, H. S., Reiss, A. L., Brown, J. E., et al. (1993). Volumetric MRI changes in basal ganglia of children with Tourette's syndrome. *Neurology, 43,* 950–956.

Singer, H. S., Szymanski, S., Giuliano, J., et al. (2002). Elevated intrasynaptic dopamine release in Tourette's syndrome measured by PET. *American Journal of Psychiatry, 159,* 1329–1336.

Singer, H. S., Tune, L. E., Butler, I. J., Zaczek, R., & Coyle, J. T. (1982). Clinical symptomatology, CSF neurotransmitter metabolites, and serum haloperidol levels in Tourette syndrome. *Advances in Neurology, 35,* 177–183.

Singh, D. N., Howe, G. L., Jordan, H. W., & Hara, S. (1982). Tourette's syndrome in a black woman with associated triple X and 9p mosaicism. *Journal of the National Medical Association, 74,* 675–682.

Stamenkovic, M., Schindler, S. D., Asenbaum, S., et al. (2001). No change in striatal dopamine re-uptake site density in psychotropic drug naive and in currently treated Tourette's disorder patients: A [^{123}I]-beta-CIT SPECT-study. *European Neuropsychopharmacology, 11,* 69–74.

State, M. W., Greally, J. M., Cuker, A., et al. (2003). Epigenetic abnormalities associated with a chromosome 18(q21–q22) inversion and a Gilles de la Tourette syndrome phenotype. *Proceedings of the National Academy of Sciences USA, 100,* 4684–4689.

Stober, G., Hebebrand, J., Cichon, S., et al. (1999). Tourette syndrome and the norepinephrine transporter gene: Results of a systematic mutation screening. *American Journal of Medical Genetics, 88,* 158–163.

Stoetter, B., Braun, A. R., Randolph, C., et al. (1992). Functional neuroanatomy of Tourette syndrome: Limbic–motor interactions studied with FDG PET. *Advances in Neurology, 58,* 213–226.

Taylor, L. D., Krizman, D. B., Jankovic, J., et al. (1991). 9p monosomy in a patient with Gilles de la Tourette's syndrome. *Neurology, 41,* 1513–1515.

Thompson, M., Comings, D. E., Feder, L., George, S. R., & O'Dowd, B. F. (1998). Mutation screening of the dopamine D1 receptor gene in Tourette's syndrome and alcohol dependent patients. *American Journal of Medical Genetics, 81,* 241–244.

TSAICG. (1999). A complete genome screen in sib pairs affected by Gilles de la Tourette syndrome. *American Journal of Human Genetics, 65,* 1428–1436.

TSAICG. (2007). Genome scan for Tourette's disorder in affected sib-pair and multigenerational families. *American Journal of Human Genetics, 80.*

van Woerkom, T., Rosenbaum, D., & Enna, S. (1982). Overview of pharmacological approaches to therapy for Tourette syndrome, In A. Friedhoff & T. Chase (Eds.), *Advances in neurology* (Vol. 35, pp. 369–375). New York: Raven Press.

van Woerkom, T. C., Roos, R. A., & van Dijk, J. G. (1994). Altered attentional processing of background stimuli in Gilles de la Tourette syndrome: A study in auditory event-related potentials evoked in an oddball paradigm. *Acta Neurologica Scandinavica, 90,* 116–123.

Verkerk, A. J., Cath, D. C., van der Linde, H. C., et al. (2006). Genetic and clinical analysis of a large Dutch Gilles de la Tourette family. *Molecular Psychiatry, 11,* 954–964.

Verkerk, A. J., Mathews, C. A., Joosse, M., Eussen, B. H., Heutink, P., & Oostra, B. A. (2003). CNTNAP2 is disrupted in a family with Gilles de la Tourette syndrome and obsessive compulsive disorder. *Genomics, 82,* 1–9.

Walkup, J. T., LaBuda, M. C., Singer, H. S., Brown, J., Riddle, M. A., & Hurko, O. (1996). Family study and segregation analysis of Tourette syndrome: Evidence for a mixed model of inheritance. *American Journal of Human Genetics, 59,* 684–693.

Wolf, S. S., Jones, D. W., Knable, M. B., et al. (1996). Tourette syndrome: Prediction of phenotypic variation in monozygotic twins by caudate nucleus D2 receptor binding. *Science, 273,* 1225–1227.

Wong, D. F., Ricaurte, G., Grunder, G., et al. (1998). Dopamine transporter changes in neuropsychiatric disorders. *Advances in Pharmacology, 42,* 219–223.

Wong, D. F., Singer, H. S., Brandt, J., et al. (1997). D2–like dopamine receptor density in Tourette syndrome measured by PET. *Journal of Nuclear Medicine, 38,* 1243–1247.

Xu, C., Ozbay, F., Wigg, K., et al. (2003). Evaluation of the genes for the adrenergic receptors alpha2A and alpha1C and Gilles de la Tourette syndrome. *American Journal of Medical Genetics, 119B,* 54–59.

Yochelson, M. R., & David, R. G. (2000). New-onset tic disorder following acute hemorrhage of an arteriovenous malformation. *Journal of Child Neurology, 15,* 769–771.

Yoon, D., Rippel, C., Kobets, A., et al. (in press). Dopaminergic polymorphisms in Tourette syndrome: Association with the DAT gene (SLC6A3). *American Journal of Medical Genetics B, Neuropsychiatric Genetics.*

Yoon, D. Y., Gause, C. D., Leckman, J. F., & Singer, H. S. (2006). Abnormal Frontal dopaminergic abnormality in Tourette syndrome: A postmortem analysis. *Annals of Neurology, 60*(Suppl.), S140.

Ziemann, U., Paulus, W., & Rothenberger, A. (1997). Decreased motor inhibition in Tourette's disorder: Evidence from transcranial magnetic stimulation. *American Journal of Psychiatry, 154,* 1277–1284.

CHAPTER 6

Neurocognitive Factors in Tourette Syndrome

SUSANNA CHANG

In recent years a growing number of studies has investigated the cognitive, neurological, and behavioral correlates of Tourette syndrome (TS), a neuropsychiatric disorder with possible dysfunction in specific basal ganglia–thalamic–cortical (BGTC) pathways (Peterson et al., 1999). The evolving clinical picture of TS is one that highlights not only disturbances in motor function but also notable impairment in cognitive domains. Characterization of neurocognitive deficits is potentially informative about the pathophysiology of TS. Although we cannot directly deduce metabolic dysfunction in brain structure from poor neurocognitive performance, impaired performance on homogenous tasks measuring a specific cognitive function can provide us with important clues for potential anatomical substrates of TS.

Much of the TS neurocognitive research to date, unfortunately, has been riddled by methodological problems, which limits the conclusions that can be drawn from the data. Common drawbacks have included small samples sizes, inconsistency in neurocognitive test measures, lack of matched control groups, failure to control for likely comorbid conditions such as attention-deficit/hyperactivity disorder (ADHD) and/or obsessive–compulsive disorder (OCD), and subject pools that have been drawn from mental health clinics rather than epidemiologically ascertained samples. Clinic-referred individuals are likely to represent more severe cases of TS, which makes generalization to the population at large more tenuous (Schultz, Carter, Scahill, & Leckman, 1999). Moreover, given the increasing evidence suggesting that individuals with ADHD and OCD have their own specific neurocognitive profile of impairments, stringent accounting for comorbidity in TS research is a necessity (Robertson & Yakely, 1993; Towbin & Riddle, 1993; Walkup, Khan, Schuerholz, Paik, Leckman, & Schultz, 1999).

The neurocognitive literature has been somewhat inconsistent in establishing a distinctive profile for TS based on the proposed BGTC neuroanatomical circuitry, particularly with respect to executive functioning, an area that has traditionally escaped ready definitions and measurements. The most consistent neurocognitive finding to date for TS has been impaired visuomotor integration skills in the context of generally intact fine motor control and visual perceptual processes. Deficits in executive functioning have been much more variable across studies, with few consistent findings emerging (Como, 2001; Schultz, Carter, et al., 1999). However, as the design and instruments of neurocognitive studies have become progressively more refined over time, experimental investigations focusing on executive and motor functions have attested to a growing relationship between neurocognitive deficits in TS and an underlying neurobiological dysfunction (Rauch & Savage, 1997; Rauch et al., 2001; see also Cerullo et al., Chapter 5, this volume).

In addition to reviewing the specific neurocognitive deficits associated with TS, this chapter also discusses issues such as comorbidity and age and gender effects, which all too often cloud the accurate interpretation of neurocognitive findings. Furthermore, the contributions of neurocognitive deficits to TS symptom presentation and the ways in which such deficits can affect response to treatment are also reviewed in this chapter.

INTELLIGENCE

The bulk of the research on the intellectual functioning of individuals with TS suggests that the overall IQ of this group does not differ significantly from that of the general population (Apter et al., 1993; Shapiro, Shapiro, Bruun, & Sweet, 1978), with IQ scores falling generally within the normal range of functioning. However, some studies have indicated lower than average IQ in clinical samples of children affected with TS (Parraga & McDonald, 1996; Sutherland, Kolb, Schoel, Whishaw, & Davies, 1982). Such studies often used samples that characterized by high degrees of comorbid disorders, and it appears likely that IQ discrepancies could be associated with confounding diagnoses such as ADHD, OCD, and learning disabilities (Dykens et al., 1990; Yeates & Bornstein, 1994). Moreover, studies examining general cognitive functioning in children with TS alone have indicated an IQ range that is normally distributed (Bornstein, 1990).

In the earlier phases of neurocognitive research, when more specific and sensitive instruments were not readily available, studies focused on the differences between Verbal (VIQ) and Performance IQ (PIQ) as rough measures of visuospatial and verbal dysfunction. Although far from consistent, some studies demonstrated that patients with TS had significantly lower PIQ than VIQ scores (discrepancy of 15 points or greater) on standardized IQ tests such as the Wechsler Intelligence Scale for Children–III (WISC-III), indicating difficulties in visuomotor and visuoperceptual tasks (Incagnoli & Kane, 1981; Shapiro, Shapiro, Young, & Feinberg, 1988). One study indicated that 40% of a sizable TS sample had a VIQ significantly greater than the PIQ (Shapiro et al., 1988), although conclusions were somewhat limited by inclusion of subjects with ADHD comorbidity. Despite such methodological limitations, there appears to be some agreement among studies that TS subjects often show a VIQ PIQ split suggestive of problems in visuospatial, perceptual, and motor abilities. Although these findings would be more compelling if comorbidity were better controlled across studies, support for these results are present in other investigations, which have reported specific deficits in visuomotor functioning and motor skills.

EXECUTIVE FUNCTIONING

Executive functions (EF) encompass a wide domain of cognitive and behavioral abilities that include planning, organization, mental tracking, sustained attention, working memory, cognitive flexibility, impulse control and self-regulation (Pennington, 1991). Given that EF at its core represents the ability to self-regulate as well as to generate and execute goal-directed behaviors, it has been logically linked to the frontal cortex and its reciprocal connections to basal ganglia structures. The cerebral cortex assumes the role of generating movements or behaviors, and the basal ganglia act broadly to inhibit competing movements that would otherwise interfere with the desired action (Mink, 2003). These circuits are modulated by the basal ganglia via direct/excitatory and indirect/inhibitory pathways. It is postulated that if the indirect pathway is disrupted, the result may be irrepressible repetitive behaviors and thoughts, similar to those observed in OCD and TS, or negative ruminations in depression (Rauch et al., 1997; Saxena et al., 2001).

Given that TS is defined by difficulties in suppressing often complex movements and vocalizations, inhibitory processes and related executive functions are natural targets of investigation. However, deficits in executive functioning have largely been variable across studies, with few consistent findings emerging (Schultz, Carter, et al., 1999). Studies using standard psychometric instruments have attempted to assess constructs such as mental flexibility (Wisconsin Card Sort), mental tracking/sequencing (Trailmaking Test), and verbal fluency (Controlled Oral Word Association Test) without any consistency in their outcome (Baren-Cohen, Cross, Crowson, & Robertson, 1994; Bornstein, 1990; Channon, Flynn, & Robertson, 1992; Ozonoff, Strayer, McMahon, & Filloux, 1994; Schultz et al., 1998). The most consistent finding to emerge has been slowed reaction time demonstrated by subjects with TS during a continuous performance task (CPT), suggesting difficulties with sustained attention (Harris et al., 1995; Shucard, Benedict, Tekokkilic, & Lichter, 1997; Silverstein, Como, Palumbo, West, & Osborn, 1995). In one study, response time delays maintained their significance compared to normal controls even when ADHD status was controlled for (Harris et al., 1995), indicating that problems in sustained attention may be a core EF-related deficit for patients with TS.

In recent years, more attention has been focused on potential response inhibition deficits associated with TS. Casey, Tottenham, and Fossella (2002) posit that cognitive control that functions to reduce conflict in processing of information is disrupted in childhood disorders such as TS, such that problems with overriding or suppressing inappropriate thought and behaviors arise. They present data indicating that children with TS show specific deficits in the inhibition of a motor response on a go/no-go task. The study also demonstrated that each of the other three experimental groups (ADHD, Schizophrenia, Sydenham chorea—medical model of OCD) showed a distinct pattern of performance on the response inhibition tasks that indicated a four-way dissociation. The TS group demonstrated difficulty with response execution task, whereas the ADHD group showed deficits on both the stimulus selection and response execution tasks. The authors suggest that the data support the involvement of specific frontosubcortical circuits in different developmental populations.

In our program we have recently investigated the neurocognitive correlates of TS and OCD in children (Chang, McCracken, & Piacentini, in press). Utilizing a neurocognitive assessment battery tapping executive functioning, memory, and visuomotor/spatial abilities, several notable differences among the three diagnostic groups (TS, OCD, and normal controls) have emerged. The TS group was less cognitively flexible on an alternation learning task, and demonstrated poorer cognitive inhibition on the Stroop interference trial than normal controls. Additionally, the TS group showed poorer divided attention abilities than the OCD group. These findings suggest that TS, at least in childhood, is associated with EF-related cognitive impairments in the areas of response inhibition, cognitive flexibility, and divided attention.

Other investigations of EF in TS have utilized visuospatial priming (VSP) as an experimental measure of response inhibition. VSP performance reflects the reaction time required to locate a visual target, which is modified (either facilitated or inhibited) if the target is immediately preceded by a "priming" visual cue (Tipper, 1985; Tipper & Baylis, 1987). Swerdlow, Magulac, Filion, and Zinner (1996) demonstrated that patients with TS, both children and adults, exhibited significantly reduced inhibition in relation to VSP facilitation. Given a visual cue that was inhibitory in nature, TS subjects still demonstrated facilitation, suggesting less inhibitory priming. Furthermore, the literature suggests that a correlation exists among normal control subjects between inhibitory priming and performance on the Stroop test, a cognitive test of response inhibition (Swerdlow, Filion, Geyer, & Braff, 1995). There are also reports of impaired Stroop interference performance in adults with TS (Georgiou, Bradshaw, Phillips, Bradshaw, & Chiu, 1995), indicating that deficits on both measures in TS groups may reflect overlap in dysfunction of frontosubcortical circuits regulating performance on these tasks.

Another series of studies with neurodevelopmentally disordered subjects, including those with TS, examined everyday problem solving on real-life-type tasks that involved generating a range of solutions to brief problem scenarios and selecting a preferred final solution (Channon, Crawford, Vakili, & Robertson, 2003; Channon, 2004). It was thought that effective problem solving involved both nonsocial executive processes, social and emotional processes, and practical and social knowledge. When asked to generate a range of possible solutions, subjects with TS produced significantly fewer solutions than a matched healthy control group, although they did not differ in average solution quality. When asked for their preferred solution, the TS group also scored below the control group in final solution quality. Examination of aspects of solution quality, problem appreciation, social appropriateness, and practical effectiveness showed that the solutions of subjects with TS were poorer on each of these indices.

The TS group was also tested with standardized psychometric instruments to assess EF (Channon et al., 2003), and the group performed worse compared to the control group only in the number of inhibitory

errors made on a Hayling test, a measure of inhibition and strategy generation (Burgess & Shallice, 1996). These two studies suggest that TS
uncomplicated by other comorbidities is associated with difficulties in
real-life-type problem solving, which relies on executive processes such
as planning, social judgment, identification of appropriate goals, and assessment of future potential consequences of different courses of action.
Moreover, subjects with TS also demonstrated mild deficits in inhibitory
aspects of executive function when assessed with more traditional cognitive instruments. Because executive impairments in TS appears to be relatively mild, whether or not it is detected in a given study may depend
on factors such as the sensitivity of the particular measure used and adequate controls for study comorbidity.

MEMORY SYSTEMS

Relatively little focus has been placed on examining memory and learning abilities in people with TS. The few studies that exist present inconsistent findings, once again making it difficult to draw any definitive
conclusions. Some studies indicate little if any impairment in general
neurocognitive functioning, including memory abilities in subjects with
TS (Bornstein, 1990, 1991a), with mild deficits likely associated with
comorbidity status. In contrast, a study by Stebbins and colleagues
(1995) demonstrated that patients with TS only were impaired on measures of strategic, working, and procedural (rotary pursuit) memory, im-
plicating deficits in both explicit and implicit memory systems. A recent
study by Channon, Pratt, and Robertson (2001) examined both implicit
and explicit memory along with executive functions in TS-only, TS +
OCD and TS + ADHD groups. Results indicate that the TS-only group
did not evidence any significant implicit or explicit memory impairment
when compared to normal controls. However, the authors note that several of the explicit memory measures (e.g., story, visual recall) approached group significance for the TS-only group and deserve further
investigation.

Rauch and colleagues (Rauch & Savage, 1997) have conducted interesting work in the area of implicit procedural memory using the serial
reaction time (SRT) paradigm with adults with TS. Their work suggests
that these patients evidence some deficits in implicit memory that are
consistent with the conceptualization of the disorder as involving frontosubcortical dysfunction (Rauch et al., 2001). Neurological conditions
with frontosubcortical involvement, such as Parkinson and Huntington
diseases, are thought to share the same cognitive impairments in execu-

tive functions, memory, and visuospatial abilities seen in patients with TS (Rauch & Savage, 1997). Further research in this area is needed to elucidate precisely what, if any, memory impairments exist in TS populations, and how they may be related to other cognitive findings for the disorder.

MOTOR FUNCTIONING

The most robust and consistent finding in the neurocognitive literature on TS is visuomotor integration (VMI) impairment. Measures of visuomotor integration—the most common being copying tasks of simple and complex geometric designs—tap multiple cognitive processes such as fine motor coordination and visuoperceptual ability, in addition to more executive skills such as motor inhibition and sustained attention. In a comprehensive review, Schultz, Carter, and colleagues (1999) noted that the overwhelming majority of studies reported visuomotor integration deficits in samples with TS when they were compared either to a normal control group or to normative table data. Typically, TS subjects evidenced performance levels on simple visuomotor integration tasks that were approximately one standard deviation below age norms, despite IQ in the normal range.

Results are more equivocal when drawing tasks are more complex and demanding, possibly requiring EF skills such as planning and organization for optimal execution (Schultz, Carter, et al., 1999). Studies utilizing the Rey–Osterrieth Complex Figure, a copying task that is influenced by EF organization as well as visuomotor integration skills, demonstrated inconsistent results, with some finding indicating significant difference between subjects with TS and normal controls, and other findings suggesting no group difference (Randolph, Hyde, Gold, Goldberg, & Weinberger, 1993; Sutherland et al., 1982). Other studies using the Rey figure attempted to account for ADHD comorbidity in evaluating VMI deficits, and found that subjects with TS without comorbid ADHD performed much better on the Rey copying task than those with ADHD (Harris et al., 1995; Schuerholz, Baumgardner, Singer, Reiss, & Denckla, 1996). However, another study indicated no differences in Rey performance between patients with TS and control subjects or between subjects with TD alone and those with comorbid ADHD (Schultz et al., 1998). Overall, such findings suggest that comorbid ADHD symptomatology may contribute to the visuomotor integration deficits observed in patients with TS, particularly given that children with ADHD alone have been shown to have VMI deficits relative to normal controls

(Frost, Moffitt, & McGee, 1989). Thus, performance of patients with TS on complex drawing tasks that demand greater EF skill may be more sensitive to ADHD status.

Studies examining fine motor skill and coordination in patients with TS indicate that performance trails age norm levels by 0.5 to 1.0 standard deviations—slightly less in magnitude but generally shown to be as consistent as visuomotor integration deficits across studies. Bornstein and colleagues tested patients with TS in a series of studies on several measures of gross and fine motor skills (Bornstein, 1990, 1991a, 1991b; Yeates & Bornstein, 1994). Results suggest that simple motor speed remains intact in patients with TS, but that fine motor skill dependent on visuoperceptual processes (e.g., as needed on the grooved pegboard test) is consistently impaired regardless of ADHD status. Moreover, studies have documented that the motor skills deficits were not affected by the actual presence of motor tics, suggesting that the impairment observed was a core deficit and not a consequence of simple tic expression (Schultz et al., 1998; Yeates & Bornstein, 1994).

Research aimed at examining visuoperceptual/visuospatial processes in patients TS has been hampered by the lack of specificity in instruments used to measure this cognitive domain. Few studies have utilized measures of visuoperceptual abilities that have not been confounded by general IQ or motor skill demands. One recent study by Schultz and colleagues (1998) attempted to examine a component process model of visuomotor integration in children with TS by assessing performance on tests that separately tapped visuomotor integration ability, motor skill, response inhibition, and perceptual/spatial ability. VMI scores were correlated with performance on fine motor skill and perceptual/spatial tasks, lending support for a component process model. However, visuoperceptual ability, fine motor skill, and response inhibition were also separate areas of weakness for the children with TS, regardless of their ADHD status. Moreover, none of the three separate component processes mentioned above could fully account for the VMI deficits observed, suggesting that the integration of visuoperceptual and motor functions is a specific area of vulnerability for children with TS.

AGE AND GENDER EFFECTS

Age Effects

In TS, tic onset typically occurs in early to mid childhood with fluctuating symptoms gradually worsening and reaching their peak severity in early adolescence (Leckman, King, & Cohen, 1999). Tics then subside substantially in number, frequency, and severity by early adulthood—a trend that is borne out by epidemiological data that indicate lower prevalence of TS among adults compared to children (Zohar, Apter, King, Pauls, Leckman, & Cohen, 1999). Although rates as high as 40% have been reported for full remission of all tic symptoms (Torup, 1962), other studies have indicated that 90% of adults still evidenced some tic symptoms according to videotaped observations (Pappert, Goetz, Louis, Blasucci, & Leurgans, 2003). However, for many patients with TS the transition to adulthood represents a significant improvement in tic disability and severity (Leckman et al., 1999; Pappert et al., 2003). Whether or not differences exist in the neurocognitive profile shown by children and adults with TS according to a developmental trajectory is not yet clear due to a lack of studies examining the issue.

A series of studies conducted by Bornstein (1990, 1991a) examined sizable samples of children and adults diagnosed with TS on an extensive battery of neurocognitive tests. Findings revealed a very similar pattern of test performance, with the majority of both children and adults exhibiting functioning within the normal range. However, a significant minority (20%) of both child and adult groups evidenced mild neurocognitive deficits in the domains of psychomotor and sensoriperceptual functions. Furthermore, in both age groups, later age at symptom onset was associated with worse neurocognitive performance, even when symptom duration was controlled for. The authors concluded that a stable pattern of mild neurocognitive abnormalities is associated with TS across the age span from childhood into adulthood. These findings are fairly consistent with reports of childhood TS being associated with mild difficulties in psychomotor and visuographic skills, attention, and select executive functions (Como, 2001). There have been fewer neurocognitive studies with adult patients with TS, and findings have been more variable; some studies report more severe impairment (Moldofsky & Lazar, 1983), and others cite more select deficits in areas such as attention (Como & Kurlan, 1989).

More recently, studies have attempted to examine specific cognitive abilities such as response inhibition in child and adult groups using more experimental paradigms. Swerdlow and colleagues (1996), using the visuospatial priming paradigm described earlier, found that relative to age-matched controls, patients with TS exhibited significant inhibitory deficits during both childhood and adulthood, and children with TS exhibited less inhibitory priming than child controls. Although the adults with TS did not demonstrate inhibitory priming compared to controls, they did show a relative deficit of inhibition versus facilitation—the same priming pattern characteristic of children with TS. The authors conclude that the normal developmental pattern of VSP across age (excessive facilitation in comparison with inhibition in children, which equalizes with age) appears to be exaggerated in patients with TS relative to controls, and that this pattern of inhibitory deficits persists in an attenuated manner into adulthood for subjects with TS. Such cognitive age effects are particularly interesting in light of the anatomical differences found in child and adult imaging studies of TS (Baumgardner et al., 1996; Gerard & Peterson, 2003; Peterson et al., 2001). Clearly, given the developmental aspects of TS, age needs to be considered appropriately in research studies utilizing longitudinal designs with age ranges that give us sufficient power to examine age effects.

Gender Effects

It is likely that gender may influence the expression of TS. The syndrome is clearly more prevalent among males than females, with most epidemiological studies citing a male–female ratio of approximately 3:1 (Singer, 1994; Zohar et al., 1999). Hence many studies of subjects with TS have been dominated by, if not limited to, males. It is unclear whether these rates are related to a higher prevalence of TS among males versus females or to greater symptom severity in males, which may, in turn, lead to higher clinical referral rates. The question of whether gender phenotypes involve differential clinical or neurobiological factors has been raised but remains to be fully explored. In their study of gender effects Santangelo and colleagues (1994) reported that males have a more frequent history of simple tics than females, along with tic onset that is more often associated with rage. In females, tic onset was more associated with compulsive-type tics compared to males. TS diagnosis was also found to occur at later ages among females than males. Although gender-related differences in the types of symptoms experienced at tic onset were found, the study concluded that overall the experience of TS appears to be similar for both groups.

The question of whether males and females with TS are also similar with regard to their neurocognitive profile remains unclear. In one of the few studies that examined gender differences in TS neurobiology, Cutting, Mazzocco, Singer, and Denckla (1997) studied children diagnosed with TS, TS + ADHD, ADHD, and normal controls on a variety of executive functioning and motor tasks. Results indicated that girls with TS only were slower than boys in that group on Letter Word Fluency, an EF task requiring speed and efficiency in memory search. Furthermore, girls with TS only performed more poorly on this task compared to girls in any of the other groups. The Letter Word Fluency task emerged as an area of deficit in the TS-only group, regardless of gender, but within that group, girls showed greater deficits than boys. A task of verbal fluency is likely mediated by left frontal lobe circuitry, which may be disrupted by the reversal of the normal left-larger-than-right pattern of asymmetry in regions of the basal ganglia and enlarged regions of the corpus callosum found in children with TS (Baumgardner et al., 1996; Mostofsky, Wendlandt, Cutting, Denckla, & Singer, 1999; Peterson et al., 1993; Singer et al., 1993). Girls typically show a greater left-versus-right brain asymmetry than boys, and demonstrate an associated strength in linguistic skill compared to boys. Therefore, the verbal fluency and memory search deficits evidenced by the TS-only girls in this study is particularly striking, and greater attention toward exploring gender-related differences in neurocognitive and neurobiological indices seems well deserved.

COMORBIDITY

Tics rarely exist in isolation in individuals with TS but tend to be accompanied by a host of other cognitive and behavioral difficulties, including most commonly the diagnoses of OCD and ADHD (Coffey & Park, 1997; Grad, Pelcovits, & Olson, 1987). (See Scahill, Sukhodolsky, & King, Chapter 4, this volume, for a full discussion of comorbidity with TS.) Although data suggest that cases of TS that meet full criteria for OCD hover around 30%, obsessive and compulsive features are much more common in patients with TS, and in some studies approach 80% (King, Leckman, Scahill, & Cohen, 1999). Similarly, the rate of ADHD in TS subjects is estimated to be 50%, with some studies citing even higher prevalence rates (Walkup et al., 1999). Data from the neuroimaging, lesion, and neurochemical literature suggest that TS, OCD, and ADHD may all result from aberrant functioning of specific BGTC pathways. The sensorimotor and limbic BGTC circuits have been implicated in TS, the orbitofrontal and limbic pathways in OCD, and the sensorimotor, orbitofrontal, and limbic circuits in ADHD (Sheppard, Bradshaw, Purcell, & Pantelis, 1999). All three conditions may be considered, in some sense, disorders of disinhibition, characterized by failure to inhibit voluntary and involuntary repetitive behaviors. Given the overlap in comorbidities, symptom profiles, and neurobiology, a better understanding of the unique and shared neurocognitive deficits associated with each of these disorders is important from both etiological and remedial perspectives (Spencer et al., 1998).

Given the frontostriatal system dysfunction suggested by imaging studies for these disorders, the functional areas to further elucidate and disentangle lie in visuospatial, executive, and memory domains. Neurocognitive studies of OCD uncomplicated by TS have primarily reported impairments in select visuospatial, executive, and visual memory functions (Savage, 1998), which are consistent with the profile of patients with corticostriatal dysfunction. ADHD investigations have also implicated a pattern of frontostriatal dysfunction, including deficits in attentional control, executive functions such as planning and organization, and verbal and visual memory (Armstrong, Hayes, & Martin, 2001; Mahone, Koth, Cutting, Singer, & Denckla, 2001). Studies of TS neurocognition have indicated that impairment exists in some but not all patients, suggesting that TS may be a heterogenous condition in which neurocognitive dysfunction exists on a spectrum that is influenced by factors such as psychiatric comorbidity (Bornstein, 1990, 1991a, 1991b; de Groot, Yeates, Baker, & Bornstein, 1997).

Neurocognitive studies have attempted to focus on what specific contributions each disorder makes to the pattern of cognitive performance in children with TS who have OCD and/or ADHD. Dykens and colleagues reported that impaired Performance IQ was related to the presence of ADHD but not to other measures of IQ or academic achievement in child groups with TS and TS + ADHD (Dykens et al., 1990). Similarly, Brand et al. (2002) found that patients with TS and comorbid ADHD evidenced poorer performance than those with TS alone with respect to verbal and performance intelligence as well as word fluency. Harris and colleagues (1995) also reported that ADHD presence in children with TS was related to impairments on an executive functioning measure relative to a TS-only group. By contrast, Schuerholz et al. (1996) compared patients with TS alone to patients with TS + ADHD and found poorer performance on verbal fluency in the TS-only group. In another study of executive functioning in subjects with TS and ADHD, Mahone and colleagues (2001) found that both ADHD and TS-only groups were largely free of executive impairment relative to controls. However, when less traditional process variables were examined, results indicated that both groups performed worse than the normal controls on the number of intrusion errors made on a verbal list-learning task, and the ADHD group performed worse than the TS group on certain aspects of a word fluency task. The authors concluded that uncomplicated TS should not routinely be considered to have significant executive function impairment, and when deficits are evident, contributions from existing comorbid disorders should be carefully evaluated.

Similar findings have been found in neurocognitive studies investigating TS samples with comorbid OCD. Bornstein (1991b) stratified a TS sample by the presence of obsessive symptoms and reported that patients with TS and obsessive symptoms demonstrated greater impairment on executive function measures relative to subjects without obsessions. Other studies have also shown that greater impairments in aspects of attention and memory are more evident in patients with TS and comorbid OCD, indicating that OCD is associated with greater cognitive dysfunction in TS (Silverstein et al., 1995; Stebbins et al., 1995).

There appears to be mounting research to suggest that comorbidities such as OCD and ADHD exacerbate the cognitive impairment found in TS. In support, de Groot and colleagues (1997) found that in subjects with TS, comorbid obsessive and obsessive plus attention symptoms were related to impaired performance on achievement and executive function measures. However, attention symptoms alone were not correlated with any cognitive impairment. The presence of both obsessive and attention problems identified those children with TS with the most severe and broadest profile of impairments. Similarly, Ozonoff, Strayer, McMahon, and Filloux (1998) assessed the ability to inhibit processing of irrelevant distracter stimuli with a negative priming task in patients with TS and OCD and/or ADHD. When they divided the sample into groups with or without comorbidity, they found that subjects with TS and comorbid conditions tended to perform more poorly than the normal control group, whereas those without comorbidity performed similar to controls. Similarly, the same pattern in cognitive performance was seen when the TS sample was divided into those subjects exhibiting numerous symptoms of TS, OCD, and ADHD, and those showing fewer and less severe symptoms. The authors concluded that neurocognitive impairment occurs generally as a function of comorbidity and symptom severity in TS.

Several studies have noted that the majority of patients with TS perform within normal limits of tests of neurocognitive functioning (Bornstein, 1990, 1991a; Randolph et al., 1993; Schultz et al., 1998). Furthermore, comorbid conditions such as OCD and ADHD have been demonstrated to greatly impact the degree of deficit observed in the subsample of patients with TS who show any clinically meaningful impairment. In considering what, if any, specific cognitive impairment may be uniquely characteristic of TS, the most compelling evidence seems to point to deficits in visuomotor integration and response inhibition. Although both TS and OCD have been shown to be associated with impairments in visuospatial processes, TS appears to be more strongly associated with difficulties in visuomotor integration, whereas OCD is related to problems in visuoperceptual processing (Schultz, Carter, et al., 1999). With regard to response inhibition abilities, Casey (2002) has shown that TS and OCD symptomatology is each associated with unique deficits in different aspects of response inhibition: TS, with the inhibition of a motor response, and OCD, with the inhibition of a behavior set (e.g., remapping from one set of responses to a new set of responses). Furthermore, Schultz, Carter, and colleagues (1999) found that visuomotor integration skill and inhibitory control, in combination were able to accurately classify 82% of a group of unaffected controls and 80% of children with TS. Despite such distinctions, the overlap among these three disorders is large with respect to comorbidity, neurobiology, and some aspects of symptom presentation. Therefore, comorbidity needs to be taken into account systematically in conducting studies of neurocognitive functioning in order to disentangle what is shared versus what is unique.

IMPACT ON SYMPTOM PRESENTATION

Chronic tic disorders in childhood have been related to a variety of problems, including aggressiveness, impulsivity, mood disturbance, poor social skills, and increased rates of family conflict (Leckman & Cohen, 1999). Often such behavioral, emotional, and social difficulties of patients with a tic disorder are far more disabling and prominent than the core tic symptoms themselves, thus complicating symptom presentation and constituting a major challenge to treatment (Hoekstra et al., 2004). How areas of cognitive impairment may contribute to the overall symptom presentation of an individual with TS is a largely unexplored subject. One study examining inhibitory deficits in patients with TS found a positive correlation among neurocognitive impairment, levels of comorbidity, and symptom severity (Ozonoff et al., 1998). Thus, subjects with TS who demonstrated greater inhibitory deficits also evidenced greater comorbidity and more severe symptoms of TS, ADHD, and OCD.

Channon and colleagues (2003) examined executive aspects of social cognition in patients with TS and without any comorbid conditions, and found that they performed more poorly compared to controls on a real-life-type interpersonal problem-solving task both in the generating a range of potential solutions and in selecting a socially appropriate and practically effective final solution. Additionally, subjects with TS performed more poorly relative to controls on a more abstract nonsocial executive function task assessing response inhibition and strategy generation. They also reported a greater number of dysexecutive problems in their everyday lives, including difficulties with emotion, personality, motivation, behavior, and cognition on a self-report questionnaire. The authors propose that a social problem-solving task may be better able to tap into the specific executive deficits that may be implicated in TS than traditional standardized measures used in most other studies. An ecologically based real-life problem-solving task would assess multiple contextual abilities such as the selection of relevant information for attention, identification of appropriate goals, sensitivity to potential future consequences of different courses of action, making reasoned judgments, and evaluating performance.

Indeed, if such complex executive abilities play a role in the profile of neurocognitive dysfunction in TS, they may well be related to the range of social, emotional, and behavioral difficulties that often characterize the disorder. Dykens et al. (1990), using the Vineland Adaptive Behavior Scales and the Child Behavior Checklist demonstrated that socialization skills emerged as a significant weakness in adaptive functioning. Other studies have shown that patients with TS may have greater behavioral difficulties in areas such as dating and forming and maintaining friendships and show socially inappropriate behaviors such as aggression and social withdrawal (Champion, Fulton, & Shady, 1988; Kurlan et al., 1996; Stokes, Bawden, & Camfield, 1991). It is unclear whether such psychosocial difficulties common to TS are etiologically related to the disorder and a potential reflection of underlying EF deficits, or are sequelae of living with a debilitating disorder and its associated symptoms (Scahill, Walker, Lechner, & Tynan, 1993). Identifying the factors that predict or lead to the emergence of associated behavioral problems and comorbid disorders may improve prevention and intervention strategies.

Brand and colleagues (2002) attempted to examine more directly the association between neurocognitive deficits in executive abilities and psychosocial functioning, controlling for ADHD comorbidity. They proposed that executive functions such as planning, attention, and cognitive flexibility may permit more adaptive coping with a tic disorder and its attendant social and behavioral difficulties. Thus, patients with TS who are more cognitively flexible may experience less distress and interference related to their condition and as a consequence have better psychosocial functioning. The study found that TS with comorbid ADHD is associated with more severe TS symptoms and worse psychosocial and cognitive functioning on tests of verbal and performance intelligence and word fluency compared to a TS-only group. However, diminished cognitive flexibility did not appear to moderate the influence of symptom severity on psychosocial functioning in the subjects with TS. The study highlights again the importance of comorbidity factors in TS. Given the data that suggest executive impairments in TS, albeit inconsistent, efforts to develop more ecologically valid measures to assess specific executive deficits in TS, especially as they may relate to the subject's psychosocial functioning, would be interesting and fruitful.

The comorbidity research clearly indicates that in patients with TS, conditions such as ADHD and OCD significantly increase the likelihood that learning problems or demonstrable cognitive impairment will be present. Studies indicate that children with TS may be more likely to evidence learning disabilities or academic deficiencies in math and written language (Como, 2001; Incagnoli & Kane, 1981; Matthews, 1988). Such disabilities, in addition to other cognitive impairments, may place a child with TS at higher risk for poor school performance and academic failure. School difficulties may also result from a variety of factors aside from cognitive impairment, such as include concentration and physical coordination problems as well as emotional distress related to the tic symptoms. The psychosocial impact of these problems is significant, and thus when cognitive impairment and related problems are suspected, they need to be addressed expeditiously. A thorough psychoeducational evaluation may help pinpoint any learning difficulties and areas of academic deficiency in children with TS who have a poor academic record despite normal intelligence. In addition, a selective neurocognitive evaluation, focused on the areas of visuomotor integration, motor skill, perceptual/spatial ability, and executive functions, may highlight any cognitive areas that may benefit from remediation. Children with TS often demonstrate, for instance, poor penmanship, which may reflect impairments in visuomotor integration and fine motor skills that are suspected to be core deficits in TS (Schultz, Carter, et al., 1999).

IMPACT ON TREATMENT RESPONSE

Only a small handful of studies has examined neurocognitive function in relation to treatment of any kind for TS. Most studies have been limited by methodologies characterized by case study design, lack of control group, and ill-defined protocols. Despite such limitations, some interesting results have emerged to suggest that neurocognitive deficits may be state, versus trait, markers of the disorder, and can be ameliorated with effective treatment. Case studies have demonstrated that extracranial application of electromagnetic fields in the picotesla range intensity have reversed the visuoconstructional and visuomotor deficits observed in children with TS (Sandyk, 1995, 1997). In a more rigorous study that randomized children with TS into one of three treatment conditions (pimozide, haloperidol, or no-medication control group), findings demonstrated that pimozide treatment was superior to haloperidol with regard to tic improvement, and that it was associated with greater positive change in memory search efficiency compared to the no-drug condition (Salle, Sethuraman, & Rock, 1994). (See Harrison, Schneider, & Walkuop, Chapter 7, this volume, for a detailed discussion of medication treatment.) Such studies, although few in number, present the provocative idea that cognitive deficits associated with TS may improve with effective treatment, but clearly findings need to be replicated with more rigorously designed studies that examine in detail the relationship among cognitive functioning, symptom severity, and treatment response.

Such work has already begun with OCD, a disorder that shares many characteristics with TS (Bolton, Raven, Madronal-Luque, & Marks, 2000; Hollander, Shiffman, Cohen, Rivera-Stein, Rosen, et al., 1990; Sanz, Molina, Martin-Loeches, Calcedo, & Rubia, 2001; Thienenmann & Koran, 1995). A recent study of neurocognitive and positron emission tomography (PET) indices following serotonin reuptake inhibitor medication treatment for OCD was the first to demonstrate a significant relationship among improved performance on a neurocognitive measure, the Rey–Osterrieth Complex Figure Test, and metabolic changes in the putamen, cerebellum, and hippocampus (Kang et al., 2003). Such studies raise the question of whether neurocognitive abnormalities in TS may also be state markers that can normalize with effective treatment, rather than stable trait markers of the disease.

Another area of research that has received little attention thus far is whether neurocognitive indices may function as predictors of treatment response in patients with TS. In one of the only studies to examine this issue, Deckersbach, Rauch, Buhlmann, and Wilhelm (2006) conducted a study to evaluate cognitive impairments in inhibition as a predictor for treatment response to habit reversal therapy (HRT) or supportive psychotherapy. More specifically, before randomization to either HRT or supportive psychotherapy, patients completed a computerized measure of response inhibition, the visuospatial priming (VSP; Swerdlow et al., 1996) task. Preliminary data from this study indicate that 71% of patients treated with HRT were responders (reduction of tic severity > 30%), whereas only 13% of patients in the psychotherapy condition responded. Correlation analysis between inhibitory priming reaction times and changes in tic severity from pre- to posttreatment indicated that faster reaction times (i.e., more impairment in inhibition) indicated less response to HRT but not to supportive treatment. In both groups, negative priming was only weakly correlated with tic severity. Thus, greater deficits in inhibition at baseline predict a worse response to an effective form of treatment for TS in this study.

Data on the relationship between cognitive deficits in TS and response to specific types of treatments will help influence intervention guidelines and recommendations. For example, if the cognitive impairment observed in TS is malleable, then benefits may be gained from supplementing standard treatments with additional work targeting specific areas of cognitive deficit, such as executive functions or visuomotor integration skills. Some studies have suggested that skills such as cognitive flexibility and planning/organization may be trained on a behavioral level (Delahunty & Morice, 1996; Savage, 1998), and such programs may work in conjunction with more traditional treatment protocols to optimize functional outcomes for TS patients.

Conclusions from studies investigating comorbidity and cognitive impairment in TS suggest that increasing levels of comorbidity are associated with greater cognitive deficits (Ozonoff et al., 1998). Moreover, there is some evidence to suggest that a profile of comorbidity leads to differential treatment response. Studies examining treatment response in OCD subjects with and without tics have shown that response to cognitive-behavioral therapy does not differ between the two diagnostic groups, but that the OCD group with tics demonstrated a poorer response to SSRI than the group without tics (Himle, Fischer, Van Etten, Janeck, & Hanna, 2003; Miguel, Shavitt, Ferrao, Brotto, & Diniz, 2003). It would be productive to extend these types of investigations to include the kinds of neurocognitive predictors of treatment response that might exist for different types of TS treatments in order to better guide their selection and implementation.

The majority of those affected with tics will not require special intervention. Just as a minority of patients has tics severe enough to warrant medication treatment, the majority of subjects with TS do not demonstrate clear cognitive impairment requiring specialized services. In addition, it is often the case that symptoms associated with comorbid OCD and/or ADHD may prove more problematic and impairing and therefore need to be the initial focus of intervention. The degree of cognitive impairment present may serve as a guide for treatment selection. The growing literature on cognitive-behavioral treatments for tic disorder presents mounting evidence for positive effects (Peterson & Azrin, 1993; Piacentini & Chang, 2001; Turpin, 1983; Wilhelm et al., 2003; Woods, Miltenberger, & Lumley, 1996). However, behavioral interventions are more cognitively demanding, requiring higher levels of motivation, effort, and behavioral compliance than pharmacological treatments. A child who might be laboring under the multiple burdens of academic failure, learning disabilities, psychosocial problems, and specific cognitive deficits in the areas of inhibition and visuomotor integration may need a multimodal approach to treatment that incorporates pharmacology, behavior modification, as well as family and school interventions (Walter & Carter, 1997).

FUTURE DIRECTIONS

An abundance of opportunities exist to extend and enrich investigations into the neurocognitive correlates of TS with neurobehavioral and neuroimaging tools. Combining cognitive probe paradigms with functional imaging techniques permits researchers to examine the relationship between behavior and neuroanatomical functioning. Furthermore, applying such techniques to intervention research to study the neural mechanisms underlying treatment response (with cognitive-behavioral therapy and/or medication) not only advances our etiological understanding of the disorder, but also assists us in refining our interventions. Future investigations of TS might include the assessment of neurocognitive and functional brain abnormalities before and after treatment. In addition, cognitive measures that are more sensitive and specific to the executive and visuomotor deficits implicated in TS need to be developed so that we are better able to characterize the neurocognitive profile of TS from comorbid conditions such as OCD and ADHD. Studies that sample broadly from the age spectrum may also help us to distinguish how neurodevelopment may interact with cognitive vulnerabilities to influence symptom presentation in the patient with TS. In conclusion, the future of neurocognitive research with TS is promising, given the multidisciplinary collaborations that are possible among neurocognitive, neurobiological, and genetic domains of study.

REFERENCES

Apter, A., Pauls, D. L., Bleich, A., Zohar, A. H., Kron, S., Ratzoni, G., et al. (1993). An epidemiological study of Gilles de la Tourette's syndrome in Israel. *Archives of General Psychiatry, 50,* 734–738.

Armstrong, C. L., Hayes, K. M., & Martin, R. (2001). Neurocognitive problems in attention deficit disorder: Alternative concepts and evidence for impairment in inhibition of selective attention, *Annals of New York Academy of Science, 931,* 196–215.

Baron-Cohen, S., Cross, P., Crowson, M., & Robertson, M. (1994). Can children with Gilles de la Tourette syndrome edit their intentions? *Psychological Medicine, 24,* 29–40.

Baumgardner, T., Singer, H. S., Denckla, M. B., Rubin, M. A., Abrams, M. T., Colli, M. J., et al. (1996). Morphology of the corpus callosum in children with Tourette syndrome and attention deficit hyperactivity disorder. *Neurology, 47,* 477–482.

Bolton, D., Raven, P., Madronal-Luque, R., & Marks, I. M. (2000). Neurological and neuropsychological signs in obsessive compulsive disorder: Interaction with behavioural treatment. *Behaviour and Research Therapy, 38*(7), 695–708.

Bornstein, R. A. (1990). Neuropsychological performance in children with Tourette's syndrome. *Psychiatry Research, 33,* 73–81.

Bornstein, R. A. (1991a). Neuropsychological performance in adults with Tourette's syndrome. *Psychiatry Research, 37,* 229–236.

Bornstein, R. A. (1991b). Neuropsychological correlates of obsessive characteristics in Tourette syndrome. *Journal of Neuropsychiatry and Clinical Neuroscience, 3,* 157–162.

Bornstein, R. A., Carroll, A., & King, G. (1985). Relationship of age to neuropsychological deficit in Tourette's syndrome. *Journal of Developmental and Behavioral Pediatrics, 6*(5), 284–286.

Brand, N., Geenen, R., Oudenhoven, M., Lindenborn, B., van der Ree, A., Cohen-Dettenis,

P., et al. (2002). Brief report: Cognitive functioning in children with Tourette's syndrome with and without comorbid ADHD. *Journal of Pediatric Psychology, 27*(2), 203–208.

Burgess, P. W., & Shallice, T. (1996). Response suppression, initiation and strategy use following frontal lobe lesions. *Neuropsychologia, 34,* 263–273.

Casey, B. J., Tottenham, N., & Fossella, J. (2002). Clinical, imaging, lesion and genetic approaches toward a model of cognitive control. *Developmental Psychobiology, 40,* 237–254.

Champion, L. M., Fulton, W. A., & Shady, G. A. (1988). Tourette syndrome and social functioning in a Canadian population. *Neuroscience and Biobehavioral Review, 12,* 255–257.

Chang, S. W., McCracken, J. T., & Piacentini, J. C. (in press). Neurocognitive correlates of child obsessive compulsive disorder and Tourette syndrome. *Journal of Clinical and Experimental Neuropsychology.*

Channon, S. (2004). Frontal lobe dysfunction and everyday problem-solving: Social and non-social contributions. *Acta Psychologica, 115,* 235–254.

Channon, S., Crawford, S., Vakili, K., & Robertson, M. (2003). Real-life-type problem solving in Tourette syndrome. *Cognitive and Behavioral Neurology, 15,* 3–15.

Channon, S., Flynn, D., & Robertson, M. M. (1992). Attentional deficits in Gilles de la Tourette syndrome. *Neuropsychiatry, Neuropsychology and Behavioral Neurology, 5,* 170–177.

Channon, S., Pratt, P., & Robertson, M. (2001). Executive function, memory, and learning in Tourette's syndrome. *Neuropsychology, 17*(2), 247–254.

Coffey, B. J., & Park, K. S. (1997). Behavioral and emotional aspects of Tourette syndrome. *Neurologic Clinics, 15*(2), 277–290.

Como, P. G. (2001). Neuropsychological function in Tourette syndrome. In D. J. Cohen, C. G. Goetz, & J. Jankovic (Eds.), *Tourette syndrome* (pp. 103–111). Philadelphia: Lippincott, Williams & Wilkins.

Como, P. G., & Kurlan, R. (1989). Neuropsychological testing in Tourette's syndrome: A comparison of clinic and family populations. *Neurology, 39*(Suppl. 1), 342.

Deckersbach, T., Rauch, S., Buhlmann, U., & Wilhelm, S. (2006). Habit reversal versus supportive psychotherapy in Tourette's disorder: A randomized controlled trial and predictors of treatment response. *Behaviour Research and Therapy, 44,* 1079–1090.

de Groot, C. M., Yeates, K. O., Baker, G. B., & Bornstein, R. A. (1997). Impaired neuropsychological functioning in Tourette's syndrome subjects with co-occurring obsessive–compulsive and attention deficit symptoms. *Journal of Neuropsychiatry, 9,* 267–272.

Delahunty, A., & Morice, R. (1996). Rehabilitation of frontal/executive impairments in schizophrenia. *Australian–New Zealand Journal of Psychiatry, 30,* 760–767.

Dykens, E., Leckman, J. F., Riddle, M. A., Hardin, M. T., Schwartz, S., & Cohen, D. (1990). Intellectual, academic, and adaptive functioning of Tourette syndrome children with and without attention deficit disorder. *Journal of Abnormal Child Psychology, 18,* 607–615.

Frost, L. A., Moffitt, T. E., & McGee, R. (1989). Neuropsychological correlates of psychopathology in an unselected cohort of young adolescents. *Journal of Abnormal Psychology, 98,* 307–313.

Georgiou, N., Bradshaw, J. L., Phillips, J. G., Bradshaw, J. A., & Chiu, E. (1995). Advance information and movement sequencing in Gilles de la Tourette's syndrome. *Journal of Neurological and Neurosurgical Psychiatry, 58,* 184–191.

Gerard, E., & Peterson, B. S. (2003). Developmental processes and brain imaging studies in Tourette syndrome. *Journal of Psychosomatic Research, 55,* 13–22.

Grad, L. R., Pelcovits, D., & Olson, M. (1987). Obsessive–compulsive symptomatology in children with Tourette's syndrome. *American Academy of Child and Adolescent Psychiatry, 26,* 69.

Harris, E. L., Schuerholz, L. J., Singer, H. S., Reader, M. J., Brown, J. E., Cox, C., et al. (1995). Executive function in children with Tourette syndrome and/or attention deficit hyperactivity disorder. *Journal of the International Neuropsychological Society, 1,* 511–516.

Himle, J. A., Fischer, D. J., Van Etten, M. L., Janeck, A. S., & Hanna, G. L. (2003). Group behavioral therapy for adolescents with tic-related and non-tic-related obsessive–compulsive disorder. *Depression and Anxiety, 17,* 73–77.

Hoekstra, P. J., Steenhuis, M., Troost, P. W., Korf, J., Kallenberg, C. G. M., & Mindera, R. B. (2004). Relative contribution of attention-deficit hyperactivity disorder, obsessive–compulsive disorder, and tic severity to social and behavioral problems in tic disorders. *Developmental and Behavioral Pediatrics, 25*(4), 272–279.

Hollander, E., Shiffman, E., Cohen, B., Rivera-Stein, M. A., Rosen, W., Gorman, J. M., et al. (1990). Signs of central nervous system dysfunction in obsessive–compulsive disorder. *Archives of General Psychiatry, 47,* 27–32.

Incagnoli, T., & Kane, R. (1981). Neuropsychological functioning in Gilles de la Tourette's syndrome. *Journal of Clinical Neuropsychology, 3,* 165–171.

Kang, D. H., Kwon, J. S., Kim, J. J., Youn, T., Park, H. J., Kim, M. S., et al. (2003). Brain glucose metabolic changes associated with neuropsychological improvements after 4 months of treatment in patients with obsessive–compulsive disorder. *Acta Psychiatrica Scandinavica, 107*(4), 291–297.

King, R. A., Leckman, J. F., Scahill, L., & Cohen, D. J. (1999). Obsessive–compulsive disorder, anxiety, and depression. In J. F. Leckman & D. J. Cohen (Eds.), *Tourette's syndrome—tics, obsessions, compulsions: Developmental psychopathology and clinical care* (pp. 43–62). New York: Wiley.

Kurlan, R., Daragjati, C., Como, P. G., McDermott, M. D., Trinidad, K. S., Roddy, S., et al. (1996). Non-obscene complex socially inappropriate behavior in Tourette's syndrome. *Journal of Neuropsychiatry and Clinical Neuroscience, 8,* 311–317.

Leckman, J. F., & Cohen, D. J. (1999). Evolving models of pathogenesis. In J. F. Leckman & D. J. Cohen (Eds.), *Tourette's syndrome—tics, obsessions, compulsions: Developmental psychopathology and clinical care* (pp. 155–176). New York: Wiley.

Leckman, J. F., King, R. A., & Cohen, D. J. (1999). Tics and tic disorders. In J. F. Leckman & D. J. Cohen (Eds.), *Tourette's syndrome—tics, obsessions, compulsions: Developmental psychopathology and clinical care* (pp. 23–42). New York: Wiley.

Mahone, E. M., Koth, C. W., Cutting, L., Singer, H. S., & Denckla, M. B. (2001). Executive function in fluency and recall measures among children with Tourette's syndrome or ADHD. *Journal of the International Neuropsychological Society, 7,* 102–111.

Matthews, W. S. (1988). Attention deficits and learning disabilities in children with Tourette's syndrome. *Psychiatric Annals, 18,* 414–416.

Miguel, E. C., Shavitt, R. G., Ferrao, Y. A., Brotto, S. A., & Diniz, J. B. (2003). How to treat OCD in patients with Tourette syndrome. *Journal of Psychosomatic Research, 55,* 49–57.

Mink, J. W. (2003). The basal ganglia and involuntary movements: Impaired inhibition of competing motor patterns. *Archives of Neurology, 60*(10), 1365–1368.

Moldosfsky, H., & Lazar, L. (1983, February). *Impaired neuropsychological functioning in Gilles de la Tourette's syndrome.* Paper presented at International Neuropsychological Society, Mexico City.

Mostofsky, S. H., Wendlandt, J., Cutting, L., Denckla, M. B., & Singer, H. S. (1999). Corpus callosum measurements in girls with Tourette syndrome. *Neurology, 53*(6), 1345–1347.

Ozonoff, S., Strayer, D. L., McMahon, W. M., & Filloux, F. (1994). Executive function abilities in autism and Tourette syndrome: An information processing approach. *Journal of Child Psychology and Psychiatry, 35,* 1015–1032.

Ozonoff, S., Strayer, D. L., McMahon, W. M., & Filloux, F. (1998). Inhibitory deficits in Tourette syndrome: A function of comorbidity and symptom severity. *Journal of Child Psychiatry, 39*(8), 1109–1118.

Pappert, E. J., Goetz, C. G., Louis, E. D., Blasucci, L., & Leurgans, S. (2003). Objective assessments of longitudinal outcome in Gilles de la Tourette's syndrome. *Neurology, 61,* 936–940.

Parraga, H. C., & McDonald, H. G. (1996). Etiology of Tourette's disorder. *Journal of the American Academy of Child and Adolescent Psychiatry, 35,* 2–3.

Pennington, B. F. (1991). *Diagnosing learning disorders.* New York: Guildford Press.

Pennington, B. F., & Ozonoff, S. (1996). Executive functions and developmental psychopathology. *Journal of Child Psychology and Psychiatry, 37*(1), 51–87.

Peterson, A. L., & Azrin, N. H. (1993). Behavioral and pharmacological treatments for Tourette syndrome: A review. *Applied and Preventative Psychology, 2,* 231–242.

Peterson, B. S., Leckman, J. F., Arnsten, A., Anderson, G. M., Staib, L. H., Gore, J. C., et al. (1999). Neuroanatomical circuitry. In J. F. Leckman & D. J. Cohen (Eds.), *Tourette's syndrome—tics, obsessions compulsions: Developmental psychopathology and clinical care* (pp. 230–260). New York: Wiley.

Peterson, B. S., Riddle, M. A., Cohen, D. J., Katz, L. D., Smith, J. C., & Leckman, J. F. (1993). Reduced basal ganglia volumes in Tourette's syndrome using three-dimensional reconstruction techniques from magnetic resonance images. *Neurology, 43,* 941–949.

Peterson, B. S., Staib, L., Scahill, L., Zhang, H., Anderson, C., Leckman, J. F., et al. (2001). Regional brain and ventricular volumes in Tourette syndrome. *Archives of General Psychiatry, 58,* 427–440.

Piacentini, J., & Chang, S. (2001). Behavioral treatments for Tourette syndrome: State of the art. In D. J. Cohen, J. Jankovic, & C. Goetz (Eds.), *Advances in neurology: Tourette syndrome* (Vol. 85, pp. 319–332). Philadelphia: Lippincott, William & Wilkins.

Randolph, C., Hyde, T. M., Gold, J. M., Goldberg, T. E., & Weinberger, D. R. (1993). Tourette's syndrome in monozygotic twins: Relationship of tic severity to neuropsychological function. *Archives of Neurology, 50,* 725–728.

Rauch, S. L., & Savage, C. R. (1997). Neuroimaging and neuropsychology of the striatum. *Psychiatric Clinics of North America, 20*(4), 741–768.

Rauch, S. L., Savage, C. R., Alpert, N. M., Dougherty, C., Kendrick, A., Curran, T., et al. (1997). Probing striatal function in obsessive–compulsive disorder: A PET study of implicit sequence learning. *Journal of Neuropsychiatry and Clinical Neuroscience, 9*(4), 568–573.

Rauch, S. L., Whalen, P. J., Curran, T., Shin, L. M., Coffey, B. J., Savage, C. R., et al. (2001). Probing striato–thalamic function in obsessive–compulsive disorder and Tourette syndrome using neuroimaging methods. *Advances in Neurology, 85,* 207–224.

Robertson, M. M., & Yakeley, J. W. (1993). Obsessive–compulsive disorder and self-injurious behavior. In R. Kurlan (Ed.), *Handbook of Tourette's syndrome and related tic and behavioral disorders* (pp. 45–87). New York: Marcel Dekker.

Sallee, F. R., Sethuraman, G., & Rock, C. M. (1994). Effects of pimozide on cognition in children with Tourette syndrome: Interaction with comorbid attention deficit hyperactivity disorder. *Acta Psychiatrica Scandinavica, 90*(1), 4–9.

Sandyk, R. (1995). Improvement of right hemisphere functions in a child with Gilles de la Tourette's syndrome by weak electromagnetic fields. *International Journal of Neuroscience, 81*(3–4), 199–213.

Sandyk, R. (1997). Reversal of a visuoconstructional disorder by weak electromagnetic fields in a child with Tourette's syndrome. *International Journal of Neuroscience, 90*(3–4), 159–167.

Santangelo, S. L., Pauls, D. L., Goldstein, J. M., Faraone, S. V., Tsuang, M. T., & Leckman, J. F. (1994). Tourette's syndrome: What are the influences of gender and comorbid obsessive–compulsive disorder? *Journal of the American Academy of Child and Adolescent Psychiatry, 33*(6), 795–804.

Sanz, M., Molina, V., Martin-Loeches, M., Calcedo, A., & Rubia, F. J. (2001). Auditory P300 event related potential and serotonin reuptake inhibitor. *Psychiatry Research, 101*(1), 75–81.

Savage, C. R. (1998). Neuropsychology of obsessive–compulsive disorder: Research findings and treatment implications. In M. A. Jenike, L. Baer, & W. E. Minichiello (Eds.), *Obsessive–compulsive disorders: Practical management,* (3rd ed., pp. 254–275). St. Louis, MO: Mosby.

Saxena, S., Brody, A. L., Ho, M. L., Alborzian, S., Ho, M. K., Maidment, K. M., et al. (2001). Cerebral metabolism in major depression and obsessive–compulsive disorder occurring separately and concurrently. *Biological Psychiatry, 50,* 159–170.

Scahill, L., Walker, R., Lechner, S. N., & Tynan, K. E. (1993). Inpatient treatment of obsessive compulsive disorder: A case study. *Journal of Child and Adolescent Psychiatric Nursing, 6,* 5–14.

Schuerholz, L. J., Baumgardner, T. L., Singer, H. S., Reiss, A. L., & Denckla, M. B. (1996). Neuropsychological status of children with Tourette's syndrome with and without attention deficit hyperactivity disorder. *Neurology, 26,* 958–965.

Schuerholz, L. J., Cutting, L., Mazzocco, M. M., Singer, H. S., & Denckla, M. B. (1997). Neuromotor functioning in children with Tourette syndrome with and without attention deficit hyperactivity disorder. *Journal of Child Neurology, 12,* 438.

Schultz, R. T., Carter, A. S., Gladstone, M., Scahill, L., Leckman, J. F., Peterson, B. S., et al. (1998). Visual–motor, visuoperceptual and fine motor functioning in children with Tourette syndrome. *Neuropsychology, 12,* 134–145.

Schultz, R. T., Carter, A. S., Scahill, L., & Leckman, J. F. (1999). Neuropsychological findings. In J. F. Leckman & D. J. Cohen (Eds.), *Tourette's syndrome—tics, obsessions, compulsions: Developmental pathology and clinical care* (pp. 80–103). New York: Wiley.

Schultz, R. T., Evans, D. W., & Wolff, M. (1999). Neuropsychological models of childhood obsessive–compulsive disorder. *Child and Adolescent Psychiatric Clinics of North America, 8*(3), 513–531.

Shapiro, A. K., Shapiro, E., Bruun, R., & Sweet, R. D. (1978). *Gilles de la Tourette's syndrome.* New York: Raven Press.

Shapiro, A. K., Shapiro, E., Young, J. G., & Feinberg, T. (1988). *Gilles de la Tourette's syndrome* (2nd ed.). New York: Raven Press.

Sheppard, D. M., Bradshaw, J. L., Purcell, R., & Pantelis, C. (1999). Tourette's and comorbid syndromes: Obsessive compulsive and attention deficit hyperactivity disorder. A common etiology? *Clinical Psychology Review, 19*(5), 531–552.

Shucard, D. W., Benedict, R. H. B., Tekokkilic, A., & Lichter, D. G. (1997). Slowed reaction time during a continuous performance test in children with Tourette's syndrome. *Neuropsychology, 11,* 147–155.

Silverstein, S. M., Como, P. G., Palumbo, D. R., West, L. L., & Osborn, L. M. (1995). Multiple sources of attentional dysfunction in adults with Tourette's syndrome: Comparison with attention-deficit hyperactivity disorder. *Neuropsychology, 9,* 157–164.

Singer, H. S. (1994). Neurobiological issues in Tourette syndrome. *Brain Development, 16*(5), 353–364.

Singer, H. S., Reiss, A. L., Brown, R. N., Aylward, E. H., Shih, B. A., Chee, E., et al. (1993). Volumetric MRI changes in basal ganglia of children with Tourette's syndrome. *Neurology, 43*, 950–956.

Spencer, T., Biederman, J., Harding, M., O'Donnell, D., Wilens, T., Faraone, S., et al. (1998). Disentangling the overlap between Tourette's disorder and ADHD. *Journal of Child Psychology and Psychiatry and Allied Disciplines, 39*(7), 1037–1044.

Stebbins, G. T., Singh, J., Weiner, J., Wilson, R. S., Goetz, C. G., & Gabrieli, J. D. E. (1995). Selective impairment of memory functioning in unmedicated adults with Gilles de la Tourette's syndrome. *Neuropsychology, 9*, 329–337.

Stokes, A., Bawden, H. N., & Camfield, P. R. (1991). Peer problems in Tourette's disorder, *Pediatrics, 87*, 936–942.

Sutherland, R. J., Kolb, B., Schoel, W. M., Wishaw, I. Q., & Davies, D. (1982). Neuropsychological assessment of children and adults with Tourette syndrome: A comparison with learning disabilities and schizophrenia. In A. J. Friedhoff & T. N. Chase (Eds.), *Gilles de la Tourette syndrome: Advances in neurology* (pp. 311–321). New York: Raven Press.

Swerdlow, N. R., Filion, D., Geyer, M. A., & Braff, D. L. (1995). "Normal" personality correlates of sensorimotor, cognitive, and visuo-spatial gating. *Biology and Psychiatry, 37*, 286–299.

Swerdlow, N. R., Magulac, M., Filion, D., & Zinner, S. (1996). Visuospatial priming and latent inhibition in children and adults with Tourette's disorder. *Neuropsychology, 10*(4), 485–494.

Thienemann, M., & Koran, L. M. (1995). Do soft signs predict treatment outcome in obsessive–compulsive disorder? *Journal of Neuropsychiatry and Clinical Neuroscience, 7*(2), 18–22.

Tipper, S. P. (1985). The negative priming effect: Inhibitory effects of ignored primes. *Quarterly Journal of Experimental Psychology, 37A*, 571–590.

Tipper, S. P., & Baylis, G. C. (1987). Individual differences in selective attention: The relation of priming and interference to cognitive failure. *Personality and Individual Differences, 8*, 667–675.

Torup, E. (1962). A follow-up study of children with tics. *Acta Paediatrica Scandinavica, 51*, 261–268.

Towbin, K. E., Peterson, B. S., Cohen, D. J., & Leckman, J. F. (1999). Differential diagnosis. In J. F. Leckman & D. J. Cohen (Eds.), *Tourette's syndrome—tics, obsessions, compulsions: Developmental pathology and clinical care* (pp. 118–139). New York: Wiley.

Towbin, K. E., & Riddle, M. A. (1993). Attention deficit hyperactivity disorder. In R. Kurlan (Ed.), *Handbook of Tourette's syndrome and related tic and behavioral disorders* (pp. 89–110). New York: Dekker.

Turpin, G. (1983). The behavioural management of tic disorders: A critical review. *Advances in Behavior Research and Therapy, 5*, 203–245.

Walkup, J. T., Khan, S., Schuerholz, L., Paik, Y., Leckman, J. F., & Schultz, R. (1999). Phenomenology and natural history of tic-related ADHD and learning disabilities. In J. F. Leckman & D. J. Cohen (Eds.), *Tourette's syndrome—tics, obsessions, compulsions: Developmental pathology and clinical care* (pp. 63–79). New York: Wiley.

Walter, A. L., & Carter, A. S. (1997). Gilles de la Tourette's syndrome in childhood: A guide for school professionals. *School Psychology Review, 26*(1), 28–46.

Wilhelm, S., Deckersbach, T., Coffey, B. J., Bohne, A., Peterson, A. L., & Baer, L. (2003). Habit reversal versus supportive psychotherapy for Tourette's disorder: A randomized controlled trial. *American Journal of Psychiatry, 160*, 1175–1177.

Woods, D. W., Miltenberger, R. G., & Lumley, V. A. (1996). Sequential application of major habit-reversal components to treat motor tics in children. *Journal of Applied Behavioral Analysis, 29,* 483–493.

Yeates, K. O., & Bornstein, R. A. (1994). Attention deficit disorder and neuropsychological functioning in children with Tourette's syndrome. *Neuropsychology, 8,* 65–74.

Zohar, A. H., Apter, A., King, R. A., Pauls, D. L., Leckman, J. F., & Cohen, D. J. (1999). In J. F. Leckman & D. J. Cohen (Eds.), *Tourette's syndrome—tics, obsessions, compulsions: Developmental pathology and clinical care* (pp. 63–79). New York: Wiley.

PART II

Clinical Management
of Symptoms
and Associated Conditions

CHAPTER 7

Medical Management of Tourette Syndrome and Co-Occurring Conditions

JOYCE N. HARRISON
BENJAMIN SCHNEIDER
JOHN T. WALKUP

The medical management of Tourette syndrome (TS) depends upon a careful initial assessment and identification of tic symptoms as well as co-occurring symptoms. TS is frequently accompanied by other difficulties, including attentional deficits, learning problems, and anxiety and mood symptoms. In many cases these co-occurring problems may be of greater clinical importance than the tic symptoms. The presence of co-occurring problems also has important implications for initial treatment choices. Other chapters in this book provide important information on the assessment of tics and co-occurring conditions (see Scahill, Sukhodolsky, & King, Chapter 4; Harrison, Schneider, & Walkup, Chapter 7; Buhlmann, Deckersback, Cook, & Wilhelm, Chapter 9). This chapter begins with a general approach to the treatment of TS followed by a review of various medical treatments for TS and associated conditions. Approaches to the treatment-refractory and clinically complex patient are also addressed in this chapter.

STANDARD APPROACHES TO TREATMENT

Educating the Patient and the Family

The beginning of treatment can be a delicate process given the difficulties patients and their families experience before finding appropriate care. Most families are frightened about their child having a major neuropsychiatric disorder and often envision a grim prognosis. After the evaluation is completed, general education of the patient and family about the nature and course of the disorder is essential to address these concerns. Most patients and families are relieved to hear that the majority of persons with a tic disorder reach peak tic severity in their early teens and have consistent improvement as they move into adulthood. They are also pleased to hear that tic symptoms do not necessarily have a significant impact on longer-term function. In this regard, it is often helpful to cite examples of the patient's family (e.g., the father has tics and is doing well) or sports personalities and other public figures who have identified themselves as having TS and are doing well both personally and professionally.

Once issues regarding the tics are discussed and clarified, the focus shifts to the discussion of co-occurring conditions. One challenge for patients, families, and clinicians is to overcome the tendency to focus primarily on the tic symptoms. Tics may be more readily apparent and generally considered to be straightforward to treat with medications, whereas the co-occurring conditions, especially internalizing symptoms, are easy to overlook and may require special treatment expertise. It is also possible that other psychiatric disorders not traditionally thought to be part of tic disorders will co-occur in patients with TS. Psychoeducation regarding the role of comorbid conditions in the patient's current presentation is useful for establishing the initial treatment plan. A full discussion of co-occurring conditions with the patient and family addresses one of the major pitfalls of treatment of patients with TS, that is, to pursue tic suppression to the exclusion of the treatment of the other co-occurring conditions that are possibly more impairing. Full discussion with the family of the tics and co-occurring problems leads invariably to the next step in treatment planning: creating a hierarchy for treatment.

Creating a Hierarchy of the Clinically Impairing Conditions

Most clinicians, as part of their diagnostic assessment, create some clinical priorities for treatment; in TS, with the multitude of often complex problems, it is essential that a conscious effort be made to formulate, organize, and create hierarchies of treatment. Let's consider two examples:

(1) a child with moderate tics and severe and impairing hyperactivity—hyperactivity may be the first and most important symptom to address; and (2) a child with moderate tics and separation anxiety with school refusal—treatment with a selective serotonin reuptake inhibitor (SSRI) for his or her separation anxiety and behavioral treatment for school refusal may be more appropriate than treatment with neuroleptics for tic suppression.

TREATMENT OF THE MOST IMPAIRING CONDITIONS

This section focuses on the basic strategies for tic suppression and treatment of commonly co-occurring disorders. Particular emphasis is placed on the complexities of clinical treatment. It should be remembered that there is no cure for tics and that the goal of treatment is the reduction of tic severity and associated distress. Doses suggested are approximate based on the authors' review of the literature. (For a comprehensive review, see Sandor, 2003; Scahill, Chappell, King, & Leckman, 2000; Silay & Jankovic, 2005.)

Typical Neuroleptics

The typical neuroleptics (i.e., haloperidol, pimozide, and fluphenazine) are the best-evaluated and most potent agents for tic suppression and only agents indicated for tic suppression. It is hypothesized that the blockade of postsynaptic dopamine type 2 receptors accounts for their efficacy. Dopamine receptor antagonists significantly reduce tic frequency and severity in the vast majority of cases. Despite this well-demonstrated efficacy, in clinical practice, typical neuroleptics are probably used less frequently than in the past because patients do not find that the benefit outweighs the side effect burden. However, it is not clear at this time which patients will benefit without side effects, so making a decision to not use typical neuroleptics in advance of a treatment trial may not be wise. A carefully conducted treatment trial may be very useful for a patient and family to understand both the benefits and the nature of the side effects associated with the typical neuroleptics.

Haloperidol

Early reports of successful treatment of TS with haloperidol were published over 40 years ago (Seignot, 1961). Clinical trials and extensive clinical experience with haloperidol suggest that relatively low doses are sufficient to control tics in most patients with TS, and low doses minimize side effects. For haloperidol, doses in the range of 1–5 mg/day are usually adequate. Starting doses are low (0.25–0.5mg/day), with small increases in the dose (0.25–0.5 mg/day) every 5 to 7 days until tic symptoms are less impairing. Most often, neuroleptics are given at bedtime, but with low doses, some patients may require twice-a-day dosing for good tic control.

Typical side effects of haloperidol include sedation, weight gain, extrapyramidal symptoms (akathesia, dystonic reactions, dyskinesia), cognitive dulling and the common anticholinergic side effects. Children with TS may have a heightened vulnerability to subtle neuroleptic side effects such as clinical depression, separation anxiety, panic attacks, school avoidance, and aggressive outbursts (Bruun, 1988).

Dosage reduction is the best response to most side effects, although the addition of medications such as benzotropine for the extrapyramidal symptoms can be useful. Dosage reductions in those children with TS who have taken neuroleptics long term may be complicated by withdrawal dyskinesias and significant tic worsening or rebound (Carpenter, Leckman, Scahill, & McDougle, 1999). Withdrawal dyskinesias are choreoathetoid movements of the orofacial region, trunk, and extremities that appear after neuroleptic discontinuation or dosage reduction and tend to resolve in 1–3 months. Tic worsening above pretreatment baseline level (i.e., rebound) can last up to 1–3 months after discontinuation or dosage reduction. Concerns have also been expressed about the risk of tardive dyskinesia, which is similar in character to withdrawal dyskinesia. Tardive dyskinesia most often develops during the course of treatment or is "unmasked" with dosage reductions. There have been case reports of tardive dyskinesia in patients with TS, but overall the risk appears to be relatively low in children and adolescents, ranging from 1 to 4.8% (Golden, 1985; Mennesson et al., 1998; Riddle, Hardon, Towbin, Leckman, & Coen, 1987). The onset of anxiety, which is clearly related to neuroleptic treatment, is more common than tardive dyskinesia (Bruun, 1988; Linet, 1985; Mikkelsen, Detlor, & Cohen, 1981).

Pimozide

Pimozide is a potent and specific blocker of dopamine D2 receptors. It is considered an alternative to haloperidol because it has comparable efficacy with fewer sedative and extrapyramidal side effects. Pimozide has calcium channel blocking properties that may increase the risk for QTc prolongation; however, doses in the treatment range are not often associated with significant of QTc prolongation. The coadministration of other medications that affect cardiac conduction, such as the tricyclic antidepressants (TCAs), is generally contraindicated. Also, the risk for cardiac conduction abnormalities may increase when pimozide is combined with drugs that inhibit cytochrome P450 3A4 (Desta, Kerbusch, & Flockhart, 1999). Electrocardiograms at baseline, during the dose titration phase, and annually during treatment with pimozide are recommended for adequate management of patients (Kurlan, 1997; Scahill et al., 2000; Singer, 2005).

Beginning treatment with 0.5–1 mg/day is prudent, although with pimozide's long half-life, every-other-day dosing can be used to decrease the effective daily dose. The dosage may be increased in 0.5–1 mg increments every 5–7 days until symptoms are controlled. Most patients experience clinical benefit with few side effects in the range of 1–4 mg/day. Higher doses can be associated with more side effects.

There have been several comparison studies of haloperidol and pimozide. Historically, haloperidol has been considered to be more potent, with most drug-to-drug comparison studies using pimozide doses about twice those of haloperidol. In a recent crossover study with 22 patients, pimozide showed superior efficacy, with 40% improvement over baseline as compared to 27% with haloperidol. However, in this study, haloperidol was no more effective than placebo, which contrasts with earlier studies (Sallee, Nesbitt, Jackson, Sine, & Sethuraman, 1997). Follow-up studies of up to 15 years suggest that patients are more likely to remain on pimozide than haloperidol (Regeur, Pakkenberg, Fog, & Pakkenberg, 1986; Sandor, Musisi, Moldsofsky, & Lang, 1990). In a comparison study of pimozide, haloperidol, and no drug in patients with TS and attention-deficit/hyperactivity disorder (ADHD), pimozide at 1–4 mg/day was useful in decreasing tics and improving some aspects of cognition that are commonly impaired in ADHD (Sallee & Rock, 1994). The potential to have an impact on both TS and attentional symptoms with a single agent is an advantage that pimozide may have over other neuroleptics.

Fluphenazine

Fluphenazine is a typical neuroleptic that has both dopamine D1 and D2 receptor-blocking activity. In spite of the fact that clinical experience suggests that it has somewhat fewer side effects than haloperidol, it has been less widely used for treatment of tics than haloperidol or pimozide. A controlled trial of haloperidol, fluphenazine, and trifluoperazine found that there was comparable efficacy for tic reduction, but the fluphenazine was the best tolerated (Borison et al., 1982). In an open trial of 21 patients who had a poor response to haloperidol, 52% had a better response to fluphenazine than to haloperidol. The side effect profile of fluphenazine was superior to haloperidol, with a mean dose of fluphenazine 7mg/day (Goetz, Tanner, & Klawans, 1984). In a naturalistic follow-up of 41 patients treated for at least a year, fluphenazine was reported to be safe and effective without a single occurrence of tardive dyskinesia (Silay, Vuong, & Jankovic, in press; Scahill, Erenberg, & the Tourette Syndrome Practice Parameter Workshop, 2006). Fluphenazine is slightly less potent than haloperidol, so starting doses are somewhat higher (0.5–1 mg/day) as are treatment doses (3–5 mg/day).

Atypical Neuroleptics

Newer atypical neuroleptics are characterized by a combined affinity for 5HT-2 and D2 receptors, so they may have fewer extrapyramidal side effects and a lower risk of tardive dyskinesia than the typical neuroleptics. The differences in efficacy appear to be related to the relative potency of dopamine blockade. There is growing evidence of their efficacy in tic suppression, and they are gradually replacing haloperidol and pimozide as the mainstay in the treatment of tics (Sandor, 2003).

Risperidone

Of the atypicals, risperidone has been the most extensively studied; there were initial case reports followed by open-label studies (Lombroso, Scahill, & Chappell, 1995; Brunn & Budman, 1996a; Robertson, Scull, Eapen, & Trimble, 1996). More recently, two randomized, double-blind placebo-controlled trials have demonstrated risperidone's efficacy in reducing tics at doses of 2.5 mg/day (range 1–6 mg/day; Scahill et al., 2003; Dion, Annable, Sandor, & Chouinard, 2002). In randomized double-blind comparison trials, risperidone was found to have equal efficacy with clonidine and was superior to pimozide in reducing tic severity (Gaffney et al., 2002; Gilbert, Balterson, Sethuraman, & Sallee, 2004).

Side effects have included sedation, increased appetite and weight gain, increased prolactin levels, and acute social phobia. Extrapyramidal symptoms occur much less frequently than with haloperidol or pimozide. Depression and dysphoria have been reported in adults and adolescents treated with risperidone for TS (Margolese, Annable, & Dion, 2002).

Olanzapine

There is emerging evidence for the clinical effectiveness of olanzapine, which has modest D2 affinity, in the treatment of TS. Case reports and open-label studies suggest good efficacy and tolerability (Stamenkovic et al., 2000; Budman, Gayer, Lesser, Shi, & Bruun, 2001; Lucas, Shi, & Bruun, 2002). A 52-week double-blind crossover study of olanzapine (5 or 10 mg) versus pimozide (2 or 4 mg) found that olanzapine was superior to pimozide in terms of tic reduction, sedation, and patient preference (Onofrj, Paci, & D'Andreamatteo, 2000). A single-blind pilot study of 10 patients (ages 7–13) with a primary diagnosis of TS and aggression, found significant reduction of tic severity and aggression with olanzapine. The small sample size limits the clinical significance of these findings. Also, given the lesser potency, it is unclear if higher relative doses are required for tic suppression than for other indications, resulting in greater potential for side effects, especially weight gain.

Ziprasidone

Ziprasidone is a newer atypical with 5HT-2 and D2 blocking properties and 5HT-1A agonist and norepinephrine and serotonin reuptake blocking effects, which may contribute to its anxiolytic and antidepressant effects. In an 8-week double-blind multisite study of 28 children and adolescents with tic disorder, ziprasidone at a mean dose of 28.2 mg in two divided doses was significantly better than placebo in decreasing tic severity and frequency (Sallee et al., 2000). There were relatively few side effects reported, with transient sedation the most common. There were no significant changes in weight or cardiac conduction.

Quetiapine

Preliminary case reports suggest that quetiapine may be clinically effective for tic suppression but requires relatively high doses (200–500mg/day) (Darraga & Darraga, 2001). This may be due to its relatively low D2 blockade activity. These findings are based on only two cases and need to be interpreted with caution.

Aripiprazole

Aripiprazole is a novel atypical antipsychotic currently used for the treatment of schizophrenia. It is a potent dopamine partial agonist that acts as an antagonist at D2 receptors under hyperdopaminergic conditions and as an agonist under hypodopaminergic conditions. It has been hypothesized that the lack of complete dopamine blockade may result in fewer side effects. Recent case reports of efficacy of aripiprazole in patients with TS are promising (Bubl, Perloy, Tebartz, & Van Elst, 2006). Within 2 weeks of treatment with 15 mg/day of two adults with TS, the frequency and severity of vocal tics decreased rapidly in one patient, and motor tics almost disappeared completely in both patients (Kastrup, Schlotter, Plewnia, & Bartels, 2005). Data from early studies of aripiprazole in patients with schizophrenia suggest that it is safe and well tolerated, with no evidence of weight gain, marked sedation, or extrapyramidal symptoms (Kane et al., 2002; Pigott et al., 2003). However, one study found more insomnia, tremor, akathesia, vomiting, and nausea in the patients treated with aripiprazole than placebo (Pigott et al., 2003). In a brief trial of 5 youths with pervasive developmental disorder, aripiprazole was well tolerated (Stigler, Posey, & McDougle, 2004). Controlled trials that are currently underway are clearly needed to establish the efficacy of aripiprazole for TS.

Summary

Although early reports suggest the atypical neuroleptics are effective, large-scale trials have not been completed and comparison trials have not been conducted. Side effects, however, have dampened the enthusiasm for the atypicals in the treatment of TS. Weight gain is most problematic with olanzapine, quetiapine, risperidone, and less of a problem with ziprasidone (Alison & Casey, 2001). A study of the risk of QTc prolongation suggests that close electrocardiographic monitoring is warranted when prescribing ziprasidone to children (Blair, Scahill, State, & Martin, 2005). Atypical antipsychotics have been associated with increased glucose levels and new onset diabetes; asymptomatic hypoglycemia has been associated with treatment with olanzapine (Wirshing et al., 1998; Budman et al., 2001). Table 7.1 provides a summary of antipsychotic medications used for tic suppression.

Other Dopamine-Modulating Agents

Pergolide

Agonist activity on presynaptic dopamine neurons results in decreased dopamine release and may therefore result in decreased tic severity in patients with TS. A number of small open studies of dopamine agonists and a small randomized placebo-controlled trial ($n = 24$) of pergolide, a mixed D1–D2–D3 dopamine agonist used for Parkinson's disease and restless legs syndrome, have been promising. In two double-blind placebo-controlled studies, pergolide treatment was significantly more effective in reducing tic severity compared to placebo and was well tolerated, with few adverse events (Gilbert et al., 2000, 2003). Three children with

TABLE 7.1. Antipsychotic Medications Used for Tic Suppression

Generic name	Brand name	Daily dosage (mg/day)	Side effects	Comments
Typical neuroleptics				
Haloperidol	Halidol	1–5	Sedation, weight gain, extrapyramidal symptoms	Good efficacy but side effects problematic
Pimozide	Orap	2–8	QTc prolongation, sedation, extrapyramidal symptoms	Good efficacy, fewer problematic side effects
Fluphenazine	Prolixin	1.5–10	Sedation, extrapyramidal symptoms, weight gain	Comparable to haloperidol but less widely used
Atypical neuroleptics				
Risperidone	Risperidol	1–3	Sedation, weight gain, elevated prolactin	Good efficacy
Olanzapine	Zyprexa	5–10	Sedation, weight gain	Weight gain problematic
Ziprasidone	Geodon	10–80	Weight gain, sedation, ?QTc	Some evidence for efficacy
Quetiapine	Seroquel	200–500	Sedation, weight gain	Requires relatively higher doses for tic suppression
Aripiprazole	Abilify	10–20	Insomnia, akathesia, tremor	Only case reports of efficacy

TS who had failed to improve on several neuroleptic trials improved with pergolide (Chianchetti, Fratta, Pisano, & Minafra, 2005). However, pergolide use may be limited by reports of ergot-induced pleural, retroperitoneal, or pericardial fibrosis, vasospasm, and cardiotoxicity in Parkinson's treatment (Scahill et al., 2006).

Sulpiride and Tiapride

Sulpiride and tiapride are substituted benzamides that are not available in the United States but are commonly used in Europe as first-line treatment of tics. Like pimozide, they are unique in their combination of relatively specific dopamine D2 receptor-blocking activity and the potential for reduced extrapyramidal symptoms and tardive dyskinesia. In an uncontrolled retrospective study of 63 patients with TS, ages 10–68, 60% demonstrated a positive response to sulpiride (Robertson, Schnieder, & Lees, 1990). More recently, two case reports have documented the efficacy of amisulpride, which is unique in that it reportedly binds preferentially to the limbic system, thereby providing some clinical advantages over other atypicals (Fountoulakis, Iacovides, & St. Kaprinis, 2004). In a controlled trial of 27 children with TS, tiapride was superior to placebo in tic reduction at doses ranging from 5 to 6 mg/kg/day (Eggers, Rothenberger, & Berghaus, 1988). It is unlikely that these agents will become available in the United States.

Tetrabenazine

Tetrabenazine has a long history of use in TS and other movement disorders. It is a non-neuroleptic that is a weak postsynaptic antagonist of dopamine and depletes presynaptic dopamine by interfering with reuptake and storage. In a small open-label trial of 17 patients with TS, 65% had modest tic reduction (Jankovic & Orman, 1988). A larger, more recent open study of tetrabenazine, which included 47 patients with TS, reported significant tic reduction in two-thirds of patients (Jankovic & Beach, 1997). Side effects included drowsiness, parkinsonism, insomnia, depression, nervousness and anxiety, and akathisia. It is currently only available in the United States as an investigational drug.

Levodopa, Talipexole, Ropinirole, Metoclopromide

A small single-blind pilot study of six patients with TS who had never been treated with a neuroleptic were given 150 mg of levodopa after carbidopa pretreatment. All showed significant reduction in tic severity on both subjective and objective measures (Black & Mink, 2000). A placebo-controlled study using the partial dopamine agonist talipexole showed no positive effect on tics or improvement of problems with side effects of dizziness and nausea (Goetz, Stebbins, & Thelen, 1994). Relatively low doses (0.25 to 0.5 mg) of ropinirole, a nonergoline D2/D3 agonist, used in an open-label study of 15 patients with TS improved tics (Anca, Giladi, & Korczyn, 2004).

Metoclopramide is a dopamine agonist traditionally used to treat gastroesophageal reflux. A double-blind, placebo-controlled study of 27 children and adolescents with TS reported 39% tic reduction as compared to 13% with placebo (Nicolson, Craven-Thuss, Smith, McKinley, & Castellanos, 2005).

Alpha-Adrenergic Agonists

Clonidine

There is a long history of the use of the antihypertensive agent clonidine for suppression of tics and ADHD symptoms. A preponderance of evidence supports the use of clonidine, an α-2-adrenergic agonist as a potentially effective treatment for patients with TS. Clonidine may reduce mild to moderate tics and improve attention (Sandor, 2003). Whereas controlled trials have shown that some patients benefit, the overall effect of clonidine for tic suppression and ADHD is more modest than that achieved with the "gold standards" (haloperidol and the stimulants, respectively) for these conditions (Goetz, 1993; Tourette Syndrome Study Group, 2002).

Given clonidine's mild side effect profile, it is often the first-line treatment for tic suppression, especially in those children with TS and ADHD. Initial dose is 0.025 mg/day and increased in increments of 0.025–0.05 mg/day every 3–5 days or as side effects (sedation) allow. Usual effective treatment doses are in the range of 0.1–0.3 mg/day and are given in divided doses 4–6 hours apart. Higher doses are associated with side effects, primarily sedation, and are not necessarily more effective. The onset of action is slower for tic suppression (3–6 weeks) than for ADHD symptoms. Side effects, in addition to sedation, include irritability, headaches, decreased salivation, and hypotension and dizziness at higher doses. Owing to clonidine's short half-life, some patients experience mild withdrawal symptoms between doses. Although symptomatic drop in blood pressure is generally not a problem with clonidine, patients and families need to be educated about the potential for rebound increases in blood pressure, heart rate, tics, and anxiety with abrupt discontinuation or missed doses (Leckman et al., 1986; Cantwell, Swanson, & Connor, 1997). Blood pressure and pulse should be measured at baseline and monitored during dose adjustment. Specific guidelines for blood pressure monitoring during follow-up have not been established (Scahill, Erenberg, and the Tourette Syndrome Practice Parameter Work Group, 2006). Baseline and follow-up electrocardiograms have been recommended in some practice guidelines (American Academy of Child and Adolescent Psychiatry, 1997).

Clonidine is also available in a transdermal patch (Catapres-TTS) which provides a more stable clinical effect, fewer side effects for some patients, and avoids multiple daily doses (Burris, 1993). Children are usually stabilized on oral doses before they are switched to the patch. Local skin irritation to the patch material occurs in about half of patients and may ultimately result in discontinuation. A variety of strategies has been used clinically to reduce the risk of rash, but none has been tested. During strenuous activities, patches may fall off. Patients lose benefit if the patch falls off; also, that fell off (and were not appropriately disposed of) have been ingested by younger siblings and pets, who experienced toxic lowering of blood pressure and resulting complications (Broderick-Cantwell, 1990).

Guanfacine

Guanfacine is an α-2-adrenergic agonist that has been suggested as a better tolerated alternative to clonidine. In nonhuman primates, guanfacine appears to bind preferentially with α-2-adrenergic receptors in prefrontal cortical regions—areas associated with attentional and organizational functions (Arnsten & van Dyck, 1997). On the basis of these animal models, it is hypothesized that guanfacine is likely to have a greater impact on attention, with significantly less sedation than is associated with the nonselective α-2-adrenergic agonist clonidine. Guanfacine's long half-life offers the advantage of twice daily dosing, which is more convenient than the multiple dosing required with clonidine. In a randomized double-blind placebo-controlled 8-week trial (n = 31) of children with tics and ADHD, guanfacine in doses up to 0.3 mg/day had an average 31% reduction in tic severity compared to no reduction on placebo. Clinically, the effect on tics is less than would be expected with neuroleptics (Scahill et al., 2001). In a second placebo-controlled trial there was a 30% reduction in tics from baseline, but this was not superior to placebo, possibly due to small sample size (Cummings, Singer, Krieger, Miller, & Mahone, 2002). In both these trials the tic severity of the subjects was reportedly mild, the usefulness of guanfacine for moderate to severe tics is unknown.

Other Agents Studied for Tic Suppression

Baclofen

Baclofen is a muscle relaxant that influences gamma-aminobutyric acid (GABA) neurotransmission. It acts presynaptically to inhibit the release of excitatory amino acids such as glutamate. In a large open-label trial, 264 children with TS were treated with 10 mg/day baclofen, increased by 10 mg increments weekly until improvement was noted or side effects appeared. Two hundred and fifty of these patients had significant decrease in tic severity; sedation was the most common side effect. Unfortunately, the subjects were not randomized, and there were no baseline or follow-up measures of the tics. In a small, randomized, placebo-controlled, double-blind study, 10 children were treated with baclofen 20 mg tid.

Baclofen was not found to be effective in reducing tic severity but did appear to have an effect on tic-related impairment (Singer, Wendlandt, Krieger, & Giuliano, 2001).

Nicotine

The possible benefit of nicotine augmentation of haloperidol treatment in patients with TS is suggested by several open-label studies of nicotine administration via transdermal patch or chewing gum. In an early study of 10 children with TS, nicotine chewing gum effectively decreased tics in 8 of the 10 children when given in conjunction with haloperidol (Sanberg et al., 1989). In another small study, 5 patients with TS chewed gum containing 2 mg of nicotine over 30 minutes; 10 patients received the gum in combination with haloperidol. The gum alone had a modest effect compared to the combined treatment, but this effect was transient. Additionally, the bitter taste and the gastrointestinal upset were not well tolerated (McConville et al., 1992).

Several studies of transdermal nicotine with and without haloperidol treatment have been undertaken (Silver & Sanberg, 1993; Silver et al., 1996). Most recently, a double-blind placebo-controlled study randomized 70 patients to 33 days of either transdermal nicotine patches or placebo patches plus "individually based optimal doses" of haloperidol at least 2 weeks before assignment. At day 19, 50% of the haloperidol dose was dropped. There was significant reduction in the clinician-rated global improvement scale in the nicotine group, but by day 19, the apparent beneficial effects of the nicotine patch on tic severity was no longer evident. Furthermore, 23% of the patients in the nicotine group and 20% of the placebo group were withdrawn because of adverse side effects or recurrence of symptoms. The most common side effects in the nicotine group were nausea (71%) and vomiting (40%) (Silver, Shytle, Sheehan, et al., 2001).

Mecamylamine

Mecamylamine, a nicotine receptor antagonist that is used as an antihypertensive, was reported in two retrospective case studies of 24 child and adult patients to significantly reduce tic severity (Sanberg et al., 1989; Silver, Shytle, Sheehan, et al., 2001). But an 8-week double-blind placebo-controlled study of 61 patients with TS showed no significant benefit of mecamylamine when used alone in doses up to 7.5 mg/day (Silver, Shytle, Sheehan, et al., 2001). The effectiveness of nicotinergic agents in augmentation of neuroleptics remains unclear and warrants further investigation.

Botulinum Toxin

There is evidence to suggest that botulinum toxin may be useful in select cases as a treatment for severe tics (Kwak, Hanna, & Jankovic, 2000). The first open-label study of 450 patients with TS reported efficacy and safety (Awaad, 1999). In two subsequent open-label studies of child and adult patients with TS, 39 of 45 patients reported at least moderate improvement (Jankovic, 1994; Kwak et al., 2000). In most cases the benefit was limited to the anatomical area of the injection. The most common side effects were excessive paralysis of injected muscles and included neck weakness, ptosis, and mild transient dysphagia. The results of a randomized double-blind placebo-controlled crossover study of 20 patients were disappointing. Although there was a 40% decrease in tic frequency as well as the urge associated with the tic, patients reported inner restlessness, an increased urge to perform the treated tic, and that the decrease in the treated tic prompted a new "replacement" tic. The patients' subjective perception was that overall the treatment did not improve their condition (Marras, Andrews, Sime, & Lang, 2001).

Delta-9-Tetrahydrocannabinol

Recent clinical trials have suggested that delta-9-tetrahydrocannibinol, the main psychoactive ingredient of cannabis, may have beneficial effects for TS. A recent randomized double-blind placebo-controlled crossover trial of a single dose of delta-9-tetrahydrocannabinol in 12 adults with TS showed improvement in tics on subjective ratings and, to a lesser extent, on objective rating of motor and vocal tics (Muller-Vahl et al., 2002). Efficacy and safety of this intervention warrant further investigation. Occasionally young adults will describe decreased tic severity while drinking alcohol or smoking marijuana. Although there may be some merit to these claims, as both are central nervous system depressants, the deleterious effects of ongoing (or even episodic) use of alcohol or smoked marijuana for tic suppression should be obvious to clinicians and is not recommended.

Infection and Autoimmune-Based Treatments

Penicillin

Several treatment studies have been undertaken based on the hypothesis that some forms of TS or obsessive–compulsive disorder (OCD) may be related to streptococcal infection. Based on the beneficial effects of penicillin prophylaxis in preventing recurrences of rheumatic fever, a similar strategy was employed in subjects meeting criteria for pediatric autoimmune neuropsychiatric disorders associated with streptococcal infections (PANDAS). Children with PANDAS ($n = 37$) were randomized to receive either 4 months of penicillin 250 mg bid followed by 4 months of placebo, or placebo then penicillin (Garvey et al., 1999). The study was flawed in a number of ways. First, infections occurred at equal rates for subjects on active drug and placebo, suggesting that the medication, dosing, and/or compliance were not adequate for prophylaxis. Second, the crossover design is readily confounded, given the potential lag time between infection and symptom presentation. For example, subjects who were infected during the placebo phase could have presented 1–2 months later with PANDAS symptoms after the crossover to penicillin and be rated as a penicillin failure. Third, subjects were not screened and followed for infection prior to enrollment into the trial. It is possible that a subject who developed an exacerbation of symptoms shortly after beginning the trial was infected before the trial actually began. Although the concept of prophylaxis is compelling, special design considerations will be required in future studies. A more recent study of antibiotic prophylaxis used a more appropriate design, but the lack of a placebo control makes it very difficult to assess whether the results were related to treatment of the natural course of the disorder. A definitive trial is still required.

Intravenous Immunoglobulin

After reports of small open trials with the immunomodulatory treatments such as plasma exchange or intravenous immunoglobulin (IVIG), a larger trial comparing these methods to sham IVIG was undertaken. Children with PANDAS ($n = 30$) were randomly assigned (1:1:1) to treatment with plasma exchange (five single-volume changes over 2 weeks), IVIG (1g/kg daily on 2 consecutive days), or placebo (saline solution given in the same manner as IVIG). Outcome assessments occurred at baseline, 1 month, and 12 months after treatment. At 1 month the IVIG and plasma exchange group demonstrated improvements in obsessive–compulsive symptoms, and the plasma exchange group demonstrated tic reductions as well. After the 1-month assessment, subjects receiving placebo were offered active treatment, and all subjects were followed up to 1 year. Subjects were reported as doing well at 1 year (Lougee et al., 2000). Although this study is encouraging, there are a number of methodological problems. First, there was no placebo control for one of the active treatments—plasma exchange. The result for the plasma exchange reflects open treatment. Second, blind raters were not used, resulting in the possibility of a compromised blind. Third, statements about long-term outcome need to be interpreted with caution because the outcome is uncontrolled after the first month of treatment—

sham IVIG subjects subsequently received active treatment and were included in the long-term outcome. Children also received medication treatments as well as additional immunotherapies, which could confound the outcome.

In a more recent small double-blind placebo-controlled study, 30 patients with tic disorder were randomized to IVIG (1g/kg on 2 consecutive days) or placebo. Symptoms were rated with the Yale Global Severity Scale (YGTSS), Yale–Brown Obsessive Compulsive Scale (YBOCS), and the Clinical Global Impressions Scale (CGI) at baseline and on weeks 2, 4, 6, and 14 posttreatment. There was no significant difference between the groups with regard to changes in tic severity (Hoekstra, Minderaa, & Kallenberg, 2004).

These findings do support ongoing investigation of these treatment methods, but given the cost, risk, and highly experimental nature of these treatments, it is recommended that patients obtain them only in the context of ongoing clinical investigations of these treatments at major medical research centers.

Table 7.2 summarizes the non-antipsychotic medications used for tic suppression.

Other Agents with Potential Efficacy

Benzodiazepines

Although there is a long history of case reports and two open-label studies of adults and children suggesting the beneficial effects of clonazepam and other benzodiazepines, there have been no systematic studies of the efficacy of clonazepam as a single agent in the treatment of TS (Gonce & Barbeau, 1977; Steingard, Goldberg, Lee, & DeMaso, 1994). Benzodiazepines appear to be most useful in decreasing comorbid anxiety in patients with TS. Clinical experience suggests that clonazepam is useful for tic reduction in selected patients, requiring 0.5–4 mg/day in two or three divided doses. Because sedation is a significant side effect at these dosages, an extended titration phase of 3–6 months may be necessary. A slow taper is required to avoid withdrawal symptoms (Goetz, 1992). Side effects that include sedation, short-term memory problems, ataxia, and disinhibition often limit the use of benzodiazepines in children (Graae, Milner, Rizzotto, & Klein, 1994).

Anticonvulsant

Levetiracetam, an antiepileptic agent with atypical mechanisms of action, was used in 60 children and adolescents with TS in a prospective

TABLE 7.2. Other Agents Used for Tic Suppression

Generic name	Brand name	Daily dosage (mg/day)	Side effects	Comments
Pergolide	Permax	0.1–0.25	Retroperitoneal or pericardial fibrosis	Low doses are most useful; higher doses likely ineffective and may be associated with significant side effects
Sulpiride		200–1000	Sedation, akathesia, depression, weight gain	Not available in the United States
Tiapride		150–500	Sedation, akathesia, depression, weight gain	Not available in the United States
Tetrabenazine		37.5–150	Extrapyramidal symptoms, depression	Likely effective; not yet available in the United States
Levodopa/carbidopa	Sinemet	150	Depression, movement disorders	Probably not useful
Talipexole		0.3–2.4	Dizziness, nausea	No efficacy, poorly tolerated
Ropinirole	Requip	0.25–0.5	None reported	Useful in one study without placebo arm
Metoclompramide	Reglan	5–40	Elevated prolactin increased appetite	Possible efficacy for tics
Clonidine	Catapres	0.1–0.3	Sedation, irritability, headache, cardiac effects, withdrawal	Useful for mild to moderate tics, and with comorbid ADHD; also available as transdermal patch
Guanfacine	Tenex	1.0–3.0	Sedation, agitation	Comparable efficacy to clonidine, milder side effects, and easier dosing

12-16

16

(*continued*)

TABLE 7.2. (*continued*)

Generic name	Brand name	Daily dosage (mg/day)	Side effects	Comments
Baclofen		10–60	Sedation	Unclear effficacy
Nicotine		2 (gum) 7–14 (patch)	Nausea, vomiting	May be useful for neuroleptic augmentation; unclear efficacy alone; poorly tolerated
Mecamylamine		2.5–7.5	Nausea	Similar to nicotine
Botulinum toxin		Injection	Neck weakness, ptosis, dysphagia	Efficacy limited to anatomical area of injection
Delta-9-tetrahydrocannabinol				
Penicillin		500		Used for PANDAS; unclear efficacy
Intravenous immunoglobulin		1 g/kg		Unclear to no efficacy for PANDAS

open-label study (Awaad, Michon, & Minarik, 2005). A starting dose of 200 mg/day was titrated over 3 weeks to 1000–2000 mg/day. All patients showed improvement in tic severity and global improvement. There is also a report of two cases of TS successfully treated with topirimate (Abuzzahab & Brown, 2001).

Miscellaneous Agents

The higher prevalence of tics in males and the exacerbating effects of anabolic steroids suggest a possible beneficial effect of medication that inhibits steroid hormones. However, the androgen receptor blocker flutamide showed little clinical benefit in a double-blind placebo-controlled crossover study of 13 adults with TS (Peterson, Zhang, Anderson, & Leckman, 1998).

Although SSRIs have been reported to be effective in co-occurring conditions commonly associated with tics, only two small, controlled studies have assessed the efficacy of SSRIs on tics. Both studies found little or no benefit of fluoxetine on tic reduction (Kurlan et al., 1993; Scahill et al., 1997), despite clinical experience that suggests that the reduction of anxiety and depression may have significant secondary benefit on tic severity.

STRATEGIES FOR SELECTING MEDICAL TREATMENTS

The Tourette Syndrome Practice Parameter Work Group (Scahill et al., 2006) has compared the percent improvement in tics from drugs evaluated in placebo-controlled trials. Their proposed approach to pharmacotherapy suggests a graduated treatment based on tic severity. Consider these guidelines:

1. Even though haloperidol appears to be the most effective for reducing tics, it is not generally used as a first line because of its side effect profile.
2. For mild tics, medication is not generally indicated.
3. For more moderate tics, guanfacine or clonidine may be considered first line, given their safety profile, and the magnitude of benefit (~30% reduction) may be adequate.
4. Botulinum toxin may be considered in patients with a tic caused by a single or small group of muscles, although treatment guidelines remain unclear.
5. For severe tics, more potent medications such as risperidone, ziprasidone, pimozide, or fluphenazine may be selected, depending on clinician preference (Scahill et al., 2006) and patient characteristics.

NONPHARMACOLOGICAL TREATMENTS
Behavioral Approaches

A variety of behavioral approaches to tic suppression has been suggested (conditioning techniques, biofeedback, relaxation therapy, hypnosis, awareness training) but few have been systematically assessed. For a full review of nonpharmacological treatments, see Peterson, Chapter 8, this volume). The behavioral technique shown to be most effective is habit reversal training, and it has become the nonpharmacological treatment of choice. For TS this treatment involves the use of a competing muscle contraction or behavioral response that opposes the tic movement. This method is usually combined with relaxation training, self-monitoring, awareness training, and positive reinforcement (see also Chang, Chapter 6; Peterson, Chapter 8, this volume). In the few published studies of habit reversal training, there were marked overall reductions in tic severity.

In an early study, treatment averaged 20 training sessions over an 8- to 11-month period. Marked tic reduction was noted at 3–4 months. Interestingly, urges or sensations experienced before the tic movements also decreased (Azrin & Peterson, 1990). More recently, a randomized controlled trial of 32 patients with TS compared habit reversal to supportive therapy (Wilheim et al., 2003). Habit reversal initially was more effective, but after 10 months there was no significant difference in tic severity between the groups. Large controlled clinical trials for both adults and children are currently underway.

Repetitive Transcranial Magnetic Stimulation

Repetitive transcranial magnetic stimulation (rTMS) is a neurophysiological intervention that involves applying varying lengths and frequencies of stimulation to specific brain areas. The motor cortex, basal ganglia, and reticular activating system are hypothesized to be involved in the pathology of TS (Kurlan, 1994; Peterson, 1995). In a pilot study of eight patients with moderately severe TS, rTMS at 110% of the motor threshold was applied over the left motor cortex or the left prefrontal cortex, using either 1 Hz or 15 Hz TMS or sham TMS (Chae et al., 2004). Tic symptoms were reported as improved over the week of the study, and all subjects completed the study with minimal side effects (headache) and no worsening of tics or other involuntary movements. It is unclear whether this improvement was a direct effect of the treatment or secondary to the effect of rTMS on co-occurring brain-based disorders. Additionally, there is controversy about whether TMS research in children should be considered minimal risk (Gilbert, Garvey, et al., 2004). A recent study using TMS to investigate motor cortex inhibitory function in TS, ADHD. and OCD questions its usefulness for TS (Gilbert, 2006); a report of 16 patients treated with 1 Hz rTMS failed to show significant improvement.

Surgical Treatment

A variety of neurosurgical procedures have been performed in an effort to treat individuals with severe, refractory TS. Target sites have included the frontal lobe (prefrontal and bimedial frontal leucotomy), the limbic system (limbic leucotomy and anterior cingulotomy, anterior capsulotomy), the thalamus and the cerebellum (Temel & Visser-Vandewalle, 2004; Sun, Krahl, Zhan, & Shen, 2005). Deep brain stimulation (DBS) is a stereotactic treatment that was developed for other movement disorders such as parkinsonism. The first trial of DBS for intractable TS occurred in 1999 (Vandewalle et al., 1999). Since then three patients have undergone bilateral thalamic stimulation, with good result (Temel &

Visser-Vandewalle, 2004). However, surgery is still considered experimental and reserved for the most severe cases. Dramatic media reports of miraculous cures need to be substantiated with very well designed and controlled clinical trials.

TREATMENT OF CO-OCCURRING PSYCHIATRIC DISORDERS IN TS

This section focuses on the special complexities of treating the commonly co-occurring psychiatric disorders such as ADHD and OCD. In general, the treatment approach in patients with TS is similar to approaches in patients without TS, but there are some differences. Again, this section specifically focuses on management of co-occurring conditions in the context of tics.

Treatment of Attention-Deficit/Hyperactivity Disorder

Nonpharmacological Approaches

The nonpharmacological approaches to ADHD in the context of TS are similar to approaches in children without TS (also see Scahill, Sukhodolsky, & King, Chapter 4, this volume). The presence of a structured environment, both at home and at school, consistent behavioral management, and a generally positive, rewarding atmosphere can produce significant improvement in ADHD symptoms. Increasingly, there are specific programs available for children with ADHD that go beyond basic positive programming and include more intensive and focused behavioral approaches. Despite advances in nonpharmacological treatments, some families and psychiatrists, for a variety of reasons, find developing and implementing behavioral programs for children with ADHD difficult and do not take full advantage of the benefits of behavioral approaches.

Pharmacological Treatments

The two major challenges in the treatment of ADHD comorbid with TS are the risk of side effects from the stimulants and desipramine, arguably two of the more potent treatment agents for ADHD, and the lack of comparable alternatives.

STIMULANTS

Initially, in the early 1970s, a number of reports of the induction or exacerbation of tics by stimulants raised concerns about the role of stimulants in TS treatment. At that time, the concern was that the stimulants could be causing tics de novo or that increases in tic severity would persist even after stimulant medications were discontinued. Following anecdotal reports in the 1970s and 1980s, two placebo-controlled trials that excluded subjects with tic disorders reported the emergence of tics in some children with ADHD (Borcherding et al., 1990; Barclay et al., 1992). Concurrent with these reports, other authors noted that tic induction or exacerbation was relatively infrequent and that the beneficial effects in some patients with TS outweighed any negative impact on tic severity (Sanchez-Ramos & Weiner, 1993).

More recently, a critical review (Erenberg, 2005) as well as several short- and long-term double-blind placebo controlled studies have been positive and support a role for stimulants in patients with ADHD and TS (Gadow & Sverd, 1990; Gadow et al., 1995; Castellanos, Giedd, & Elia, 1997). Increasingly, psychiatrists are cautiously, and with fully informed consent, using stimulant medication in selected children and adolescents with TS and ADHD. In the patient in whom tics are increased by stimulants, combined treatment with stimulants and tic-suppressing agents can be used (Gadow et al., 1995). However, the issue with tic exacerbation, if even in a few subjects, is of concern for those specific individuals.

In a recent large multicenter double-blind placebo-controlled trial, children with ADHD and chronic tic disorder ($n = 136$) were randomly assigned to clonidine alone, methylphenidate alone, clonidine plus methylphenidate, or placebo for the treatment of their ADHD (Tourette Syndrome Study Group, 2002). The results suggest that the active treatments were superior to placebo, with the combination treatment being the most effective. Interestingly, tic severity lessened in all active treatment groups, even in the methylphenidate group, suggesting either a primary impact of stimulants on tic severity or secondary effects on tic severity mediated by ADHD improvement. With respect to tic worsening as an adverse event, there was no difference between groups: for methylphenidate, 20% reported tic increases; for clonidine, 26% reported tic increase; and for placebo, 22% reported tic increases. These data suggest that early in the course of treatment it is possible that between 20–25% of patients will experience tic worsening significant enough to be considered an adverse event regardless of treatment modality. These findings also suggest that children with ADHD and tics do not invariably manifest an increase in tics upon exposure to stimulant medication but that a certain percentage may worsen as a result of the natural course of illness or due to nonspecific aspects of treatment (i.e., seeing a doctor or being in a treatment setting). Because this is the first large-scale controlled trial to document tic worsening as an adverse event, these results also suggest that uncontrolled reports of individual medications appearing to worsen tics should not be given much support; controlled trials of medications compared to placebo are required to definitively prove that medications cause more tic increase than placebo. However, even if stimulants do not appear to cause tic increases in the most rigorous conditions, informed consent prior to initiating stimulant medication should include information regarding risks for new-onset tics or tic exacerbations that may be related to the course of the disorder or nonspecific aspects of treatment that may be misattributed to medication. Table 7.3 summarizes the stimulant medications used for the treatment of ADHD.

CLONIDINE AND GUANFACINE

Clonidine and guanfacine have been reported to be useful for both tic suppression and for ADHD in open and small controlled trials. In a very early blinded placebo-controlled discontinuation trial of clonidine for children with tic disorders and ADHD ($n = 10$), the children experienced a 37% increase in the core symptoms of ADHD following withdrawal from clonidine (Hunt et al., 1985). A comparison study of clonidine and desipramine to placebo in 34 patients with TS and ADHD found that clonidine was no better than placebo after 6 weeks of treatment (Singer et al., 1995). In an open-label study of 24 patients comparing clonidine alone, methylphenidate alone, and clonidine plus methylphenidate, all groups showed improvement of ADHD symptoms after 3 months of treatment (Connor, Barkley, & Davis, 2000). The side effect noted in these trials is predictable—sedation. In perhaps the largest comparative study of clonidine, clonidine plus methylphenidate, and placebo, both (clonidine and the combination of clonidine and methylphenidate), were effective in reducing ADHD and tic symptoms (Tourette Syndrome Study Group, 2002). Although there are little data to support concern for combining clonidine and methylphenidate, the historical controversy (Wilens et al., 1999) may still result in clinicians' unwillingness to use these medications in combination. It is important to note the absence of cardiac toxicity in children on combined medication in this study.

One small open-label study and one randomized controlled trial of guanfacine in children and adolescents with ADHD and TS support its efficacy and safety (Chappell et al., 1995; Scahill et al., 2001). In the largest trial to date, 34 youths with ADHD and TS were randomly assigned to 8 weeks of guanfacine or placebo. Guanfacine was superior to placebo (37 vs. 8%) in reduction of the total score on the teacher-rated ADHD Rating Scale. Over half of the subjects on guanfacine were considered much or very much improved, compared with 0/17 subjects on

TABLE 7.3. Stimulant Medications Used for the Treatment of ADHD

Generic class	Brand name	Daily dosage (mg/day)	Side effects	Comments
Amphetamine preparations				
Short-acting	Adderall Dexedrine DextroStat	2.5–40	Insomnia, decreased appetite, growth effects, weight loss, depression, cardiac effects, withdrawal and rebound	May exacerbate tics but generally useful
Intermediate-acting	Dexedrine spansules	5–40		
Long-acting	Adderall XR	5–30		
Methylphenidate preparations				
Short-acting	Focalin Methylin Ritalin	2.5–60		
Intermediate-acting	Daytrana patch Focalin XR MetadateCD Methylin ER Ritalin SR Ritalin LA	12.5–37.5 5–40		
Long-acting	Concerta	18–72		

placebo. Significant differences were also observed in omission and commission errors on a continuous performance test (Scahill et al., 2001).

TRICYCLIC ANTIDEPRESSANTS

Desipramine is a tricyclic antidepressant with prominent noradrenergic activity that has been noted to improve attention and concentration in children and adolescents with ADHD and with TS plus ADHD. Three placebo-controlled studies have demonstrated desipramine efficacy (Biederman et al., 1989; Singer et al., 1995; Spencer et al., 2002). Even though the cardiac side effects of increased heart rate and elevation in blood pressure are not usually clinically significant, many clinicians are reluctant to use desipramine due to concerns about prolonged cardiac conduction times and reports of sudden deaths in children and adolescents (Wilens et al., 1993; Riddle, Geller, & Ryan, 1993; Varley, 2001), and have used Imipramin, a less potent tricyclic antidepressant.

Nortriptyline has been used as an alternative to desipramine, but it has not been well studied. A chart review assessed the effect of nortriptyline in children and adolescents with TS and ADHD. The majority of subjects experienced moderate to marked improvement in both ADHD and tics (Wilens et al., 1993). Although the concern regarding sudden death is less with nortriptyline than desipramine, it is prudent to obtain baseline and follow-up electrocardiograms.

NEWER ANTIDEPRESSANTS

Buproprion is often used in the treatment of ADHD in children, given its long half-life and dopaminergic activity. A few studies have demonstrated its efficacy for ADHD as compared to methylphenidate and placebo (Barrickman et al., 1995; Casat, Pleasants, & Van Wyck Fleet, 1987; Casat, Pleasants, Schroeder, & Parler, 1989; Conners et al., 1996). There is little data supporting its efficacy in ADHD with tics. Some children may experience an exacerbation of tics on buproprion, but caution is warranted regarding overinterpreting this finding, given the lack of a controlled comparison with placebo in this report (Spencer et al., 1993). At higher doses than typically used to treat ADHD, buprorion may increase the risk of seizures in vulnerable individuals (Belson & Kelley, 2002).

Atomoxetine is a selective noradrenergic reuptake inhibitor (SNRI) that has demonstrated efficacy for the treatment of ADHD without tics in two double-blind placebo-controlled studies of 467 children (Michelson, 2001, 2002). It is approved for use in children and adults with ADHD. Given its mechanism of action, it is possible that atomoxetine could improve ADHD symptoms without exacerbating tic symptoms. It may be given in two divided doses to minimize adverse effects, which include irritability nausea, vomiting, loss of appetite and insomnia. Recent reports of significant liver toxicity in a very small number of patients required a labeling change.

Pindolol, a ß-blocker, was compared to methylphenidate and placebo in a controlled study of 52 children with ADHD (Buitelaar, van der Gaag, Swaab-Barneveld, & Kuiper, 1996). It effectively reduced ADHD symptoms at 20 mg/day, but troubling side effects, including nightmares and hallucinations, raise questions about its usefulness.

Deprenyl is a monoamine oxidase (MAO) inhibitor that enhances dopaminergic function in patients with Parkinson disease. A placebo-controlled crossover study of 24 children with ADHD and TS suggests that deprenyl may be effective for treating ADHD without increasing tics (Feigin et al., 1996). Table 7.4 summarizes the nonstimulant medications used for the treatment of ADHD.

TABLE 7.4. Nonstimulant Medications Used for ADHD

Generic name	Brand name	Daily dosage (mg/day)	Side effects	Comments
Noradrenergic agonists				
Clonidine	Catapres	0.1–0.3	See Table 7.2	May be useful alone or in combination; effective for impulsivity, hyperactivity, aggression, sleep difficulties
Guanfacine	Tenex	1–4	See Table 7.2	Same as clonidine
Antidepressants				
Imipramine	Tofranil	10–200	Sedation, weight gain, cardiovascular effects	Lower seizure threshold; monitor levels and EKG
Desipramine	Norpramin	10–200		
Nortryptyline	Pamelor	10–100		
Buproprion	Wellbutrin, SR, XL	37.5–150	Irritability, insomnia, seizures at high doses	May exacerbate tics
Other agents				
Atomoxetine	Strattera	10–80	Irritability, insomnia, anorexia, liver toxicity, cardiac effects	Selective noradrenergic reuptake inhibitor
Pindolol	Visken	15–40	Sedation, depression, nightmares, hallucinations	ß-blocker; may be useful for aggression

Treatment of Obsessive–Compulsive Disorder

Most clinical trials do not specifically note the efficacy of treatments for various subtypes of OCD, so that most of what is known about effective treatments for this disorder comes from studies that included all subtypes. It is possible that subtypes of OCD more commonly seen in people with tic disorders may be either more or less responsive to these interventions.

Nonpharmacological Approaches

The positive role of cognitive-behavioral therapy (CBT) of OCD is well established in adults and more recently has been systematically studied in children and adolescents. The Pediatric OCD Treatment Study (POTS) team reported on a randomized controlled multicenter trial of sertraline alone, CBT alone, combined sertraline and CBT, or pill placebo in 112 patients with OCD (Pediatric OCD Treatment Study Team, 2004). CBT alone was shown to be effective, but not as effective as CBT combined with sertraline. A recent controlled trial of 77 children and adolescents with OCD showed that cognitive-behavioral family-based treatment is as effective in reducing OCD for children and adolescents as individual treatment (Barrett, Healy-Farrell, & March, 2004). Given the success of CBT in OCD and the ability of therapists to adapt OCD treatment techniques to specific symptoms, it is likely that patients with OCD and TS would be able to benefit from CBT. (For a more complete discussion, see Buhlmann et al., Chapter 9, this volume.)

Pharmacological Treatments

The number of agents available for the treatment of OCD in patients with and without TS is increasing. Current available agents include the tricyclic antidepressant clomipramine and the specific serotonin reuptake inhibitors fluoxetine, paroxetine, sertraline, fluvoxamine, citalopram, and escitalopram. Most of these agents have specific Food and Drug Administration (FDA) indications for OCD (clomipramine fluvoxamine, sertraline, and fluoxetine), whereas others have data supporting their efficacy (paroxetine) or studies have not been done (citalopram and escitalopram). Given the likelihood that all medications in this class are effective, the choice of agent will likely hinge on a preferred medication half-life (i.e., long vs. short), side effect profile, the potential drug interactions (i.e., low vs. high) and the psychiatrist's and families' familiarity with the medication.

Clomipramine side effects, including anticholinergic effects, are similar to all of the tricyclic antidepressants: dry mouth, constipation, sedation, increased heart rate, and orthostatic changes in blood pressure. The SSRIs have a different pattern of side effects than that seen with clomipramine. SSRI side effects are generally mild. Those most commonly seen at increased rated compared to placebo are behavioral activation and gastrointestinal upset. Other side effects can include head-ache, insomnia (not related to activation), anorexia (not related to gastrointestinal upset), and sexual dysfunction. Despite the similarities among these medications, they are chemically different, especially in their metabolic pathways and patterns of drug interactions. The patterns of drug interaction are especially important because in children with complex presentations, multiple drugs are often used simultaneously. The reports of potential fatal toxicity of pimozide with some of the SSRIs underscores the need for doctors, patients, and pharmacists to think about drug interactions when developing treatment plans.

Psychiatrists frequently prescribe on the basis of their familiarity and comfort with the given medication. The increased complexity of drug interactions with the SSRIs requires medication choices to be based on specific characteristics of the patient and the metabolic and drug in-teraction profile of the medication.

It has been estimated that 30–40% of patients with OCD will show only partial response to one or more adequate trials of clomipramine or an SSRI (Tourette Syndrome Practice Parameter Work Group, 2004). A number of augmentation strategies has been used, the best being the ad-dition of CBT. Pharmacological augmentation trials, including lithium, neuroleptics, buspirone, clonazepam, liothyronin (T3), and fenflura-mine, have shown positive outcomes in open trials, but only neuroleptic augmentation has shown benefit in controlled trials (McDougle et al., 2000). Controlled trials of haloperidol combined with specific SSRIs in patients with TS and OCD demonstrated improvement in both tic and OCD symptoms (McDougle et al., 1994).

An issue of great concern recently emerged regarding the use of SSRIs in children and adolescents. In the over 20 studies of these medica-tion, involving over 4,000 children and adolescents, indication of a small but meaningful risk of suicidal ideation and behavior (suicidality emerged). In short, 4% of children on medication had suicidality events compared to 2% of children on placebo. These data resulted in the FDA mandating a warning about suicidality in each of the antidepressant medications, product labeling, the development of a medication guide that would accompany each prescription at the pharmacy, and unit dos-ing (i.e., bulk prescriptions would not be allowed). Although a complete discussion of this issue is beyond the scope of this chapter, parents and professionals are encouraged to go to the FDA website for more infor-mation. In addition, the American Academy of Child and Adolescent Psychiatry, American Psychiatric Association, and interested family and lay mental health organizations have prepared a comprehensive medica-tion guide for patients and families to read prior to taking antidepres-sants (see *www.parentsmedguide.com*). It is very important for all involved to realize that, in assessing the risk of antidepressants, patients and families must compare the risk of treatment versus the risk of treating with another form of therapy versus no treatment at all. To decide not to treat due to worry about side effects may put a patient and family in the situation of experiencing the risk of an untreated disorder, which may be substantially worse than the risk of treatment. Table 7.5 summarizes the medications used for the treatment of OCD with TS.

TREATMENT-REFRACTORY CASES

Strategies for approaching two types of treatment-refractory symptoms are discussed here: (1) patients whose symptoms are truly treatment refractory, with severe impairment related to TS and OCD, despite conventional and heroic treatments; and (2) patients whose symptoms are clinically complex and enigmatic, and whose impairment is disproportionally greater than their tic, obsessive–compulsive, or ADHD symptoms would suggest.

Treatment-Refractory Tics

Perhaps the most important "treatment" in patients with severe, incapacitating tics is a full clinical reevaluation to assess the adequacy of previous evaluations and treatment efforts. It is not uncommon for "treatment-refractory" patients to have had inadequate evaluations and treatment

TABLE 7.5. Medications Used for the Treatment of OCD with TS

Generic name	Brand name	Daily dosage (mg/day)	Side effects	Comments
Clomipramine	Anafranil	25–250	Dry mouth, constipation, sedation, increased heart rate and orthostatis	Well-documented efficacy
Fluoxetine	Prozac	10–80	Nausea, agitation, behavioral activation, sexual dysfunction, suicidal ideation	Efficacy demonstrated in all but citalopram and escitalopram
Paroxetine	Paxil	10–60		
Sertraline	Zoloft	50–200		
Fluvoxamine	Luvox	50–300		
Citalopram	Celexa	20–60		
Escitalopram	Lexapro	10–20		

trials, including inadequate dose or duration of treatment, unidentified and untreated comorbidity, including comorbidity not usually considered "part of the tic disorders," or underutilized psychosocial treatments for psychosocially responsive conditions.

Two alternative treatment strategies are available for truly treatment-refractory tics. When a single tic or a few tics are refractory and impairing, the injection of botulinum toxin into the specific muscle group can be helpful (see previous section). It is essential for the psychiatrist to work with a neurologist experienced in using this method.

Neurosurgical techniques, as discussed previously, can be considered once a detailed and exhaustive reevaluation has been completed to determine whether all other treatment options are exhausted. It is also important that patients who pursue neurosurgical approaches consider centers of clinical excellence where controlled treatment trials are ongoing. Regarding treatment in nonacademic settings, it would be optimal if the outcome of all the cases treated in this manner could be available for review in the scientific literature so that conclusions can be drawn from these complex cases.

Treatment-Refractory OCD

A similarly thorough and exhaustive reevaluation is critical for patients with TS plus OCD who present as treatment refractory. Diagnostic reevaluation focuses on whether other psychiatric disorders are present and disabling and whether the current hierarchy of clinical disability considers all conditions.

Pharmacological reevaluation is especially critical because there are an increasing number of new medications and potential medication combinations. Rather than repeated change from one antiobsessional agent to another, augmentations strategies can be considered because they take less time than changing agents and may offer synergistic benefits. Low-dose neuroleptic augmentation is the best first choice; controlled trials support the use of low-dose neuroleptics for augmentation of SSRIs in OCD and tics (McDougle et al., 1994, 2000). Lithium and T3 are proven, effective augmenters of antidepressants for depression, yet neither has proven effective in OCD. Because of the frequent overlap of OCD and major depression, lithium or T3 may be the next best choice. Lithium and T3 can be added to the SSRIs or the SSRI and neuroleptic combination. Other augmenting agents, usually medications with serotonergic agonist activity, are supported only by anecdotal evidence.

Treatment-refractory or malignant OCD has been the psychiatric disorder most frequently treated with neurosurgical interventions. The surgical approaches are somewhat better defined and the outcome in severe cases is often positive. Academic medical centers that specialize in the presurgical workup and the neurosurgical procedure are available (Mindus & Jenike, 1992). Information about more intensive treatment is available *www.ocfoundation.org*.

Clinically Complex Patients

Clinically complex patients may be severely impaired without having severe tic or OCD symptoms. The clinically complex patient is often a diagnostic dilemma, with additional diagnoses complicating the clinical picture. In addition, patients can become clinically complex when otherwise straightforward treatments are a challenge to implement.

Diagnostic Challenges in Treating the Clinically Complex Patient

In clinically complex patients, the diagnostic challenge is not an accurate assessment of tics, ADHD, or obsessive–compulsive symptoms, although this is important. In clinically complex patients, the diagnostic goal is to identify what other conditions or factors may be present that make the current treatment approaches difficult. From a strictly diagnostic point of view, it is the additional psychiatric conditions beyond TS, OCD, and ADHD that often escape clinical observation and result in diagnostic dilemmas and treatment failures. For example, anxiety and mood disorders may exacerbate and complicate the clinical picture.

Treatment Implementation

In clinically complex patients, particular difficulties with treatment implementation can occur. Most clinicians are aware of problems with treatment compliance, but clinically complex patients with TS present additional treatment dilemmas.

Clinical problems occur when the treating clinician does not have access to critical information or is not in control of the treatment process. Traditionally, clinicians develop a relationship with the patient and other major figures in the patient's life. Given the current clinical climate, a comprehensive level of involvement can be overwhelming and enormously time consuming for clinicians, resulting in poorly coordinated team efforts. One clinician's lack of awareness of important clinical issues can have a negative impact on the treatment of the patient.

Clinicians who work with children and adolescents may wish to consider changes in their treatment approaches to these patients. Experience in tertiary care centers suggests that expanded time with the parents is a critically important and efficient approach to care. Clinicians who form a treatment partnership with families, respecting and addressing their concerns, educating them about TS, training them to evaluate and manage complex behaviors, and empowering them to be an effective advocate for their child are providing good care. In working directly with families, the collection of important information regarding the family's and the patient's functioning needs to be direct and regular. Often small interventions can produce changes in family functioning that have a positive ripple effect throughout the life of the child. Although focusing on the family will not make all complex patients with TS easier to treat, less than adequate contact will certainly create barriers to clinical care.

Pharmacological Treatment Dilemmas

It is often difficult to get accurate information regarding side effects and treatment response in child patients. Parents, children, and clinicians, in spite of good collaborative effort, may have different understandings of the target symptoms, side effect profile, and what constitutes a positive clinical response. This ambiguity makes anything but the most robust clinical responses difficult to observe. Again, experience at tertiary referral centers suggests that the lack of clinical response to medication in complex patients may often be related to inadequate monitoring of medicine effects and inadequate treatment trials (Walkup, 1995).

Clinically complex patients may not have a robust response to a single medication but may require multiple medication trials to identify which medications offer the most benefit, and in which combination. Sequential treatment trials are difficult for all involved, especially children and families, who are often looking for a single powerful intervention. Clinically complex patients, however, usually require sequential trials and combined medication regimens to experience optimal benefit. With the added complexity of treatment, there is the added risk of confusion and the need for an excellent clinician–patient–family relationship. In those cases in which the relationship is not optimal, it is possible that a patient may not met the maximum clinical benefit from the pharmacological interventions.

With increasing numbers of available psychotropic medications, psychiatrists become less experienced with the range of clinical effects and side effects in individual medications. In clinically complex patients, the prescription of unfamiliar medications may be necessary but may add to the risk that a trial will be discontinued prematurely because of a doubt about a side effect. In addition, unusual side effects, such as the apathy or disinhibition syndromes (Hoehn-Saric et al., 1990, 1991) seen with some patients receiving the specific SSRIs, may go unnoticed and add to the clinical morbidity.

Whereas pharmacological interventions offer great promise, clinical experience suggests that excellent diagnostic skills, good relationships with the patient and family, time for adequate monitoring, and a keen eye for effects and side effects are necessary for benefits to be realized. Less intensive efforts may make patients appear more complex than necessary.

ACKNOWLEDGMENT

Significant portions of this chapter were previously published in J. T. Walkup and M. A. Riddle, "Tic Disorders," in A. Tasman, J. Kay and J. A. Lieberman (Eds.), *Psychiatry* (2nd ed., pp. 821–841). West Sussex, UK: Wiley. Copyright 2003 by John Wiley & Sons, Ltd. Reprinted with permission.

REFERENCES

Abuzzahab, F. S., & Brown, V. L. (2001). Control of Tourette syndrome with topiramate. *American Journal of Psychiatry, 158*, 968.

Alison, D. B., & Casey, D. E. (2001). Antipsychotic-induced weight gain: A review of the literature. *Journal of Clinical Psychiatry, 62*(Suppl. 7), 22–31.

American Academy of Child and Adolescent Psychiatry. (1997). Practice parameters for the assessment and treatment of children, adolescents and adults with attention-deficit hyperactivity disorder. *Journal of the American Academy of Child and Adolescent Psychiatry, 36*(Suppl.), 95S–121S.

Anca, M. H., Giladi, N., & Korczyn, A. D. (2004). Ropinirole in Gilles de la Tourette syndrome. *Neurology, 62*, 1626–1627.

Arnsten, A. F. T., & van Dyck, C. H. (1997). Monoamine and acetylcholine influences on higher cognitive functions in non-human primates: Relevance to the treatment of Alzheimers disease. In J. D. Brioni & M. W. Decker (Eds.), *Pharmacological treatment of Alzheimer's disease: Molecular and neurobiologic foundations* (pp. 63–86). New York: Wiley.

Awaad, Y. (1999). Tics in Tourette syndrome: Multimodal, developmental intervention. *Journal of Clinical Neurology, 14*, 316–319.

Awaad, Y., Michon, A. M., & Minarik, S. (2005). Use of levetiracetam to treat tics in children and adolescents with Tourette syndrome. *Movement Disorders, 20*(6), 714–718.

Azrin, N. H., & Peterson, A. L. (1990). Treatment of Tourette syndrome by habit reversal: A waiting list control group comparison. *Behavior Therapy, 21*, 305–318.

Barclay, R. A., McMurray, M. B., Edelbrock, C. S., et al. (1992). Side effects of methylphenidate in children with attention deficit hyperactivity disorder: A systematic placebo-controlled evaluation. *Pediatrics, 86*, 184–192.

Barrett, P., Healy-Farrell, L., & March, J. S. (2004). Cognitive-behavioral family treatment of childhood obsessive–compulsive disorder: A controlled trial. *Journal of the American Academy of Child and Adolescent Psychiatry, 43*(1), 46–62.

Barrickman, L., Perry, P., Allen, A., et al. (1995). Buproprion versus methylphenidate in the treatment of attention-deficit hyperactivity disorder. *Journal of the American Academy of Child and Adolescent Psychiatry, 34,* 649–657.

Belson, M. G., & Kelley, T. R. (2002). Buproprion exposures: Clinical manifestations and medical outcome. *Journal of Emergency Medicine, 23,* 223–230.

Biederman, J., Baldessarini, R. J., Wright, V., et al. (1989). A double-blind placebo-controlled study of desipramine in the treatment of ADD: I. Efficacy. *Journal of the American Academy of Child and Adolescent Psychiatry, 28,* 777–784.

Black, K. J., & Mink, J. W. (2000). Response to levodopa challenge in Tourette syndrome. *Movement Disorders, 15,* 1194–1198.

Blair, J., Scahill, L., State, M., & Martin, A. (2005). Electrocardiographic changes in children and adolescents treated with ziprasidone: A prospective study. *Journal American Academy of Child and Adolescent Psychiatry, 44,* 73–79.

Borcherding, B. G., Keysor, C. S., Rapoport, J. L., et al. (1990). Motor/vocal tics and compulsive behaviors on stimulant drugs: Is there a common vulnerability? *Psychiatry Research, 33,* 93–94.

Borison, R. L., Ang, L., Chang, S., Dysken, M., Comaty, J. E., & Davis, J. M. (1982). New pharmacological approaches in the treatment of Tourette syndrome. *Advances in Neurology, 35,* 377–382.

Broderick-Cantwell, J. J. (1999). Case study: Accidental clonidine patch overdose in attention hyperactivity disorder patients. *Journal of the American Academy of Child and Adolescent Psychiatry, 38*(1), 95–98.

Bruun, R. D. (1988). Subtle and under recognized side effects of neuroleptic treatment in children with Tourette disorder. *American Journal of Psychiatry, 145,* 3–74

Bruun, R. D., & Budman, C. L. (1996a). Neuroleptic-induced behavior disorders in patients with Tourette syndrome. In M Richardson & G. Haughland (Eds.), *The uses of neuroleptics in children* (pp. 185–198). Washington, DC: American Psychiatric Press.

Bruun, R. D., & Budman, C. L. (1996b). Risperidone as a treatment for Tourette syndrome. *Journal of Clinical Psychiatry, 57,* 31.

Bubl, E., Perlov, E., & Tebartz Van Elst, L. (2006). Aripiperazole in patients with Tourette syndrome. *World Journal of the Biological Psychiatry, 7*(2), 123–125.

Budman, C. L., & Gayer, A. (2001). Low blood glucose and olanzapine. *American Journal of Psychiatry, 158,* 500–501.

Budman, C. L., Gayer, A., Lesser, M., Shi, Q., & Bruun, R. D. (2001). An open-label study of the treatment efficacy of olanzapine for Tourette disorder. *Journal of Clinical Psychiatry, 62,* 290–294.

Buitelaar, J. K., van der Gaag, R. J., Swaab-Barneveld, H., & Kuiper, M. (1996). Pindolol and methylphenidate in children with attention deficit hyperactivity disorder: Clinical efficacy and side effects. *Journal of Child Psychology and Psychiatry, 37,* 587–595.

Burd, L., Kerbeshian, J., Fisher, W., & Gascon, G. (1986). Anticonvulsant medications: An iatrogenic cause of tic disorders. *Canadian Journal of Psychiatry, 31,* 419.

Burris, J. F. (1993). The USA experience with the clonidine transdermal therapeutic system. *Clinical Autonomic Research, 3,* 391–396.

Cantwell, D. P., Swanson, J., & Connor, D. F. (1997). Case study: Adverse response to clonidine. *Journal of the American Academy of Child and Adolescent Psychiatry, 36,* 539–544.

Carpenter, L. L., Leckman, J. F., Scahill, L., & McDougle, C. J. (1999). Pharmacologic and other somatic approaches to treatment. In D. J. Cohen & J. F. Leckman (Eds.), *Tourette syndrome—tics, obsessions, compulsions: Developmental psychopathology and clinical care* (pp. 370–398). New York: Wiley.

Casat, C. D., Pleasants, D. Z., Schroeder, D. H., & Parler, D. W. (1989). Buproprion in children with attention-deficit disorder. *Psychopharmacology Bulletin, 25*(2), 198–201.

Casat, C. D., Pleasants, D. Z., & Van Wyck Fleet, J. (1987). A double-blind trial of buproprion in children with attention-deficit disorder. *Psychopharmacology Bulletin, 23*(1), 120–122.

Castellanos, F. X., Giedd, J. N., & Elia, J. (1997). Controlled stimulant treatment of ADHD and comorbid Tourette syndrome: Effects of stimulant and dose. *Journal of the American Academy of Child and Adolescent Psychiatry, 34*, 1140–1146.

Chae, J., Nahas, Z., Wasserman, E., et al. (2004). A pilot safety study of repetitive transcranial magnetic stimulation (rTMS) in Tourette syndrome. *Cognitive Behavioral Neurology, 17*, 109–117.

Chappell, P. B., Riddle, M. A., Scahill, L., et al. (1995). Guanfacine treatment of comorbid attention-deficit hyperactivity disorder in Tourette syndrome: Preliminary clinical experience. *Journal of the American Academy of Child and Adolescent Psychiatry, 34*, 1140–1146.

Chianchetti, C., Fratta, A., Pisano, T., & Minafra, L. (2005). Pergolide improvement in neuroleptic-resistant Tourette cases: Various mechanisms causing tics. *Journal of the Neurological Sciences, 26*(2), 137–139.

Conners, C. K., Casat, C. D., Gualtieri, C. T., et al. (1996). Buproprion hydrochloride in attention-deficit disorder with hyperactivity. *Journal of the American Academy of Child and Adolescent Psychiatry, 34*, 1314–1321.

Connor, D. F., Barkley, R. A., & Davis, H. T. (2000). A pilot study of methylphenidate, clonidine or the combination in ADHD comorbid with aggressive oppositional defiant or conduct disorder. *Clinical Pediatrics, 39*, 15–25.

Cummings, D. D., Singer, H. S., Krieger, M., Miller, T. L., & Mahone, E. M. (2002). Neuropsychiatric effects of guanfacine in children with mild Tourette syndrome: A pilot study. *Clinical Neuropharmacology, 25*(6), 325–332.

Desta, Z., Kerbusch, T., & Flockhart, D. A. (1999). Effect of clarithromycin on the pharmacokinetics and pharmacodynamics of pimozide in healthy poor and extensive metabolizers of cytochrome P450 2D6 (CYP2D6). *Clinical Pharmacology and Therapeutics, 65*(1), 10–20.

Dion, Y., Annable, L., Sandor, P., & Chouinard, G. (2002). Risperidone in the treatment of Tourette syndrome: A double-blind placebo-controlled trial. *Journal of Clinical Psychopharmacology, 22*(1), 31–39.

Eggers, C. H., Rothenberger, A., & Berghaus, U. (1988). Clinical and neurobiologic findings in children suffering from tic disease following treatment with tiapride. *European Archives of Psychiatry and Neurological Science, 237*, 223–229.

Erenberg, G. (2005). The relationship between Tourette syndrome, attention deficit hyperactivity disorder, and stimulant medication: A critical review. *Seminars in Pediatric Neurology, 12*(4), 217–221.

Feigin, A., Kurlan, R., McDermott, M. P., et al. (1996). A controlled trial of deprenyl in children with Tourette syndrome and attention deficit hyperactivity disorder. *Neurology, 46*, 965–968.

Fountoulakis, K. N., Iacovides, A., & St. Kaprinis, G. (2004). Successful treatment of Tourette disorder with amisulpride. *Annals of Pharmacotherapy, 38*, 901.

Gadow, K. D., & Sverd, J. (1990). Stimulants for ADHD in child patients with Tourette syndrome: The issue of relative risk. *Journal of Developmental and Behavioral Pediatrics, 11*, 269–271.

Gadow, K. D., Sverd, J., Sprafkin, J., et al. (1995). Efficacy of methylphenidate for attention-deficit hyperactivity disorder in children with tic disorder. *Archives of General Psychiatry, 52,* 444–455.

Gaffney, G. R., Perry, P. J., Lund, B. C., et al. (2002). Risperidone versus clonidine in the treatment of children and adolescents with Tourette syndrome. *Journal of the American Academy of Child and Adolescent Psychiatry, 41,* 330–336.

Garvey, M. A., Perlmutter, S. J., Allen, A. J., et al. (1999). A pilot study of penicillin prophylaxis for neuropsychiatric exacerbations triggered by streptococcal infections. *Biological Psychiatry, 45,* 1564–1571.

Gilbert, D. L. (2006). Motor cortex inhibitory function in Tourette syndrome, attention deficit disorder, and obsessive compulsive disorder: Studies using transcranial magnetic stimulation. *Advances in Neurology, 99,* 107–114.

Gilbert, D. L., Batterson, J. R., Sethuraman, G., & Sallee, F. R. (2004). Tic reduction with risperidone versus pimozide in a randomized, double-blind crossover trial. *Journal of the American Academy of Child and Adolescent Psychiatry, 43,* 206–214.

Gilbert, D. L., Dure, L., Sethuraman, G., et al. (2003). Tic reduction with pergolide in randomized controlled trial in children. *Neurology, 60,* 606–611.

Gilbert, D. L., Garvey, M. A., Bansal, A. S., et al. (2004). Should transcranial magnetic stimulation research in children be considered minimal risk? *Clinical Neurophysiology, 115,* 1730–1739.

Gilbert, D. L., Sethuraman, G., Sine, L., et al. (2000). Tourette syndrome improvement with pergolide in a randomized, double-blind crossover trial. *Neurology, 54,* 1310–1315.

Goetz, C. G. (1992). Clonidine and clonazepam. *Advances in Neurology, 58,* 245–251.

Goetz, C. G. (1993). Clonidine. In R. Kurlan (Ed.), *Handbook of Tourette syndrome and related tic and behavioral disorders* (pp. 377–388). New York: Marcel Dekker.

Goetz, C. G., Stebbins, G. T., & Thelen, J. A. (1994). Talipexole and adult Gilles de la Tourette syndrome: Double-blind, placebo-controlled clinical trial. *Movement Disorders, 9,* 315–317.

Goetz, C. G., Tanner, C. M., & Klawans, H. L. (1984). Fluphenazine and multifocal tic disorders. *Archives of Neurology, 41,* 271–272.

Golden, G. S. (1985). Tardive dyskinesia in Tourette syndrome. *Pediatric Neurology, 1,* 192–194.

Gonce, M., & Barbeau, A. (1977). Seven cases of Gilles de la Tourette syndrome: Partial relief with clonazepam: A pilot study. *Canadian Journal of Neurological Sciences, 3,* 279–283.

Graae, F., Milner, J., Rizzotto, L., & Klein, R. G. (1994). Clonazepam in childhood anxiety disorders. *Journal of the American Academy of Child and Adolescent Psychiatry, 33,* 372–376.

Hoehn-Saric, R., Harris, G. J., Pearlson, G. D., et al. (1991). A fluoxetine-induced frontal lobe syndrome in an obsessive–compulsive patient. *Journal of Clinical Psychiatry, 52,* 131.

Hoehn-Saric, R., Lipsey, J. R., McLeod, D. R., et al. (1990). Apathy and indifference in patients on fluvoxamine and fluoxetine. *Journal of Clinical Psychopharmacology, 10,* 343.

Hoekstra, P. J., Minderaa, R. B., & Kallenberg, C. G. (2004). Lack of effect of intravenous immunoglobulins on tics: A double-blind placebo-controlled study. *Journal of Clinical Psychiatry, 65,* 537–542.

Holtman, M., Korn-Merker, E., & Boenigk, H. E. (2000). Carbemazepine-induced combined phonic and motor tic in a boy with Down's syndrome. *Epileptic Disorders, 2,* 39.

Hunt, R. D., Minderaa, R. B., Cohen, D. J., et al. (1985). Clonidine benefits children with attention-deficit disorder and hyperactivity: Report of a double-blind placebo cross-over therapeutic trial. *Journal of the American Academy of Child and Adolescent Psychiatry, 24,* 617.

Jankovic, J. (1994). Botulinum toxin in the treatment of dystonic tics. *Movement Disorders, 9,* 347–349.

Jankovic, J., & Beach, J. (1997). Long-term effects of tetrabenazine in hyperkinetic movement disorders. *Neurology, 48,* 358–362.

Jankovic, J., & Orman, J. (1988). Tetrabenazine therapy of distonia, chorea, tics, and other dyskinesias. *Neurology, 38,* 391–394.

Kane, J. M., Carson, W. H., Saha, A. R., et al. (2002). Efficacy and safety of aripiprazole and haloperidol versus placebo in patients with schizophrenia and schizoaffective disorder. *Journal of Clinical Psychiatry, 63,* 763–771.

Kastrup, A., Schlotter, W., Plewnia, C., & Bartels, M. (2005). Treatment of tics in Tourette syndrome with aripiprazole. *Journal of Clinical Psychopharmacology, 25,* 94–96.

King, R. A., Scahill, L., Lombroso, P. J., & Leckman, J. (2003). Tourette syndrome and other tic disorders. In A. Martin, L. Scahill, D. Charney, & J. F. Leckman (Eds.), *Pediatric psychopharmacology: Principles and practice* (pp. 526–542). New York: Oxford University Press.

Kurlan, R. (1994). Hypothesis II: Tourette syndrome is part of a clinical spectrum that includes normal brain development. *Archives of Neurology, 51,* 1145–1150.

Kurlan, R. (1997). Treatment of tics. *Neurologic Clinics, 15,* 403–409.

Kurlan, R., Como, P. G., Deeley, C., et al. (1993). A pilot controlled study of fluoxetine for obsessive–compulsive symptoms in children with Tourette syndrome. *Clinical Neuropharmacology, 16,* 167–172.

Kurlan, R., Kersun, J., Behr, J., et al. (1989). Carbamazepine-induced tics. *Clinical Neuropharmacology, 12,* 298.

Kwak, C. H., Hanna, P. A., & Jankovic, J. (2000). Botulinum toxin in the treatment of tics. *Archives of Neurology, 57,* 1190–1193.

Leckman, J. F., Ort, S., Caruso, K. A., et al. (1986). Rebound phenomena in Tourette syndrome after abrupt withdrawal of clonidine. Behavioral, cardiovascular, and neurochemical effects. *Archives of General Psychiatry, 43,* 1168–1176.

Linet, L. S. (1985). Tourette syndrome, pimozide and school phobia: The neuroleptic separation anxiety syndrome. *American Journal of Psychiatry, 142,* 613–615.

Lombroso, P. J., Scahill, L. D., Chappell, P. B., et al. (1995). Tourette syndrome: A multigenerational, neuropsychiatric disorder. *Advances in Neurology, 65,* 305–318.

Lougee, L., Perlmutter, S. J., Nicolson, R., et al. (2000). Psychiatric disorders in first-degree relatives of children with pediatric autoimmune neuropsychiatric disorders associated with streptococcal infections (PANDAS). *Journal of the Academy of Child and Adolescent Psychiatry, 39,* 1120–1126.

Lucas Taracena, M. T., & Montanes, R. F. (2002). Olanzapine in Tourette syndrome: A report of three cases. *Actas Espanolas de Psiquiatria, 30,* 129–132.

Margolese, H. C., Annable, L., & Dion, Y. (2002). Depression and dysphoria in adult and adolescent patients with Tourette syndrome treated with risperidone. *Journal of Clinical Psychiatry, 63,* 1040–1044.

Marras, C., Andrews, D., Sime, E., & Lang, A. E. (2001). Botulinum toxin for simple motor tics: A randomized double-blind, controlled clinical trial. *Neurology, 56,* 605–610.

McConville, B. J., Sanberg, P. R., Fogelson, M. H., et al. (1992). The effects of nicotine plus haloperidol compared to nicotine only and placebo nicotine only in reducing tic severity and frequency in Tourette disorder. *Biological Psychiatry, 15,* 832–840.

McDougle, C. J., Epperson, C. N., Pelton, G. H., et al. (2000). A double-blind, placebo-controlled study of risperidone addition in serotonin reuptake inhibitor-refractory obsessive–compulsive disorder. *Archives of General Psychiatry, 57,* 794–801.

McDougle, C. J., Goodman, W. K., Leckman, L. F., et al. (1994). Haloperidol addition in fluvoxamine refractory obsessive–compulsive disorder: A double-blind placebo-controlled trial in patients with and without tics. *Archives of General Psychiatry, 51,* 302–308.

Mennesson, M., Klink, B. A., & Fortin, A. H. (1998). Case study: Worsening Tourette's disorder or withdrawal dystonia? *Journal of the American Academy of Child and Adolescent Psychiatry, 37*(7), 785–788.

Michelson, D., Allen, A. J., Busner, J., et al. (2002). Once daily atomoxetine treatment for children and adolescents with attention-deficit hyperactivity disorder: A randomized, placebo-controlled study. *American Journal of Psychiatry, 159,* 1896.

Michelson, D., Faries, D., Wernicke, J., et al. (2001). Atomoxetine in the treatment of children and adolescents with attention-deficit hyperactivity disorder: A randomized placebo-controlled dose-response study. *Pediatrics, 108,* E83.

Miguel, E. C., Shavitt, R. G., Ferrao, Y. A., et al. (2003). How to treat OCD in patients with Tourette syndrome. *Journal of Psychosomatic Research, 55,* 49–57.

Mikkelsen, E. J., Detlor, J., & Cohen, D. J. (1981). School avoidance and social phobia triggered by haloperidol in patients with Tourette disorder. *American Journal of Psychiatry, 139,* 1572–1575.

Mindus, P., & Jenike, M. A. (1992). Neurosurgical treatment of malignant obsessive–compulsive disorder. *Psychiatric Clinics of North America, 15,* 921–938.

Muller-Vahl, K. R., Schneider, U., Koblenz, A., et al. (2002). Treatment of Tourette syndrome with delta-9–tetrahydrocannabinol(THC): A randomized crossover trial. *Pharmacopsychiatry, 35,* 57–61.

Neglia, J. P., Glaze, D. G., & Zion, T. E. (1984). Tics and vocalizations in children treated with carbamazepine. *Pediatrics, 73,* 941.

Nicholson, R., Craven-Thuss, B., Smith, J., McKinlay, B. D., & Castellanos, F. X. (2005). A randomized double-blind, placebo-controlled trial of metoclopramide for the treatment of Tourette's disorder. *Journal of the American Academy of Child and Adolescent Psychiatry, 44*(7), 640–646.

Onofrj, M., Paci, C., D'Andreamatteo, G., & Toma, L. (2000). Olanzapine in severe Gilles de la Tourette syndrome: A 52-week double-blind crossover study vs. low-dose pimozide. *Journal of Neurology, 247,* 443–446.

Parraga, H. C., & Parraga, M. I. (2001). Quetiapine treatment in patients with Tourette syndrome. *Canadian Journal of Psychiatry, 46,* 184–185.

Pediatric OCD Treatment Study Team. (2004). Cognitive-behavior therapy, sertraline, and their combination for children and adolescents with obsessive–compulsive disorder: The Pediatric OCD Treatment Study (POTS) Team. *Journal of the American Medical Association, 292*(16), 1969–1976.

Peterson, B. S. (1995). Neuroimaging in child and adolescent neuropsychiatric disorders. *Journal of the American Academy of Child and Adolescent Psychiatry, 34,* 1560–1576.

Peterson, B. S., Zhang, H., Anderson, G. M., & Leckman, J. F. (1998). A double-blind placebo-controlled, crossover trial of an antiandrogen in the treatment of Tourette syndrome. *Journal of Clinical Psychopharmacology, 18,* 324–331.

Pigott, T. A., Carson, W. H., Saha, A. R., et al. (2003). Aripiprazole for the prevention of relapse in stabilized patients with chronic schizophrenia: A placebo-controlled 26-week study. *Journal of Clinical Psychiatry, 64,* 1048–1056.

Regeur, L., Pakkenberg, B., Fog, R., & Pakkenberg, H. (1986). Clinical features and long-term treatment with pimozide in 65 patients with Gilles de la Tourette syndrome. *Journal of Neurology, Neurosurgery and Psychiatry, 49,* 791–795.

Riddle, M. A., Geller, B., & Ryan, N. (1993). Another sudden death in a child treated with desipramine. *Journal of the American Academy of Child and Adolescent Psychiatry, 32*, 792–797.

Riddle, M. A., Hardin, M. T., Towbin, K. E., Leckman, J. F., & Cohen, D. J.(1987) Tardive dyskinesia following haloperidol treatment in Tourette syndrome. *Archives of General Psychiatry, 44*, 98.

Robertson, M. M., Schnieden, V., & Lees, A. J. (1990). Management of Gilles de la Tourette syndrome using sulpiride. *Clinical Neuropharmacology, 13*, 229–235.

Robertson, M. M., Scull, D. A., Eapen, V., & Trimble, M. R. (1996). Risperidone in the treatment of Tourette syndrome: A retrospective case study. *Journal of Psychopharmacology, 10*, 317–320.

Sallee, F. R., Kurlan, R., Goetz, C. G., et al. (2000). Ziprasidone treatment of children and adolescents with Tourette syndrome: A pilot study. *Journal of the American Academy of Child and Adolescent Psychiatry, 39*, 292–299.

Sallee, F. R., Nesbitt, L., Jackson, C., Sine, L., & Sethuraman, G. (1997). Relative efficacy of haloperidol and pimozide in children and adolescents with Tourette disorder. *American Journal of Psychiatry, 154*, 1057–1062.

Sallee, F. R., & Rock, C. M. (1994). Effects of pimozide on cognition in children with Tourette syndrome: Interaction with comorbid attention deficit hyperactivity disorder. *Acta Psychiatrica Scandinavica, 90*, 4–9.

Sanberg, P. R., McConville, B. J., Fogelson, H. M., et al. (1989). Nicotine potentiates the effects of haloperidol in animals and in patients with Tourette syndrome. *Biomedicine and Pharmacotherapy, 43*, 19–23.

Sanchez-Ramos, J. R., & Weiner, W. J. (1993). Drug-induced tics. In R. Kurlan (Ed.), *Handbook of Tourette syndrome and related tic and behavioral disorders* (pp. 183–197). New York: Marcel Dekker.

Sandor, P. (2003). Pharmacologic management of tics in patients with TS. *Journal of Psychosomatic Research, 55*, 41–48.

Sandor, P., Musisi, S., Moldofsky, H., & Lang, A. (1990). Tourette syndrome: A follow-up study. *Journal of Clinical Psychopharmacology, 10*, 197–199.

Scahill, L., Chappell, P. B., Kim, Y. S., et al. (2001). A placebo-controlled study of guanfacine in the treatment of children with tic disorders and attention deficit hyperactivity disorder. *American Journal of Psychiatry, 158*, 1067–1074.

Scahill, L., Chappell, P. B., King, R. A., & Leckman, J. F. (2000). Pharmacological treatment of tic disorders. *Child and Adolescent Psychiatric Clinics of North America, 9*, 99–117.

Scahill, L., Erenberg, G., & the Tourette Syndrome Practice Parameter Work Group. (2006). Contemporary assessment and pharmacotherapy of Tourette syndrome. *NeuroRx, 3*(2), 192–206.

Scahill, L., Leckman, J. F., Schultz, R. T., et al. (2003). A placebo-controlled trial of risperidone in Tourette syndrome. *Neurology, 60*, 1130–1135.

Scahill, L., Riddle, M. A., King, M. A., et al. (1997). Fluoxetine had no marked effect on tic symptoms in patients with Tourette syndrome: A double-blind placebo-controlled study. *Journal of Child and Adolescent Psychopharmacology, 7*, 75.

Seignot, M. J. N. (1961). A case of tic of Gilles de la Tourette cured by R-1625. *Annales Medico-Psychologiques, 119*, 578–579.

Silay, Y. S., & Jankovic, S. (2005). Emerging Drugs in Tourette Syndrome. *Expert Opinion on Emerging Drugs, 10*(2), 365–380.

Silay, Y. S., Vuong, K. D., & Jankovic, J. (in press). The efficacy and safety of fluphenazine in patients with Tourette syndrome.

Silver, A. A., & Sanberg, P. R. (1993). Transdermal nicotine patch and potentiation of haloperidol in Tourette syndrome. *Lancet, 342*, 182.

Silver, A. A., Shytle, R. D., Philip, M. K., et al. (1996). Case study: Long-term potentiation of neuroleptics with transdermal nicotine in Tourette syndrome. *Journal of the Academy of Child and Adolescent Psychiatry, 35*, 1631–1636.

Silver, A. A., Shytle, R. D., Philip, M. K., et al. (2001). Transdermal nicotine and haloperidol in Tourette disorder: A double-blind placebo-controlled study. *Journal of Clinical Psychiatry, 62*, 707–714.

Silver, A. A., Shytle, R. D., Sheehan, K. H., et al. (2001). Multicenter, double-blind, placebo-controlled study of mecamylamine monotherapy for Tourette disorder. *Journal of the Academy of Child and Adolescent Psychiatry, 40*, 1103–1110.

Singer, H. S. (2005). Tourette syndrome: From behavior to biology. *Lancet Neurology, 4*(3), 149–159.

Singer, H. S., Brown, J., Quaskey, S., et al. (1995). The treatment of attention-deficit hyperactivity disorder in Tourette syndrome: A double-blind placebo-controlled study with clonidine and desipramine. *Pediatrics, 95*, 74–81.

Singer, H. S., Wendlandt, J., Krieger, M., & Giuliano, J. (2001). Baclophen treatment in Tourette syndrome: A double-blind placebo-controlled, crossover trial. *Neurology, 56*, 599–604.

Snijders, A. H., Bloem, B. R., Orth, M., Rothwell, J. C., Trimble, M. R., & Robertson, M. M. (2005). Video assessment of rTMS for Tourette syndrome. *Journal of Neurology, Neurosurgery and Psychiatry, 76*(12), 1743–1744.

SoterodeMenezes, M. A., Rho, J. M., Murphy, P., et al. (2000). Lamotrigine-induced tic disorder: Report of five pediatric cases. *Epilepsia, 41*, 962.

Spencer, T., Biederman, J., Coffey, B., et al. (2002). A double-blind comparison of desipramine and placebo in children and adolescents with chronic tic disorder and comorbid attention-deficit/hyperactivity disorder. *Archives of General Psychiatry, 59*, 649–656.

Spencer, T., Biederman, J., & Steingard, R. (1993). Buproprion exacerbates tics in children with attention-deficit hyperactivity disorder and Tourette syndrome. *Journal of the American Academy of Child and Adolescent Psychiatry, 32*, 211–214.

Stamenkovic, M., Schindler, S. D., Aschauer, H. N., et al. (2000). Effective open-label treatment of Tourette disorder with olanzapine. *International Clinical Psychopharmacology, 15*, 23–28.

Steingard, R. J., Goldberg, M., Lee, D., & DeMaso, D. R. (1994). Adjunctive clonazepam treatment of tic symptoms in children with comorbid tic disorders and ADHD. *Journal of the American Academy of Child and Adolescent Psychiatry, 32*, 350–353.

Stevens, R. J., Bassel, C., & Sandor, P. (2004). Olanzepine in the treatment of aggression and tics in children with Tourette syndrome: A pilot study. *Journal of Child and Adolescent Psychopharmacology, 14*, 255–266.

Stigler, K. A., Posey, D. J., & McDougle, C. J. (2004). Aripiprazole for maladaptive behavior in pervasive developmental disorders. *Journal of Child and Adolescent Psychopharmacology, 14*, 455–463.

Sun, B., Krahl, S. E., Zhan, S., & Shen, J. (2005). Improved capsulotomy for refractory Tourette's syndrome. *Stereotactic Functional Neurosurgery, 83*(2–3), 55–56.

Temel, Y., & Visser-Vandewalle, V. (2004). Research review: Surgery in Tourette syndrome. *Movement Disorders, 19*, 3–14.

Tourette Syndrome Study Group. (2002). Treatment of ADHD in children with Tourette syndrome: A randomized controlled trial. *Neurology, 58*, 527.

Vandewalle, V., van der Linden, C., Groenewegen, H. J., et al. (1999). Stereotactic treatment of Gilles de la Tourette syndrome by high frequency stimulation of the thalamus. *Lancet, 353*, 724.

Varley, C. K. (2001). Sudden death related to selected tricyclic antidepressants in children: Epidemiology, mechanisms, and clinical implications. *Paediatric Drugs, 3*, 613–627.

Walkup, J. T. (1995). Clinical decision making in child and adolescent psychopharmacology. *Child and Adolescent Psychiatric Clinics of North America, 4*, 23–39.

Wilens, T. E., Biederman, J., Geist, D. E., et al. (1993). Nortriptyline in the treatment of ADHD: A chart review of 58 cases. *Journal of the American Academy of Child and Adolescent Psychiatry, 32*, 343–349.

Wilens, T. E., Spencer, T. J., Swanson, J. M., et al. (1999). Combining methylphenidate and clonidine: A clinically sound medication option. *Journal of the American Academy of Child and Adolescent Psychiatry, 38*, 614–622.

Wilheim, S., Deckersbach, T., Coffey, B., et al. (2003). Habit reversal versus supportive therapy for Tourette disorder: A randomized controlled trial. *American Journal of Psychiatry, 160*, 1175–1177.

Wirshing, D. A., Spellberg, B. J., Erhart, S. M., et al. (1998). Novel antipsyhotics and new onset diabetes. *Biological Psychiatry, 44*, 778–783.

CHAPTER 8

Psychosocial Management of Tics and Intentional Repetitive Behaviors Associated with Tourette Syndrome

ALAN L. PETERSON

This chapter reviews the psychosocial management of tics and intentional repetitive behaviors associated with Tourette syndrome (TS) and chronic tic disorders. Extensive literature reviews of research on nonpharmacological treatments for TS and tic disorders have been published previously (see Azrin & Peterson, 1988a; Carr & Chong, 2005; Houlihan, Hofschulte, & Patten, 1993; Peterson & Azrin, 1993; Peterson, Campise, & Azrin, 1994; Turpin, 1983). This chapter provides an update on this research and specific details on the procedures involved in evidenced-based interventions. Although a variety of nonpharmacological interventions are discussed (e.g., contingency management/function-based treatments, massed practice, relaxation training, hypnosis, self-monitoring, exposure with response prevention, and habit reversal [HR]), a particular emphasis is given to HR—the one behavioral treatment with the most scientific evidence for its efficacy.

OVERVIEW OF NONPHARMACOLOGICAL INTERVENTIONS

In most health care settings, pharmacotherapy is considered the first-line treatment for the multiple motor and vocal tics associated with TS. Primary care physicians, neurologists, and psychiatrists are the medical providers most likely to evaluate and treat patients with TS, and these physicians are most likely to use drugs as the primary treatment approach. Although little research is available on the pharmacological treatment of chronic motor or vocal tic disorders, there is a large body of research literature to support the pharmacological treatment of TS (see Lavenstein, 2003; Robertson & Stern, 2000; Sandor, 2003). (Scahill, Sukhodolsky, and King, Chapter 4, this volume) notes the significant benefits of pharmacotherapy, as well as its limitations. For example, few patients find that medications totally eliminate their tics. Likewise, some TS medications are associated with a range of unwanted side effects that can result in poor compliance or in early termination of treatment. For example, long-term use of some medications, such as haloperidol, can lead to additional movement disorders such as tardive dyskinesia or what has been termed neuroleptic-induced tardive Tourette (Reid, 2004). Given these problems—and the fact that some parents to do not like to medicate their children—alternative and adjunctive treatments may be useful. Psychosocial treatments have been developed to fill this need. The best researched of all psychosocial interventions are behavioral treatments.

PSYCHOSOCIAL TREATMENT OF TS AND TIC DISORDERS

A variety of psychosocial treatment approaches has been evaluated in over 60 published studies of nonpharmacological treatments for TS and tic disorders. Nine published studies have focused specifically on chronic vocal tics (Bados Lopez & Olle, 1984; Fuata & Griffiths, 1992; O'Brien & Brennan, 1979; Roane, Piazza, Cercone, & Grados, 2002; Wagaman, Miltenberger, & Williams, 1995; Watson & Heindl, 1996; Watson & Sterling, 1998; Woods & Twohig, 2002; Woods, Twohig, Roloff, & Flessner, 2003) and two on eye-blinking tics (Azrin & Peterson, 1989; Gross & Mendelson, 1982). Behavioral treatment approaches have included contingency management/function-based interventions, massed practice, relaxation training, hypnosis, exposure and response prevention, and HR. All behavioral therapies should be embedded within a psychoeducational and supportive context.

Psychoeducation/Supportive Therapy

Education about tic disorder and the provision of support and reassurance to patients and their families have been described as the cornerstone for all other treatment interventions (Peterson & Cohen, 1998).

Most individuals present for treatment of tics during a period of symptom exacerbation or following a less than adequate response to prior intervention(s). Educating patients and families about the natural course of tic disorders (e.g., waxing and waning nature, peak severity typically in late childhood, often followed by gradual improvement during adolescence) and the potential benefits of psychosocial treatment often serves to reduce anxiety and provide positive expectations about the current treatment. In addition, helping the individual to identify personal strengths and providing support and reassurance about the current situation and treatment prospects serve to enhance both self-efficacy, especially in those experiencing shame or distress due to their illness, and motivation for other behavioral intervention such as HR training.

Contingency Management/Function-Based Interventions

One set of behavioral treatments has attempted to systematically understand and alter external (outside the person) events that may increase or decrease tics. Typically, this approach is conducted in two ways: by broadly reinforcing tic-free periods, or by delivering aversive stimuli contingent on tics. This type of intervention is known as "general contingency management." Using tokens to reinforce the absence of tics would be one example of a contingency-management-based intervention.

A more specialized type of contingency management procedure is known as "function-based intervention." When conducting function-based treatments, an attempt is made to identify specific environmental events that have been found to increase or decrease tics for a given individual. These specific environmental variables are then altered in the service of producing tic reduction. Although both standard contingency management and function-based interventions use the environment to create tic reduction, function-based interventions are tailored specifically to the individual's unique situation, whereas the general procedures are broadly applied without regard to the child's unique situation. Below, each of these is described in more detail.

General Contingency Management Procedures

Contingency management has been employed in over 20 published studies of behavioral treatments for TS and tic disorders. These published reports include both case studies and single-subject design research. Contingency management is based on operant learning theory and assumes that tics are maintained or exacerbated by the consequences that follow them. Therefore, tics have the potential to be modified by the contingencies that surround them.

Positive reinforcement is one form of contingency management that has been evaluated in the form of praise, monetary rewards, and preferred activities for the reduction or absence of tics. Positive reinforcement or the differential reinforcement of other (DRO) behaviors has been evaluated in 11 studies of children with tic disorders (Barr, Lovibond, & Katsavos, 1972; Browning & Stover, 1971; Doleys & Kurtz, 1974; Hollandsworth & Bausinger, 1978; Miller, 1970; Rosen & Wesner, 1973; Sand & Carlson, 1973; Schulman, 1974; Tophoff, 1973; Varni, Boyd, & Cataldo, 1978; Wagaman et al., 1995; Watson & Heindl, 1996; Watson & Sterling, 1998). One of these studies included two subjects (Browning & Stover, 1971). All of the remaining studies included single participants. Each of these studies included reinforcement as one of several behavioral treatment components; none of them evaluated the use of reinforcement alone. Decreases in tic frequency at the end of treatment were found in 8 of the 11 studies (Browning & Stover, 1971; Doleys & Kurtz, 1974; Miller, 1970; Rosen & Wesner, 1973; Schulman, 1974; Tophoff, 1973; Varni et al., 1978; Watson & Sterling, 1998). At follow-up, improvement was maintained in seven of the studies (Browning & Stover, 1971; Doleys & Kurtz, 1974; Miller, 1970; Rosen & Wesner, 1973; Tophoff, 1973; Varni et al., 1978; Watson & Sterling, 1998). However, the actual percent reduction in tics specifically attributable to contingency management for these studies is confounded by the addition of other treatment components.

Only two studies have examined the specific effects of reinforcement on tic expression (Himle & Woods, 2005; Woods & Himle, 2004). Although neither was designed as a treatment study, both allow researchers to examine the responsivity of tics to reinforcement. In both studies, children with TS were placed in a room where they were told that their movements were being recorded by a "tic detector," which was a small box placed in an observation room with the child. The "tic detector" was actually an operant token dispenser with a small camera mounted on top to provide the illusion that the machine had tic-detecting capabilities. The children were told that the machine would deliver a token for every 10 seconds he or she could go without having a tic. Results of these first two studies showed that the children had fewer tics (i.e., 60–70% reductions from baseline) when reinforced for tic-free periods as compared to periods when they were told not to suppress tics (but still thought the machine was watching them), and periods when they were told to suppress tics but in which the machine did not deliver tokens. One fear about using reinforcement to reduce tics is that such a procedure may create a "rebound" in tics after the contingency is removed. However, Himle and Woods (2005) found no evidence so support this concern.

Punishment is another form of contingency management that has been evaluated as a behavioral treatment component (in the form of electric shock) in seven studies (Barr et al., 1972; Clark, 1966), white noise (Doleys & Kurtz, 1974), or time out (Browning & Stover, 1971; Canavan & Powell, 1981; Lahey, McNees, & McNees, 1973; Varni et al., 1978). One study (Browning & Stover, 1971) failed to show a decrease in tics with the contingent punishment. All of the other studies demonstrated decreases in tic frequency at the end of treatment. Decreases in tic frequency were temporary in three of the studies using punishment (Barr et al., 1972; Canavan & Powell, 1981; Lahey et al., 1973), and there was difficulty in generalization. Barr et al. (1972) reported that tics were only reduced when a shock electrode was connected to the subject's finger. Upon removal of the electrode, tics returned to the baseline frequency. Similarly, Lahey et al. (1973) found that coprolalia was reduced using time out in a school setting. However, the coprolalia quickly returned to baseline levels when the contingencies were removed. Out of the seven published studies employing punishment for the treatment of tics, only two of the studies found that improvement was maintained at follow-up (Doleys & Kurtz, 1974; Varni et al., 1978).

In summary, general contingency management in the form of positive reinforcement and punishment has been found to be somewhat effective in reducing tics in TS and chronic tic disorders. The results are partially confounded in that the contingencies were used as part of multicomponent treatment programs, and they have not been evaluated as individual treatment components. Therefore, whereas positive reinforcement such as praise and encouragement is highly recommended as a component of treatment for patients with TS, especially children, punishment is not recommended for a number of reasons. First, the ethics of using punishment procedures in lieu of effective nonaversive procedures is questionable. Second, the client may begin to associate punishment with the person delivering the consequences, not the target behavior, an association that could have the unintended consequence of shaping the person to tic only in the absence of the punisher. Finally, punishment may paradoxically increase tic behavior by heightening anxiety or other tic-increasing factors.

Function-Based Interventions

Moving beyond broadly applied contingency management, function-based interventions attempt to understand the specific environmental events that make tics more or less likely to happen. After understanding how specific environmental events impact tics for an individual, the clinician develops a plan to systematically alter these events in the service of tic reduction. Although the technologies for the functional assessment of tics and the development of the resulting function-based assessments are in their infancy, the procedure is generally conducted in interview form, with the clinician asking the patient what external (i.e., outside the body) or internal (i.e., inside the body) antecedent events make tics more or less likely to happen. After identifying a list of environmental contexts wherein tics are made more or less frequent, the clinician takes the list of tic-exacerbating situations and identifies the consequences in those situations that may be reinforcing tics. After this list of antecedents and consequences is completed, the clinician seeks to modify the environment in the service of tic reduction.

For example, it may be determined that tics are more likely to occur at home than at school. When asked specifically about home situations in which tics are most likely to occur, it is determined that they are most likely to occur when the family is watching television. Further probing may indicate that the tics are more likely to occur when the child is watching television around others than when alone. Asking about consequences in this situation, it is discovered that the child's parents frequently attend to the child's tics as they occur by asking the child if he or she is "okay." In a function-based treatment, the clinician may attempt to minimize the amount of television to which the child is exposed, and to ask the parents to refrain from reassuring the child when he or she tics. It is unlikely that this function-based treatment will completely eliminate the tic, but the goal is not necessarily elimination; it is effective management.

In the existing literature, there are very few reports of functional analysis and function-based interventions for tics (Carr, Sidener, Sidener, & Cummings, 2005; Watson, Dufrene, Weaver, Butler, & Meeks, 2005; Watson & Sterling, 1998), although other studies consider the specific impact of environmental events on tic expression (e.g., Silva, Munoz, Barickman, & Friedhoff, 1995; Woods, Watson, Wolfe, Twohig, & Friman, 2001). Nevertheless, the Watson and Sterling paper provides a good example of a function-based treatment of tics. In this study, a 4-year-old girl with a coughing tic received a functional assessment, which indicated that social attention was maintaining the coughing tic. The behavioral treatment involved withholding parental attention when the little girl coughed (extinction) combined with attention in the form of verbal statements contingent upon no coughing (DRO) and a subsequent tangible reinforcement condition (candy). This function-based treatment approach resulted in the elimination of the coughing tic, and complete elimination of the tic was maintained at the 6-month follow-up point. Although the function-based approaches are in their infancy, they have led to profound changes in the treatment of many disorders (e.g., Hanley, Iwata, & McCord, 2003), and it is possible that a similar approach can have a large impact on tic expression.

Massed Practice

Massed practice (MP) has been evaluated in over 20 published studies for the treatment of tic disorders and TS. In MP the patient purposefully performs the tic as quickly, accurately, and with as much effort as possible for a specified period of time (e.g., 15 minutes) interspersed with brief periods of rest (e.g., 2 minutes of performing the tic, 1 minute of rest). This practice continues a number of times per day, through the course of treatment. Out of approximately 20 published studies of MP for tics, about half of them reported that tics were reduced at the end of treatment (Browning & Stover, 1971; Clark, 1966; Miller, 1970; Nicassio, Liberman, Patterson, Raminez, & Saunder, 1972; Savicki & Carlin, 1972; Storms, 1985; Tophoff, 1973; Walton, 1961, 1964; Yates, 1958). However, a number of other studies reported no reduction tics (Barr et al., 1972; Canavan & Powell, 1981; Lahey et al., 1973; O'Brien & Brennan, 1979; Sand & Carlson, 1973). A few studies even found an increase in tics (Feldman & Werry, 1966; Hollandsworth & Bausinger, 1978; Teoh, 1974; Turpin & Powell, 1984). Interestingly, one study using MP for coprolalia reported an increase in the clarity of curse words (Hollandsworth & Bausinger, 1978).

Out of the 10 studies reporting reduced tics with MP, only 5 of them included sufficient data to determine the degree of effectiveness (Browning & Stover, 1971; Clark, 1966; Nicassio et al., 1972; Savicki & Carlin, 1972; Storms, 1985). These studies reported that tics were reduced by an average of about 58%. Only one controlled group study has been published (Azrin, Nunn, & Frantz, 1980) in which 22 subjects with motor and vocal tics were randomly assigned to either an HR (n = 10) or MP (n = 12) group. The results indicated that MP reduced tics by 33% on the first day, and at a 4-week follow-up, 2 out of 12 patients (17%) were tic free. In summary, MP does not have strong empirical support for use as a treatment for tics and is therefore not recommended.

Relaxation Training

A wide variety of relaxation training approaches has been evaluated in research studies, including progressive muscle relaxation training (Jacobson, 1938; Bernstein & Borkovec, 1973), autogenic training (Schultz & Luthe, 1959), the relaxation response (Benson, 1975), and behavioral relaxation postures (Schilling & Poppen, 1983; Poppen, 1988). Relaxation training has been used as a behavioral intervention in 15 studies of TS and tic disorders (Azrin & Peterson, 1988b, 1989, 1990; Bergin, Waranch, Brown, Carson, & Singer, 1998; Canavan & Powell, 1981; Franco, 1981; Friedman, 1980; Michultka, Blanchard, & Rosenblum, 1989; O'Brien & Brennan, 1979; Peterson & Azrin, 1992; Rosen & Wesner, 1973; Savicki & Carlin, 1972; Thomas, Abrams, & Johnson, 1971; Tophoff, 1973; Turpin & Powell, 1984). However, most of these studies have used relaxation training in combination with one or more behavioral treatments. Only two studies have evaluated the independent effectiveness of relaxation training (Bergin et al., 1998; Peterson & Azrin, 1992). The study by Peterson and Azrin (1992) found that relaxation training reduced tics in TS patients by an average of 32%. However, this study was a laboratory investigation and only measured the immediate change in tic frequency as a result of a single-session of relaxation training.

In contrast, Bergin et al. (1998) studied 23 children with TS recruited from a university-based clinic. Participants were randomized and blocked according to initial tic severity and the presence of attention-deficit/hyperactivity disorder (ADHD) into either relaxation therapy or a minimal therapy control condition (awareness and quiet time training). The relaxation training treatment consisted of weekly, hour-long, individual relaxation training sessions for 6 weeks. Outcome was measured by using five established tic severity scales. Sixteen participants (seven relaxation training, nine control) completed the 3-month study. At 6 weeks, the relaxation training group had greater reduction in TS symptoms, but the values failed to reach statistical significance. There was no difference between groups at the 3-month follow-up evaluation.

In summary, the results of the Bergin et al. (1998) study and a number of additional single-subject design studies suggest that relaxation training may have some merit for the treatment of TS and tic disorders, although the overall effect size is relatively low. Tic frequencies were often significantly reduced and were sometimes nonexistent during the relaxed state. However, the reductions were often temporary, with tics returning to baseline levels after a few minutes or hours. Additional research is warranted to further evaluate the potential efficacy of relaxation training for tic disorders. Research should specifically target the evaluation of different types of relaxation exercises and more intensive relaxation training with documented regular home practice.

Hypnosis

Two studies have evaluated the use of hypnosis for the treatment of TS (Culbertson, 1989; Young & Montano, 1988). Culbertson (1989) evaluated a four-step hypnotherapy model for the treatment of an adolescent male with TS. The treatment included nine sessions of progressive relaxation, fingertip temperature feedback, an eye-roll procedure, and visual imagery. The results indicated that motor and vocal tics were minimal to nonexistent at the end of treatment.

The largest hypnosis study (Young & Montano, 1988) included a combination of HR, relaxation training, and hypnosis for the treatment of three patients with TS. In this study, tics were reduced by 94–100% for all three patients by the end of treatment. However, because neither of these studies (Culbertson, 1989; Young & Montano, 1988) was controlled, and both included additional behavioral treatment components, it is difficult to determine the specific contribution of hypnosis for the treatment of TS and tics. As such, there appears to be insufficient data, to date, to recommend hypnosis as an independent treatment for TS and tic disorders.

Self-Monitoring and Awareness Training

Self-monitoring is the systematic observation and recording of target behaviors. Self-monitoring is a behavioral strategy that is often used as an assessment technique but also has been demonstrated to be a potent treatment component. Patients are instructed to use a wrist counter, small notebook, or other device to record the occurrence of each of their tics for a specified period of time. Some published research indicates that this procedure alone can lead to reductions in tics. Four case studies ($n = 1$ for each study) have been conducted in which self-monitoring was used as the primary treatment procedure (Billings, 1978; Hutzell, Platzek, & Logue, 1974) or as a major treatment component (Savicki & Carlin, 1972; Thomas et al., 1971). Only one study included a sample of more than a single participant (Peterson & Azrin, 1992; $n = 6$). This study included six participants with TS and employed a modified counterbalanced design. Self-monitoring was evaluated over two trials for each subject. The results indicated that self-monitoring reduced tic behavior by an average of 44% over two trials with each participant. However, the efficacy of self-monitoring in reducing tics was decreased over the two trials from –54% during the first trial to –33% during the second trial, suggesting that the efficacy of self-monitoring may not last.

Awareness training is a modified version of self-monitoring in which a clinician, parent, or spouse assists in the identification, description, and monitoring of tics. Increasing a patient's knowledge of the frequency and specificity of tics through awareness training is designed to help increase the accuracy of self-monitoring of tics. One study evaluated the effectiveness of awareness training alone in treating multiple tics

(Wright & Miltenberger, 1987). In this study a young adult was assessed using a multiple baseline across behaviors design. The results showed that the awareness training was very effective in suppressing both head and facial tics and that the treatment effects generalized outside the clinic setting. Follow-up data showed that reductions in tics were maintained at the 8-month follow-up point.

In summary, all six studies that have evaluated self-monitoring or awareness training for TS and tics have found significant reductions in tics. However, the results of the study by Peterson and Azrin (1992) suggest that the effectiveness of self-monitoring may decrease over time. Exactly why this simple procedure works is unclear. Reductions in tics with self-monitoring or awareness training may be a result of reactivity and the increased awareness of tics. Likewise, there is some evidence that the act of self-monitoring may serve as a competing behavior in some cases (e.g., Woods, Miltenberger, & Lumley, 1996). The potential long-term efficacy of self-monitoring has not been evaluated. Nevertheless, self-monitoring and awareness training typically are recommended as part of a standard assessment and treatment program for tic disorders.

Exposure with Response Prevention

Exposure with response prevention has been demonstrated to be effective for the treatment of compulsive behaviors associated with obsessive–compulsive disorder (OCD; Jenike, 2001; Riddle, 1998). This treatment approach is also the newest approach to be evaluated for the treatment of TS (Woods, Hook, Spellman, & Friman, 2000; Verdellen, Keijsers, Cath, & Hoogduin, 2004). In the first study, Woods et al. (2000) evaluated the use of exposure with response prevention for the treatment of a 16-year-old male with TS. The adolescent had a complex motor tic that involved the frequent touching of others. The authors hypothesized that this tic might also be considered a compulsive behavior. The results showed that exposure with response prevention resulted in a significant decrease in touching attempts, overt anxiety, and subjective anxiety across time.

The second study (Verdellen et al., 2004) evaluated exposure with response prevention versus HR in 43 participants with TS. The outcome measures included the Yale Global Tic Severity Scale and 15-minute recordings of tic frequency completed in both the clinic and home settings. Exposure with response prevention resulted in statistically significant improvements on all outcome measures, and no significant differences were found between treatment conditions on any of the outcome measures. These two studies suggest that exposure with response prevention may be a promising new treatment approach for TS and tic disorders.

Habit Reversal

HR is the most extensively researched behavioral treatment for tic and habit disorders and has been evaluated in about 30 published studies (see previous reviews by Azrin & Peterson, 1988a; Carr & Chong, 2005; Houlihan et al., 1993; Peterson & Azrin, 1993; Peterson et al., 1994; Turpin, 1983). Eleven studies have evaluated HR treatment for TS (Araki & Nakai, 1990; Azrin & Peterson, 1988b, 1990; Carr, 1995; Carr & Bailey, 1996; Clarke, Bray, Kehle, & Truscott, 2001; Deckersbach, Rauch, Buhlmann, & Wilhelm, 2006; Peterson & Azrin, 1992; Tolchard, 1995; Verdellen et al., 2004; Wilhelm et al., 2003). Seventeen studies have investigated HR for chronic motor tic disorders (Araki & Okuma, 1985; Azrin & Nunn, 1973; Azrin et al., 1980; Azrin & Peterson, 1989; Bados Lopez & Olle, 1984; Cloutier, 1985; Finney, Rapoff, Hall, & Christopherson, 1983; Gross & Mendelson, 1982; Miltenberger & Fuqua, 1985; Miltenberger, Fuqua, & McKinley, 1985; O'Brien & Brennan, 1979; O'Connor, Gareau, & Borgeat, 1997; Ollendick, 1981; O'Connor et al., 2001; Sharenow, Fuqua, & Miltenberger, 1989; Woods et al., 1996; Zikis, 1983). HR treatment for vocal tics as been studied in two investigations (Woods & Twohig, 2002; Woods et al., 2003).

Although most of the HR studies have included single-participant research designs, seven studies employed randomized between-subjects research designs (Azrin et al., 1980; Azrin & Peterson, 1990; Deckersbach et al., 2006; O'Connor et al., 1997, 2001; Verdellen et al., 2004; Wilhelm et al., 2002). Azrin et al. (1980) conducted the first randomized trial to evaluate the efficacy of HR specifically for the treatment of chronic tic disorders. This study included 22 participants randomly assigned to either HR ($n = 10$) or MP ($n = 12$) treatment. Participants had a wide range of simple and complex motor and vocal tics, and HR was used to treat each participant's major or most disruptive tic. The results indicated that the HR group had a self-reported reduction in tics of 84% on the first day. At an 18-month follow-up, there was a 97% reduction in tics and 80% of the patients were tic-free. As noted earlier, MP led to a 33% reduction in tics, and at a 4-week follow-up, 17% of patients were tic-free. A primary limitation of this study is that the outcome was based on patient self-report.

HR was also used in a randomized group treatment outcome study of TS (Azrin & Peterson, 1990). This study employed a randomized wait-list control group design and evaluated the efficacy of the HR for 14 participants with TS. Participants were matched on age, medication usage, and tic frequency and were randomly assigned to an immediate or delayed treatment group. Tic frequency was measured in the clinic using videotapes taken through a one-way mirror and at home by unobtrusive direct observations by the participant's spouse or parent. Results showed tics to be reduced in the immediate treatment group by 89% in the clinic and by 92% at home at the 12-month follow-up point. Tic frequency in the control group remained relatively stable during the 3-month wait-list period and then achieved a similar reduction in tics after treatment. The frequency of tics recorded in the clinic decreased by 52% the first month, 65% the second month, and 93% at the end of treatment. Analyses showed that the reduction occurred for both vocal tics and motor tics, with no evidence of symptom substitution.

O'Connor et al. (1997, 2001) conducted two studies of HR treatment for chronic tic disorders. In the first study (O'Connor et al., 1997), 14 patients were nonrandomly assigned to be treated with HR alone (n = 7) or in combination with cognitive-behavioral therapy (CBT; n = 7). Both treatment approaches significantly reduced tics, and there was no significant benefit with the addition of CBT. The second study (O'Connor et al., 2001) included 47 participants randomly assigned to an HR treatment as compared to a wait-list control condition that subsequently received HR. The results indicated that after 4 months of treatment, 65% of participants reported between 75 and 100% control over their tics and 52% rated 75–100% control at the 2-year follow-up.

The first fully randomized parallel-group design study to compare HR to a control condition for the treatment of TS was conducted by Wilhelm et al. (2003). This study included 32 patients with TS randomly assigned to 14 sessions of either HR or supportive psychotherapy. Three patients (two, HR; one, supportive psychotherapy) dropped out before session 8 and were excluded from data analyses. Outcome was measured in terms of changes in tic severity and functional impairment. The results indicated that the tic severity, measured using the Yale Global Tic Severity Scale (YGTSS; Leckman et al., 1989), significantly decreased in the HR group (n = 16) at posttreatment (–35%) and as maintained at the 10-month follow-up point (–31%) as compared to the supportive psychotherapy group (n = 13; post = +1%; follow-up = –11%). Similar findings were found for the functional impairment measures for HR (post = –58%; follow-up = –41%) as compared to the supportive psychotherapy condition (post = –16%; follow-up = –17%). Using a nearly identical design, similar results were found by Deckersbach et al. (2006), who also showed that those with low pretreatment response inhibition scores responded more poorly to HR.

In another recent study, Verdellen et al. (2004) evaluated the efficacy of HR as compared to exposure with response prevention in 43 patients with TS. Outcome measures included the YGTSS, 15-minute tic frequency counts monitored in the clinic setting, and 15-minute home-based tic frequency counts. The results indicated that both treatment

conditions resulted in statistically significant improvements on all outcome measures ($p < 0.001$). No significant differences were found between the treatment conditions on any of the outcome measures.

Several studies have evaluated modifications of the original HR protocol (Miltenberger, Fuqua, & Woods, 1998; Woods & Miltenberger,
1995). Some have suggested that awareness training and competing response training may be the most important components of HR for the
treatment of motor tics (Azrin & Peterson, 1989; Miltenberger &
Fuqua, 1985; Miltenberger et al., 1985; Ollendick, 1981). However, one
study (Woods et al., 1996) found that tics were significantly reduced or
eliminated with (1) awareness training alone, (2) awareness training plus
self-monitoring, and (3) the combination of awareness training, competing response training, and social support. Another study (Sharenow et
al., 1989) investigated the contingent use of a dissimilar competing response (behavior not incompatible with the target behavior) for three
participants with motor tics and found that this type of competing response also resulted in a reduction in tics. However, the study also found
that the use of a similar competing response further reduced tics for one
out of three participants. Overall, these results seem to indicate that different components of HR may play a more important role for different
patients. Therefore, the use of the full HR treatment program is most
likely to reduce tics for most patients.

The overall results of the studies employing both within- and
between-subjects research designs indicate that HR is an effective treatment for TS and chronic motor and vocal tic disorders. These studies
have found that HR was effective for vocal and motor tics, children as
well as adults, for patients receiving TS medications as well as those not
doing so, for tic severity as well as tic frequency, and with no evidence of
symptom substitution. Additionally, the treatment effect size for HR is
generally comparable with most drug studies of TS (Peterson & Azrin,
1993).

Description of the HR Protocol

HR is a comprehensive behavioral therapy treatment that includes five
primary components—awareness training, relaxation training, competing response training, contingency management, and generalization
training—and several other behavioral treatment procedures (Azrin &
Nunn, 1973, 1977). For the treatment of TS and tic disorders, the HR
competing response is the most distinctive feature of this treatment approach. The competing response for most motor tics is the isometric
tensing of muscles opposite to the tic movements. The opposing muscles
are contracted for a brief period of time contingent on the urge to have a

tic. The following is a detailed description of the HR treatment protocol. For one tic, the HR protocol can be implemented in one or two sessions. However, a typical course of HR involves 3 to 10, 1-hour sessions, with booster sessions as needed. Prior to the initiation of HR therapy it is helpful to provide a brief description of the entire treatment package to the patient and to obtain his or her informed consent for treatment.

HR Awareness Training

The initial step in HR is awareness training, which focuses on increasing the patient's awareness of the frequency of tics, the environmental variables that influence tics, the different types of tics, and the specific movements involved in each tic. Awareness training consists of five procedures: response description, response detection, early warning, self-monitoring, and situation awareness.

RESPONSE DESCRIPTION

The first procedure in awareness training is *response description*, in which the patient learns to describe the topography of the tic behaviors. This treatment involves having the provider, patient, and sometimes a significant other (e.g., parent or spouse) identify all of the different types of tics that are emitted and develop a detailed description of each. A list of tics (e.g., head shake) and a written description for each (e.g., the head is shaken back and forth horizontally one or more times) is developed. Often it is useful to use a mirror or videotape of the patient to help in the identification and description of the tics.

The procedure of response description helps ensure that the individual is aware of all of the tics currently being emitted and the specific movement or movements involved in each tic. It would seem logical that most individuals would already be fully aware of their tics, but because some individuals may have 10 or more different types of tics and may emit over 1,000 tics per hour (see Azrin & Peterson, 1988b), it is not uncommon for some individuals to be unaware of both the presence and frequency of some of their tics.

The use of a videotape taken prior to the initiation of treatment is the best way to complete the response description. However, as mentioned earlier in this chapter, tics are sometimes temporarily reduced because of the patient's awareness of the videotaping process (Goetz, Leurgans, & Chmura, 2001). One useful strategy is to explain the important benefit of the videotapes and to ask for the patient's permission to obtain the videotapes unobtrusively as part of the assessment and treatment process. It is most useful if the videotape can be obtained through a one-way mirror so it is even less evident as to exactly when the videotaping is occurring. It is also helpful to explain the importance of videotaping the occurrence of tics and how the patient's awareness of the videotaping process may actually result in a temporary reduction of tics.

Some critics of HR have suggested that having patients focus on their tics may somehow make the tics worse or may be distressing to the individuals. However, there is no scientific evidence to support these criticisms, and there are several suggestions to reduce any concerns that a patient may have prior to the initiation of this part of treatment. Patients with tic disorders are sometimes reluctant to view themselves on a videotape or in a mirror. Therefore, prior to the initiation of the response description procedure, it is helpful to review and describe the importance and utility of the procedure and how the effectiveness of the HR treatment requires the patient to be keenly aware of all tic movements. Patient consent should always be obtained prior to obtaining any videotape. An additional benefit of reviewing the videotape is that it can actually help increase patient motivation for treatment.

RESPONSE DETECTION

The second part of awareness training is *response detection*. During this procedure, the therapist first verbally notes the occurrence of tics as they occur. For individuals with a low frequency of tics, the therapist can note the occurrence of any tic that occurs. For high-frequency tics, it is usually best if the response detection is limited to a specified target tic. The occurrence of each tic can be noted in several ways, depending on the preference of the patient. Perhaps the easiest method is to simply state the name of the type of tic as it occurs. For example, the therapist might say "head . . . head . . . head" to indicate the occurrence of three head-shaking tics. Alternatively the therapist might raise his or her index finger upon the occurrence of each tic, or use an audible hand counter that will not only indicate the occurrence of a tic, but also keep count of the total number of tics that occur during a specified period of time. It is important that response detection be done in a sensitive and nonjudgmental manner and not in a way that might be perceived by the patient as annoying or nagging. In the procedure of response detection is continued for several minutes until the therapist believes the patient is ready to progress to the next phase of treatment.

The second phase of response detection involves switching roles with the patient and having him or her note the occurrence of each tic. The patient notes the occurrence of each tic (or the target tic) in a manner similar to what was used when the therapist was noting the occurrence of the tics. This procedure is continued until the patient is able to successfully detect each tic as it occurs.

EARLY WARNING

The next portion of awareness training is *early warning*. This procedure involves having the patient pay attention to the earliest signs and symptoms (e.g., premonitory urges) that a tic is about to occur. These premonitory urges are then noted in a manner similar to that used in response detection. Both clinical reports and controlled research have indicated that most individuals are aware of a feeling, urge, or premonitory sensation just prior to the occurrence of a tic (Banaschewski, Woerner, & Rothenberger, 2003; Bliss, 1980; Bullen & Hemsley, 1983; Kwak, Dat Vuong, & Jankovic, 2003). The accurate identification of a premonitory sensation is important for the later use of the competing response procedure. Spending a longer period of time focused on early warning may be required for children, especially those who are younger (6–10 years old).

SELF-MONITORING

Self-monitoring is another part of awareness training and includes the recording of the frequency and type of tic. This procedure is usually used even before the start of treatment. Self-monitoring helps provide the initial baseline tic frequency for each different type of tic. Additionally, self-monitoring has been found to result in at least a modest reduction in tic frequency.

During self-monitoring the patient is instructed to record the occurrence of each tic for a specified duration each day. In most cases, it is best to focus on one tic at a time, unless the individual has an overall low rate of tics. In that case more than one tic can be recorded at a time. Each tic is usually recorded separately because it helps to identify which tics are most frequent and because different HR procedures may be used for each tic. The duration of the recording period must be adjusted depending on the frequency of tics. For high-frequency tics, a 10-minute self-monitoring period each day will usually suffice. For low-frequency tics, patients can keep records for longer periods of time.

Tics may be recorded in several ways. One of the simplest methods is the use of a hand-held counter or a wrist counter. Another method is to record tics in a notebook, recording sheet, index card, or personal digital assistant (PDA). When recording a single type of tic, handwritten "slash" marks can be written on a recording sheet, index card, or PDA. For the recording of multiple, low-frequency tics an abbreviated code can be developed for each patient (e.g., E = eye tic; H = head tic; S = shoulder shrug). The patient then records the code for each tic as it occurs (e.g., *E E H S E H H* to represent a series of eye, head, and shoulder tics).

Self-monitoring is often a homework assignment to be completed between treatment sessions to help evaluate progress. The use of self-monitoring should be flexibly changed as the individual progresses through the HR treatment protocol. Once the competing response training portion of the treatment has started, the self-monitoring homework should focus on the tics that are the current focus of the competing responses.

SITUATION AWARENESS

In situation awareness training, the patient tries to identify the antecedents that most reliably predicted the occurrence of the tics. This procedure helps the patient become more aware of the situations in which tics occur most frequently. Information gathered during self-monitoring is helpful in implementing this procedure. The patient identifies the external cues such as situations, persons, and places in which tics are increased or decreased. By becoming aware of the situations in which tics are more frequent, patients can then implement the appropriate procedures immediately upon entering the situations or even prior to doing so.

HR Relaxation Training

Patients with TS and tic disorders should be taught relaxation training as a general procedure to help reduce muscular tension and decrease the frequency and severity of tics. Several procedures have been demonstrated to be effective in producing muscular relaxation, including progressive muscular relaxation (Bernstein & Borkovec, 1973), deep breathing (Cappo & Holmes, 1984), visual imagery (Suinn, 1975), and self-statements of relaxation (Schultz & Luthe, 1959). A thorough review of the basic relaxation training techniques is not provided here because they have been detailed elsewhere (Benson, 1975; Bernstein & Borkovec, 1973; Poppen, 1988). Lichstein (1988) provides an excellent review of the relaxation training literature.

The potential efficacy of relaxation training is often limited by therapist failure to spend adequate time in treatment sessions focused on teaching, reviewing, and refining the relaxation strategies. Three to four complete 45-minute treatment sessions, with daily home practice between treatment sessions, are often required to obtain the full benefit of this treatment component. The effects of relaxation can be enhanced with the use of cue-controlled relaxation (Goldfried, 1971) or applied relaxation (Arntz, 2003; Linton & Gotestam, 1984; Ost & Breitholtz, 2000). For tic disorders, the premonitory sensation or urge to have a tic can be used as a cue to implement a brief, applied relaxation exercise. This strategy can be further enhanced if it is incorporated during or immediately after a competing response. An example of a cue-controlled or applied relaxation exercise is to have the patient take several slow, deep, rhythmic breaths. At the end of each exhalation the individual can focus on letting all of his or her muscles become as relaxed as possible. Self-statements of relaxation, such as repeating the words *calm* or *just relax*, can also enhance the cue-controlled relaxation exercise. Cue-controlled or applied relaxation exercises are designed to be easily incorporated into ongoing activities and to be performed for only a brief period of time (e.g., 1 minute). The usual result is that individuals do not get as relaxed as they might if performing a longer relaxation exercise, such as a 20-minute progressive muscle relaxation. However, cue-controlled or applied relaxation may "take the edge off" or reduce muscular tension or urges to have a tic just enough to prevent a tic from occurring.

HR Competing Response Training

The primary HR component is the *competing response*. The goal is to identify a competing behavior or response that, when performed, will prevent the tic from occurring. The competing response is designed to be (1) opposite to, or incompatible with, the tic movement, (2) maintained for a brief period of time (about 1 minute), (3) socially inconspicuous, and (4) compatible with normal, ongoing activities.

The competing response for most motor tics involves the isometric tensing of the muscles that are opposite to the tic movement. The patient is instructed to tense the muscles just tight enough so that the tic movement cannot occur, even when he or she is instructed to attempt to perform the tic movement intentionally. Some tics require competing responses other than isometric tensing of muscles, such as the use of a rhythmic deep breathing pattern for vocal tics or a rhythmic soft eye-blinking technique for eye tics. For unusual tics the therapist and patient must sometimes collaborate to try to identify a particular competing response that will prevent the tic from occurring.

As mentioned previously, there is some evidence that the competing response does not specifically have to be opposite the tic movement to result in a reduction in tics (Sharenow et al., 1989). Therefore, the identification of a competing response that is exactly opposite to the tic may be less important than identifying one that will simply disrupt the tic sequence. Another alternative to the isometric muscular tension competing response is to use a relaxed, more natural, and graceful variation of the original tic. This strategy may include trying to modify the tic so that only a part of the tic movement is expressed. The tic movement can then gradually be faded out completely. To employ the competing response, the patient implements the specific incompatible procedure for about 1 minute or until the premonitory urge dissipates (whichever is longer), whenever there is an urge to have a tic or immediately after the actual occurrence of a tic.

A brief description of some of the competing responses that have been found to be effective with tics follows:

- *Backward Head Jerk Tic*: The isometric tensing of the neck muscles while pulling the chin slightly down and in, and maintaining the head in an eyes-forward position.
- *Head Shake Tic*: Isometric contraction of the neck muscles with the eyes forward until the head can be maintained in a still position.
- *Shoulder Shrug Tic*: Isometric contraction of the shoulder muscles to push the shoulder downward and strengthen the muscles that work in opposition to the upward jerking movement.
- *Forward Shoulder Jerk Tic*: Push the shoulder down and tense the arm and elbow against the side of the torso; the hands can be clasped together in front of the waist area to make the competing response appear more natural.
- *Lip Pucker Tic*: Place lips together and press together lightly.
- *Eye-Blink or Eye-Squint Tic*: Systematic, voluntary, soft blinking that is consciously maintained at a rate of one blink per 3–5 seconds; frequent downward shifting of gaze about every 5–10 seconds.
- *Finger or Hand Tic*: If standing, fold hands together in front of abdomen and press hands together. If sitting, place hand on thigh with fingers lightly spread and press down on thigh.
- *Vocal Tic*: Slow, rhythmic, deep breathing through the nose while keeping the mouth closed. Exhalation should be just longer than an inhalation (e.g., 5 seconds of inhalation and 7 seconds of exhalation). The flow of air should not stop when shifting from inhalation to exhalation, and vice versa. Combine the breathing with cue-controlled or applied relaxation by letting all of the muscles become progressively more relaxed with each exhalation.
- *Sniffing or Snorting Tic*: Part lips slightly and breathe through the mouth in a manner similar to that for vocal tics.
- *Eyebrow Raising Tic*: Pull the eyebrows slightly downward, using just enough tension in the forehead muscles to prevent the eyebrows from rising upward.

- *Elbow-Flapping Tic*: Hold elbow against the side of the body and press the elbow against the side of the torso.

It is helpful to use a mirror during the practice of the competing response. The goal is to identify a competing response that will prevent the occurrence of a tic while remaining inconspicuous to others. Initially, the priority should be given to the prevention of the tic. Shaping the competing response into one that is inconspicuous can be accomplished as treatment progresses. For complex tics or intentional repetitive behaviors, the competing response should be implemented at the start of the behavior chain or the initial portion of the tic sequence.

A hierarchy of tics should be created prior to initiation of the competing response. The tic that is the most frequent or most disruptive is usually treated first. By treating the most frequent or disruptive tics first, it is often found that the effects generalize and other tics are reduced as well. However, there may be some benefit from starting with a less frequent tic so that the patient can have a successful experience. In most cases, at least one treatment session is devoted to training the individual to employ the competing response procedure for a particular tic, both during the session and during the following week in the real-world setting. Subsequent sessions begin with a review of homework, progress, and the procedures reviewed during the previous session. Each different type of tic is treated, one at a time, until a specific competing response has been established for each tic.

The patient is often involved in trying to determine the specific competing response that will work for each tic. The patient is also instructed on how to generalize the competing response procedure to new tics, should they arise. This is an important feature, considering that waxing, waning, and changing of symptoms is common in TS. One of the goals of the competing response training should be to teach patients the general model or strategy of the procedure so that they can use it independently in the future if any other tics should arise. Reviewing the possible competing responses for any type of tic the patient has ever had, including tics that were not occurring at the start of treatment, can help facilitate maintenance. Another strategy is to review competing responses for common types of tics that are often seen in other individuals with tic disorders, even though they may not have been emitted in the past by the patient.

Finally, it is sometimes difficult for patients with TS to determine if and when a new tic may be emerging. For example, sniffing or coughing may be associated with a common cold or may be the emergence of a new vocal tic. The most useful approach is to assume that if it looks like a tic or sounds like a tic, then treat it like a tic. If potentially emerging tics can be "nipped in the bud," they are much easier to treat and can prevent the development of new tics. The use of this procedure may be why previous research studies have failed to identify any symptom substitution or the emergence of new tics upon the treatment of other tics.

HR Contingency Management

In contingency management or social support training (Miltenberger et al., 1998), the parents or significant others are instructed to prompt the patient to use the competing response when necessary and to provide praise for the successful use of the procedure. Little improvement will result from behavioral therapy if the patient is not highly motivated to eliminate the tics. Contingency management helps ensure that the patient is as motivated as possible to perform all of the procedures. Family members and close friends should support and reinforce the patient by providing favorable comments on the improved appearance of the patient when they notice tic-free periods or significant reductions in tics.

Contingency management is especially important with children, who may not be as motivated to reduce the frequency or severity of tics. The child's family members and teachers are instructed to praise the child for performing the HR exercises and for improved appearance. For children who present as, or become, unmotivated or uncooperative, a token economy (Ayllon & Azrin, 1968) should be developed to provide a comprehensive contingency management program. Parents and teachers can also prompt the child by manually guiding the child through the required exercises whenever the child fails to initiate the exercises him- or herself.

As patients improve, they are encouraged to participate in enjoyable or pleasurable social activities that were previously avoided because of the social disruptiveness of their tics. For many individuals, this social component is the strongest natural reinforcement available for reducing or eliminating tics. Visiting a museum, going to a concert, or taking a trip to the library are examples of activities that may have previously been avoided because of socially disruptive tics.

HABIT INCONVENIENCE REVIEW

The patient's motivation can be further increased by using the *habit inconvenience review*. During this procedure the patient reviews all of the ways in which the tics have been inconvenient or embarrassing. The therapist and patient review in detail the inconveniences, embarrassment, disruption, and difficulties that have resulted from the tic behavior. The therapist and patient then review the potential benefits and advantages of reducing or eliminating tics. This information on the negative aspects of tics and the positive aspects of controlling tics is then written on an index card or Post-it note or in a similar format for frequent review by the patient. This card can be carried by the patient or placed in a location where it is seen on a regular basis and reviewed frequently as a cognitive strategy to increase his or her motivation to perform the exercises. It is also useful to review these inconveniences on a weekly basis, because their gradual reduction can be reinforcing.

HR Generalization Training

The initial focus of treatment is to help a patient learn to control tics in the clinic setting. However, the ultimate goal is to be able to generalize these behavioral strategies to real-world settings. The *public display* and *symbolic rehearsal* procedures can be helpful ways of generalizing the treatment effect outside the clinic setting.

PUBLIC DISPLAY

In the public display procedure the patient is encouraged to go into situations in which the tics were likely to occur in the past and to practice the competing response to control the tics. One goal of this procedure is to generate social approval from significant others.

SYMBOLIC REHEARSAL

The final phase of treatment involves symbolic rehearsal, which utilizes the list of situations obtained previously from the patient in the situation awareness procedure. The patient is asked to imagine being in common tic-eliciting situations and detecting the urge to emit a tic. The patient is then asked to perform a competing response for one of the tics. He or she is instructed to imagine successfully controlling the tics in high-risk situations in order to promote generalization.

PARAMETERS OF CLIENT APPROPRIATENESS

To Treat or Not to Treat?

One decision to be considered by health care providers, patients, and the parents of children with TS is whether or not to treat TS and motor or vocal tic disorders. Patient preference, family member perspective, and social impact are all factors to consider prior to the initiation of treatment. The preference of the patient should be the primary factor related to whether or not to treat an individual with TS and tic disorders. Some individuals with fairly mild tics are significantly distressed by them and are highly motivated to pursue whatever treatments might be available to reduce or eliminate their tics. Other individuals with rather disruptive tics have learned to tolerate their tic symptoms and may even consider their tics to be part of "who they are." These individuals are usually not interested in treatment. The potential risks and benefits of both pharmacological and behavioral treatments for TS should always be reviewed with patients (and parents, in the case of children) prior to the initiation of treatment.

The impact of the tics on others, such as parents, teachers, classmates, coworkers, and spouses, is also a factor that may influence the decision to treat or not treat. Tolerance and acceptance of tic symptoms by patients as well as significant individuals around them can be beneficial in decreasing the potential impact of tics. Conversely, some tics, such as coprolalia, can be significantly disruptive in social situations such as classrooms, work sites, or other public settings where there are established standards for acceptable social behavior. In these cases, the social impact of the tic symptoms should be discussed with, and considered by, the patient in determining potential treatment options. In the case of children, these factors become even more important because of the potential for lack of social awareness, depending on the developmental level of the child. Some of the most difficult cases are ones in which a child has no concern about his or her tics, whereas the parents are highly distressed and want the tics eliminated at almost any cost. In such cases, skills and training in child and adolescent psychology and family therapy are often useful in helping families make decisions regarding whether or not to treat tic symptoms in children.

Client Variables and Suitability for Behavioral Treatments

Although the use of HR and other psychosocial interventions for tics has been reported across the broad spectrum of age and intellectual function, the impact of these and other client factors on response to treatment has yet to be systematically evaluated. Theoretically, treatments placing greater emphasis on the recognition and extinction of the premonitory urge (e.g., HR training and exposure plus response prevention) would be less appropriate for very young or cognitively impaired children, given the level of cognitive development necessary to self-monitor and the fact that children below ages 8–10 are less consistent in their ability to recognize these urges (Woods, Piacentini, Himle, & Chang, 2005). However, anecdotal reports suggest that it is possible to use HR in youngsters as young as 6 in the presence of greater parental involvement. Although two controlled HR trials have included 6- and 7-year-old children (Azrin & Peterson, 1990; Verdellen et al., 2004, respectively), findings were not broken down by age, so it is not known whether these youngsters responded to treatment or not. Given that contingency management and, too a lesser extent, HR and exposure-based treatments can be time consuming and require some level of parental involvement, a chaotic family environment, poor parental motivation, and/or increased rates of parental psychopathology may limit the efficacy of these treatments. Likewise, the recent finding by Deckersbach et al. (2006) suggests that those with poor response inhibition may not do as well with HR.

SUMMARY AND RECOMMENDATIONS FOR FUTURE DIRECTIONS

Overall there is strong scientific evidence for the behavioral, psychosocial, or nonpharmacological treatment of TS and chronic tic disorders. Behavioral treatments, especially HR, have been shown to significantly reduce tics, and a number of studies have demonstrated that the improvement continues up to a year after the completion of treatment. Some research also supports the use of relaxation training, self-monitoring, and reinforcement for the treatment of TS and chronic tic disorders. Exposure with response prevention is the most recently studied behavioral treatment for tic disorders and holds promise as a useful treatment approach.

Nevertheless, additional research on the efficacy of the behavioral procedures is required. Division 12 (clinical psychology) of the American Psychological Association has developed guidelines with which psychological treatments can be evaluated for their level of empirical support in the scientific literature (Task Force on Promotion and Dissemination of Psychological Procedures, 1995; Chambless & Hollon, 1998). These guidelines can be used to classify psychological treatments as either "well-established" or "probably efficacious," based on the number and types of published studies that exist to support them. Given these guidelines in relation to the existing body of research on HR, the treatment would be classified as "probably efficacious." HR also meets most of the criteria to be classified as a "well-established" treatment. However, the lack of large-scale randomized clinical trial currently limits HR from being considered a "well-established" treatment. To address this issue, a large, multisite, NIMH-funded randomized clinical trial is currently underway by many authors in this book. This study is a collaborative effort of the Tourette Syndrome Association and researchers from UCLA (John Piacentini and Susanna Chang), Harvard University/Massachusetts General Hospital (Sabine Wilhelm and Thilo Deckersbach), Johns Hopkins

University (John Walkup and Golda Ginsburg), Yale University (Lawrence Scahill), the University of Wisconsin–Milwaukee (Douglas Woods), and the University of Texas Health Sciences Center at San Antonio (Alan Peterson). If the results of this multisite collaborative study are similar to those found in previous published research, HR would then be classified as a "well established" treatment.

In addition to the lack of a large, well-controlled trial, very limited scientific data are currently available on the comparative or combined efficacy of behavior therapy and medication treatments of tic disorders. Most behavioral studies have found that tic symptoms are improved whether or not an individual is currently taking a medication for their tics, although no randomized controlled trial has specifically investigated this aspect of treatment. The current data suggest that behavioral treatments can be beneficial as an addition or alternative to medication treatments. Future research should investigate individual and combined efficacy of behavioral and pharmacological treatments for TS and chronic tic disorders. (For detailed information on the use of medication, see Harrison, Schneider, & Walkup, Chapter 7, this volume.)

Further limitations with behavioral approaches to the treatment of tics, which must be addressed with future research and professional training, are as follows. First, behavioral treatment approaches require implementation by therapists with a fairly high degree of training and clinical experience in behavior therapy. Second, there are relatively few providers who are both knowledgeable of, and trained in, the use of HR for the treatment of tic disorders. Third, the use of behavior therapy for the treatment of tic disorders demands a significant amount of treatment time, especially as compared to medication treatments. It is hoped that in the next few years, many of these issues can begin to be addressed in order to establish the parameters of HR effectiveness and develop structured training programs that will disseminate the technology to those in the field.

REFERENCES

Araki, H., & Nakai, Y. (1990). Behavior therapy for a woman suffering from Gilles de la Tourette's syndrome for 20 years. *Japanese Journal of Behavior Therapy, 16,* 27–36.

Araki, R., & Okuma, H. (1985). Multiple tics and snapping scapulae treated effectively with habit-reversal: Importance of competing response training. *Japanese Journal of Behavior Therapy, 11,* 51–56.

Arntz, A. (2003). Cognitive therapy versus applied relaxation as treatment of generalized anxiety disorder. *Behaviour Research and Therapy, 41,* 633–646.

Ayllon, T., & Azrin, N. H. (1968). *The token economy: A motivational systam for therapy and rehabilitation.* Englewood Cliffs, NJ: Prentice-Hall.

Azrin, N. H., & Nunn, R. G. (1973). Habit reversal: A method of eliminating nervous habits and tics. *Behaviour Research and Therapy, 11*, 619–628.

Azrin, N. H., & Nunn, R. G. (1977). *Habit control in a day.* New York: Pocket Books.

Azrin, N. H., Nunn, R. G., & Frantz, S. E. (1980). Habit reversal vs. negative practice treatment of nervous tics. *Behavior Therapy, 11,* 169–178.

Azrin, N. H., & Peterson, A. L. (1988a). Behavior therapy for Tourette's syndrome and tic disorders. In D. J. Cohen, R. D. Bruun, & J. F. Leckman (Eds.), *Tourette's syndrome and tic disorders: Clinical understanding and treatment* (pp. 237–255). New York: Wiley.

Azrin, N. H., & Peterson, A. L. (1988b). Habit reversal for the treatment of Tourette syndrome. *Behaviour Research and Therapy, 26,* 347–351.

Azrin, N. H., & Peterson, A. L. (1989). Reduction of an eye tic by controlled blinking. *Behavior Therapy, 20,* 467–473.

Azrin, N. H., & Peterson, A. L. (1990). Treatment of Tourette syndrome by habit reversal: A waiting-list control group comparison. *Behavior Therapy, 21,* 305–318.

Bados Lopez, A., & Olle, N. P. (1984). A case study: Elimination of an exhalation tic through the sequential application of progressive muscular relaxation and habit reversal. *Revista de Analisis del Comportamiento, 2,* 339–346.

Banaschewski, T., Woerner, W., & Rothenberger, A. (2003). Premonitory sensory phenomena and suppressibility of tics in TS: Developmental aspects in children and adolescents. *Developmental Medicine and Child Neurology, 45,* 700–703.

Barr, R. F., Lovibond, S. H., & Katsaros, E. (1972). Gilles de la Tourette's syndrome in a brain-damaged child. *Medical Journal of Australia, 2,* 372.

Benson, H. (1975). *The relaxation response.* New York: Avon Books.

Bergin, A., Waranch, H. R., Brown, J., Carson, K., & Singer, H. S. (1998). Relaxation therapy in Tourette syndrome: A pilot study. *Pediatric Neurology, 18,* 136–142.

Bernstein, D. S., & Borkovec, T. D. (1973). *Progressive relaxation training.* Champaign, IL: Research Press.

Billings, A. (1978). Self-monitoring in the treatment of tics: A single-subject analysis. *Journal of Behavior Therapy and Experimental Psychiatry, 9,* 339–342.

Bliss, J. (1980). Sensory experiences in Gilles de la TS. *Archives of General Psychiatry, 37,* 1343–1347.

Browning, R. M., & Stover, D. O. (1971). *Behavior modification in child treatment: An experimental and clinical approach.* Chicago: Aldine–Atherton.

Bullen, J. G., & Hemsley, D. R. (1983). Sensory experience as a trigger in Gilles de la Tourette's syndrome. *Journal of Behavior Therapy and Experimental Psychiatry, 14,* 197–201.

Canavan, A. G. M., & Powell, G. E. (1981). The efficacy of several treatments of Gilles de la Tourette's syndrome as assessed in a single case. *Behaviour Research and Therapy, 19,* 549–556.

Cappo, B. M., & Holmes, D. S. (1984). The utility of prolonged respiratory exhalation for reducing physiological and psychological arousal in non-threatening and threatening situations. *Journal of Psychosomatic Research, 28,* 265–373.

Carr, J. E. (1995). Competing responses for the treatment of Tourette syndrome and tic disorders. *Behaviour Research and Therapy, 33,* 455–456.

Carr, J. E., & Bailey, J. S. (1996). A brief behavior therapy protocol for Tourette syndrome. *Journal of Behavior Therapy and Experimental Psychiatry, 27,* 33–40.

Carr, J. E., & Chong, I. M. (2005). Habit reversal treatment of tic disorders: A methodological critique of the literature. *Behavior Modification, 29,* 858–875.

Carr, J. E., Sidener, T. M., Sidener, D. W., & Cummings, A. R. (2005). Functional analysis and habit-reversal treatment of tics. *Behavioral Interventions, 20,* 185–202.

Chambless, D. L., & Hollon, S. D. (1998). Defining empirically supported therapies. *Journal of Consulting and Clinical Psychology, 66,* 7–18.

Clark, D. F. (1966). Behaviour therapy of Gilles de la Tourette's syndrome. *British Journal of Psychiatry, 112,* 771–778.

Clarke, M. A., Bray, M. A., Kehle, T. J., & Truscott, S. D. (2001). A school-based intervention designed to reduce the frequency of tics in children with Tourette's syndrome. *School Psychology Review, 30,* 11–22.

Cloutier, J. (1985). Elimination of a nervous tic through habit reversal. *Technologie et Therapie du Comportement, 8,* 153–159.

Culbertson, F. M. (1989). A four-step hypnotherapy model for Gilles de la Tourette's syndrome. *American Journal of Clinical Hypnosis, 31,* 252–256.

Deckersbach, T., Rauch, S., Buhlmann, U., & Wilhelm, S. (2006). Habit reversal versus supportive psychotherapy in Tourette's disorder: A randomized controlled trial and predictors of treatment response. *Behaviour Research and Therapy, 44,* 1079–1090.

Doleys, D. M., & Kurtz, P. S. (1974). A behavioral treatment program for the Gilles de la TS. *Psychological Reports, 35,* 43–48.

Feldman, R. B., & Werry, J. S. (1966). An unsuccessful attempt to treat a ticquer by massed practice. *Behaviour Research and Therapy, 4,* 111–117.

Finney, J. W., Rapoff, M. A., Hall, C. L., & Christopherson, E. R. (1983). Replication and social validation of habit reversal treatment for tics. *Behavior Therapy, 14,* 116–126.

Franco, D. P. (1981). Habit reversal and isometric tensing with motor tics. *Dissertation Abstract International, 42,* 3418B.

Friedman, S. (1980). Self-control of the treatment of Gilles de la Tourette's syndrome: Case study with 18–month follow-up. *Journal of Conferences in Clinical Psychology, 48,* 400–402.

Fuata, P., & Griffiths, R. A. (1992). Cognitive behavioural treatment of a vocal tic. *Behaviour Change, 9,* 14–18.

Goetz, C. G., Leurgans, S., & Chmura, T. A. (2001). Home alone: methods to maximize tic expression for objective videotape assessments in Gilles de la TS. *Movement Disorders, 16,* 693–697.

Goldfried, M. R. (1971). Systematic desensitization as training in self-control. *Journal of Consulting and Clinical Psychology, 37,* 228–234.

Gross, A. M., & Mendelson, A. N. (1982). Elimination of an eye-blink tic using self-administered overcorrection. *Behavioral Engineering, 8,* 1–4.

Hanley, G. P., Iwata, B. A., & McCord, B. E. (2003). Functional analysis of problem behavior: A review. *Journal of Applied Behavior Analysis, 36,* 147–185.

Himle, M. B., & Woods, D. W., & (2005). An experimental evaluation of tic suppression and the tic rebound effect. *Behaviour Research and Therapy, 43,* 1443–1451.

Hollandsworth, J. G., & Bausinger, L. (1978). Unsuccessful use of massed practice in the treatment of Gilles de la TS. *Psychological Reports, 43,* 671–677.

Houlihan, D., Hofschulte, L., & Patten, C. (1993). Behavioral conceptualizations and treatments of Tourette's syndrome: A review and overview. *Behavioral Residential Treatment, 8,* 111–131.

Hutzell, R. R., Platzek, D., & Logue, P. E. (1974). Control of symptoms of Gilles de la Tourette's syndrome by self-monitoring. *Journal of Behavior Therapy and Experimental Psychiatry, 5,* 71–76.

Jacobson, E. (1938). *Progressive relaxation* (2nd ed.). Chicago: University of Chicago Press.

Jenike, M. A. (2001). An update on obsessive–compulsive disorder. *Bulletin of the Menninger Clinic, 65,* 4–25.

Kwak, C., Dat Vuong, K., & Jankovic, J. (2003). Premonitory sensory phenomenon in Tourette's syndrome. *Movement Disorders, 18,* 1530–1533.

Lahey, B. B., McNees, M. P., & McNees, M. C. (1973). Control of an obscene "verbal tic" through time out in an elementary classroom. *Journal of Applied Behavioral Analysis, 6,* 101–104.

Lavenstein, B. L. (2003). Treatment approaches for children with Tourette's syndrome. *Current Neurological and Neurosciences Report, 3,* 143–188.

Leckman, J. F., Riddle, M. A., Hardin, M. T., Ort, S. I., Swartz, K. L., Stevenson, J., et al. (1989). The Yale Global Tic Severity Scale (YGTSS): Initial testing of a clinician-rated scale of tic severity. *Journal of the American Academy of Child and Adolescent Psychiatry, 28,* 566–573.

Lichstein, K. L. (1988). *Clinical relaxation strategies.* New York: Wiley.

Linton, S. J., & Gotestam, K. G. (1984). A controlled study of the effects of applied relaxation and applied relaxation plus operant procedures in the regulation of chronic pain. *British Journal of Clinical Psychology, 23,* 291–299.

Michultka, D. M., Blanchard, E. B., & Rosenblum, E. L. (1989). Stress management and Gilles de la Tourette's syndrome. *Biofeedback and Self-Regulation, 14,* 115–123.

Miller, A. L. (1970). Treatment of a child with Gilles de la Tourette's syndrome using behavior modification techniques. *Journal of Behavior Therapy and Experimental Psychiatry, 1,* 319–321.

Miltenberger, R. G., & Fuqua, R. W. (1985). A comparison of contingent vs. non-contingent competing response practice in the treatment of nervous habits. *Journal of Behavior Therapy and Experimental Psychiatry, 16,* 195–200.

Miltenberger, R. G., Fuqua, R. W., & McKinley, T. (1985). Habit reversal with muscle tics: Replication and component analysis. *Behavior Therapy, 16,* 39–50.

Miltenberger, R. G., Fuqua, R. W., & Woods, D.W. (1998). Applying behavior analysis to clinical problems: Review and analysis of habit reversal. *Journal of Applied Behavioral Analysis, 31,* 447–469.

Nicassio, F. J., Liberman, R. P., Patterson, R. L., Raminez, E., & Saunder, N. (1972). The treatment of tics by negative practice. *Journal of Behavior Therapy and Experimental Psychiatry, 3,* 281–287.

O'Brien, J. S., & Brennan, J. H. (1979). The elimination of a severe long term facial tic and vocal distortion with multi-facet behavior therapy. *Journal of Behavior Therapy and Experimental Psychiatry, 10,* 257–261.

O'Connor, K. P., Brault, M., Robillard, S., Loiselle, J., Borgeat, F., & Stip, E. (2001). Evaluation of a cognitive-behavioral program for the management of chronic tic and habit disorders. *Behaviour Research and Therapy, 39,* 667–681.

O'Connor, K. P., Gareau, D., & Borgeat, F. (1997). A comparison of a behavioural and a cognitive-behavioural approach to the management of chronic tic disorders. *Clinical Psychology and Psychotherapy, 4,* 105–117.

Ollendick, T. H. (1981). Self-monitoring and self-administered overcorrection: The modification of nervous tics in children. *Behavior Modification, 5,* 75–84.

Ost, L. G., & Breitholtz, E. (2000). Applied relaxation vs. cognitive therapy in the treatment of generalized anxiety disorder. *Behaviour Research and Therapy, 38,* 777–790.

Peterson, A. L., & Azrin, N. H. (1992). An evaluation of behavioral treatments for Tourette syndrome. *Behaviour Research and Therapy, 30,* 167–174.

Peterson, A. L., & Azrin, N. H. (1993). Behavioral and pharmacological treatments for Tourette syndrome: A review. *Applied and Preventive Psychology, 2,* 231–242.

Peterson, A. L., Campise, R. L., & Azrin, N. H. (1994). Behavioral and pharmacological treatments for tic and habit disorders: A review. *Developmental and Behavioral Pediatrics, 15,* 430–441.

Peterson, B., & Cohen, D. (1998). The treatment of Tourette's syndrome: Multimodal, developmental intervention. *Journal of Clinical Psychiatry, 59*(Suppl. 1), 62–72.

Poppen, R. (1988). *Behavioral relaxation training and assessment.* New York: Pergamon Press.

Reid, S. D. (2004). Neuroleptic-induced tardive Tourette treated with clonazepam: A case report and literature review. *Clinical Neuropharmacology, 27,* 101–104.

Roane, H. S., Piazza, C. C., Cercone, J. J., & Grados, M. (2002). Assessment and treatment of vocal tics associated with Tourette's syndrome. *Behavior Modification, 26,* 482–498.

Robertson, M. M., & Stern, J. S. (2000). Gilles de la TS: Symptomatic treatment based on evidence. *European Child and Adolescent Psychiatry, 9*(Suppl. 1), 160–175.

Rosen, M., & Wesner, C. (1973). A behavioral approach to Tourette's syndrome. *Journal of Canadian Clinical Psychology, 41,* 303–312.

Sand, P. L., & Carlson, C. (1973). Failure to establish control over tics in the Gilles de la Tourette's syndrome with behavior therapy techniques. *American Journal of Psychiatry, 122,* 665–670.

Sandor, P. (2003). Pharmacological management of tics in patients with TS. *Journal of Psychosomatic Research, 55,* 41–48.

Savicki, V., & Carlin, A. S. (1972). Behavioral treatment of Gilles de la Tourette's syndrome. *International Journal of Child Psychotherapy, 1,* 97–109.

Schilling, D. J., & Poppen, R. (1983). Behavioral relaxation training and assessment. *Journal of Behavior Therapy and Experimental Psychiatry, 14,* 99–107.

Schulman, M. (1974). Control of tics by maternal reinforcement. *Journal of Behavior Therapy and Experimental Psychiatry, 5,* 95–96.

Schultz, J. H., & Luthe, W. (1959). *Autogenic therapy: Vol 1. Autogenic methods.* New York: Grune & Stratton.

Sharenow, E. L., Fuqua, R. W., & Miltenberger, R. G. (1989). The treatment of muscle tics with dissimilar competing response practice. *Journal of Applied Behavior Analysis, 22,* 35–42.

Silva, R. R., Munoz, D. M., Barickman, J., & Friedhoff, A. J. (1995). Environmental factors and related fluctuation of symptoms in children and adolescents with Tourette's disorder. *Journal of Child Psychology and Psychiatry, 36,* 305–312.

Storms, L. (1985). Massed negative practice as a behavioral treatment for Gilles de la Tourette's syndrome. *American Journal of Psychotherapy, 39,* 277–281.

Suinn, R. M. (1975). Anxiety management training for general anxiety. In R. Suinn & R. Weigel (Eds.), *The innovative psychological therapies: Critical and creative incidents* (pp. 66–70). New York: Harper & Row.

Task Force on Promotion and Dissemination of Psychological Procedures. (1995). Training in and dissemination of empirically validated psychological treatments. *The Clinical Psychologist, 48*(1), 2–23.

Teoh, J. L. (1974). Gilles de la Tourette's syndrome: A study of the treatment of six cases by mass negative practice and with haloperidol. *Singapore Medical Journal, 15,* 139–146.

Thomas, E. J., Abrams, K. S., & Johnson, J. B. (1971). Self-monitoring and reciprocal inhibition in the modification of multiple tics of Gilles de la Tourette's syndrome. *Journal of Behavior Therapy and Experimental Psychiatry, 2,* 159–171.

Tolchard, B. (1995). Treatment of Gilles de la Tourette's syndrome using behavioural psychotherapy: A single case example. *Journal of Psychiatric Mental Health Nursing, 2,* 233–236.

Tophoff, M. (1973). Massed practice, relaxation and assertion training in the treatment of Gilles de la Tourette's syndrome. *Journal of Behavior Therapy and Experimental Psychiatry, 4,* 71–73.

Turpin, G. (1983). The behavioral management of tic disorders: A critical review. *Advances in Behaviour Research and Therapy, 5,* 203–245.

Turpin, G., & Powell, G. E. (1984). Effects of massed practice and cue-controlled relaxation on tic frequency in Gilles de la Tourette's syndrome. *Behaviour Research and Therapy, 22*, 165–178.

Varni, J. W., Boyd, E. F., & Cataldo, M. F. (1978). Self-monitoring, external reinforcement, and time-out procedures in the control of high rate tic behaviors in a hyperactive child. *Journal of Behavior Therapy and Experimental Psychiatry, 9*, 353–358.

Verdellen, C. W., Keijsers, G. P., Cath, D. C., & Hoogduin, C. A. (2004). Exposure with response prevention versus habit reversal in Tourettes's syndrome: A controlled study. *Behaviour Research and Therapy, 42*, 501–511.

Wagaman, J. R., Miltenberger, R. G., & Williams, D. E. (1995). Treatment of a vocal tic by differential reinforcement. *Journal of Behavior Therapy and Experimental Psychiatry, 26*, 35–39.

Walton, D. (1961). Experimental psychology and the treatment of a ticquer. *Journal of Child Psychology and Psychiatry, 2*, 148–155.

Walton, D. (1964). Massed practice and simultaneous reduction in drive level: Further evidence on the efficacy of this approach to the treatment of tics. In H. J. Eysenck (Ed.), *Experiments in behaviour therapy* (pp. 96–113). London: Pergamon Press.

Watson, T. S., Dufrene, B., Weaver, A., Butler, T., & Meeks, C. (2005). Brief antecedent assessment and treatment of tics in the general education classroom. *Behavior Modification, 29*, 839–857.

Watson, T. S., & Heindl, B. (1996). Behavioral case consultation with parents and teachers: An example using differential reinforcement to treat psychogenic cough. *Journal of School Psychology, 34*, 365–378.

Watson, T. S., & Sterling, H. E. (1998). Brief functional analysis and treatment of a vocal tic. *Journal of Applied Behavior Analysis, 31*, 471–474.

Wilhelm, S., Deckersbach, T., Coffey, B. J., Bohne, A., Peterson, A. L., & Baer, L. (2003). Habit reversal versus supportive psychotherapy for Tourette's disorder: A randomized controlled trial. *American Journal of Psychiatry, 160*, 1175–1177.

Woods, D. W., & Himle, M. B. (2004). Creating tic suppression: Comparing the effects of verbal instruction to differential reinforcement. *Journal of Applied Behavior Analysis, 37*, 417–420.

Woods, D. W., Hook, S. S., Spellman, D. F., & Friman, P. C. (2000). Case study: Exposure and response prevention for an adolescent with Tourette's syndrome and OCD. *Journal of the American Academy of Child and Adolescent Psychiatry, 39*, 904–907.

Woods, D. W., & Miltenberger, R. G. (1995). HR: A review of applications and variations. *Journal of Behavior Therapy and Experimental Psychiatry, 26*, 123–131.

Woods, D. W., Miltenberger, R. G., & Lumley, V. A. (1996). Sequential application of major habit reveral components to treat motor tics in children. *Journal of Applied Behavior Analysis, 29*, 483–493.

Woods, D. W., Piacentini, J., Himle, M., & Chang, S. (2005). Premonitory Urge Tics for Scale (PUTS): Initial psychometric results and examination of the premonitory urge phenomenon in youths with tic disorders. *Developmental and Behavioral Pediatrics, 26*, 397–403.

Woods, D. W., & Twohig, M. P. (2002). Using habit reversal to treat chronic vocal tic disorder in children. *Behavioral Interventions, 17*, 159–168.

Woods, D. W., Twohig, M. P., Flessner, C. A., & Roloff, T. J. (2003). Treatment of vocal tics in children with TS: Investigating the efficacy of habit reversal. *Journal of Applied Behavioral Analysis, 36*, 109–112.

Woods, D. W., Watson, T. S., Wolfe, E., Twohig, M. P., & Friman, P. C. (2001). Analyzing the influence of tic-related conversation on vocal and motor tics in children with Tourette's syndrome. *Journal of Applied Behavior Analysis, 34*, 353–356.

Wright, K. M., & Miltenberger, R. G. (1987). Awareness training in the treatment of head and facial tics. *Journal of Behavior Therapy and Experimental Psychiatry, 18,* 269–274.

Yates, A. J. (1958). The application of learning theory to the treatment of tics. *Journal of Abnormal Social Psychology, 56,* 175–182.

Young, M. H., & Montano, R. T. (1988). A new hypnobehavioral method for the treatment of children with Tourette's disorder. *American Journal of Clinical Hypnosis, 31,* 97–106.

Zikis, P. (1983). Habit reversal treatment of a 10 year old schoolboy with severe tics. *Behavior Therapist, 6,* 50–51.

CHAPTER 9

Psychosocial Management of Comorbid Internalizing Disorders in Persons with Tourette Syndrome

ULRIKE BUHLMANN
THILO DECKERSBACH
LAURA COOK
SABINE WILHELM

Comorbid internalizing disorders, including obsessive–compulsive disorder (OCD), other anxiety disorders, and mood disorders, are among the most common complicating factors experienced by individuals with Tourette syndrome (TS) and other chronic tic disorders. In many cases, it is these comorbid difficulties and not the tics themselves that precipitate treatment-seeking behaviors. Similar to other complicating factors, individuals presenting with a tic disorder complicated by internalizing comorbidity require a detailed and comprehensive assessment of their complete clinical picture. Regardless of whether or not TS is the primary diagnosis, it is usually recommended that clinicians focus initial intervention efforts on the symptoms that are most distressing and/or disruptive with regard to the patient's social, familial, and academic/occupational functioning. That is, an optimal treatment plan should provide a comprehensive yet hierarchical approach for addressing the patient's tics and comorbid anxiety and/or depressive symptoms.

COMORBID OCD

OCD is a common psychiatric disorder that affects 1–3% of both the adult (Regier et al., 1993) and child/adolescent (Rapoport et al., 2000) populations. The comorbidity of OCD and TS is bidirectional yet unbalanced. Although 20–60% of children and adults with TS also meet diagnostic criteria for comorbid OCD (Coffey & Park, 1997; Kadesjo & Gillberg, 2000; Leckman, Walker, Goodman, Pauls, & Cohen, 1994), only 7–37% of individuals with OCD have been found to meet criteria for TS (Miguel, Rosario-Campos, Shavitt, Hounie, & Mercadente, 2001). Most individuals with OCD exhibit multiple types of obsessions (i.e., recurrent, intrusive thoughts, images, or urges with various contents, including aggressive, sexual, superstitious, illness-related, or religious themes) and compulsions (i.e., repetitive behaviors such as hand washing, checking, or mental acts such as silent prayer or counting; American Psychiatric Association, 1994). In addition, some compulsions may occur in the absence of preceding obsessions. These compulsions often involve the need for touching and rubbing and often resemble the complex motor tics experienced by patients with TS. Among adults, the age of onset in OCD usually varies between early adolescence to adulthood, with males usually having an earlier onset than females (13–15 years of age vs. 20–24 years of age; Rasmussen & Eisen, 1990). Most child-onset cases first appear between the ages of 6 and 11 (Hanna, 1995; Rapoport et al., 2000), although onsets as young as ages 1–2 have been observed clinically. Interestingly, more males than females report prepubertal onset of OCD, whereas this gender difference disappears in adulthood (e.g., Geller et al., 1998; Swedo et al., 1989).

Similarities and Differences between TS and OCD

Differentiating OCD from tic symptoms can be difficult especially given the significant rates of overlap between these two disorders. Although simple tics (e.g., eye blinking, head and arm jerking) are not often mistaken for symptoms of OCD due to their brevity, purposelessness, and involuntary nature, more complex tics, such as repeating or touching to achieve a just right feeling, may be virtually indistinguishable from compulsions (Mansueto & Keuler, 2005). Although individuals with TS are likely to experience the urge to tic simply without any additional rationale (e.g., "I have the urge to turn my head to the right . . . I don't know why, I can't explain it . . . I just have to do it"), those with OCD can usually explain why they perform a particular compulsion, for example, saying that hand washing many times is necessary because of illness concerns. Whereas most individuals with TS describe their symptoms as involuntary, some experience their tics as a voluntary response to a premonitory urge (Leckman, Walker, & Cohen, 1993; Woods, Piacentini, Himle, & Chang, 2005). In fact, a growing body of evidence suggests that the functional relationship between premonitory sensation and tic expression may be similar to the relationship between obsession and compulsion in OCD, in that dissipation of the sensation/obsession contingent on performance of the tic/compulsion, serves to negatively reinforce these latter behaviors (Evers & van de Wetering, 1994; Shapiro & Shapiro, 1982). OCD in the presence of comorbid TS, often referred to as tic-related or Tourettic OCD, is characterized by a higher rate of touching, tapping, repeating, and sensory obsessions and compulsions, as opposed to contamination and cleaning-related symptoms, may represent an intermediate phenotype between the two disorders (Hanna et al., 2002; Leckman et al., 2000; Mansueto & Keuler, 2005). Differentiating TS symptoms (e.g., urges and tics) from the obsessions and compulsions associated with OCD is important given the greater likelihood of individuals with TS to act on their symptoms, as compared to those with OCD. Moreover, as is shown below, obsessions and compulsions typically require different pharmacological and behavioral treatment strategies than tics.

Treatment Approaches for OCD

Exposure with response prevention (ERP) has been shown to be effective for OCD across the age span and is considered the psychological technique of choice for this disorder (Jenike, 2004; Piacentini, March, & Franklin, 2006). Specifically, ERP involves repeated confrontations with situations that provoke distress while encouraging the patient to abstain from any anxiety-reducing rituals. For example, a patient with OCD who has contamination fears will be encouraged not to engage in any hand-washing rituals after touching a trash can in order to allow the associated anxiety to decrease through the classical conditioning process known as "extinction." ERP can be conducted in real-life or imagined situations, involving the exposure to the feared object in the absence of overt danger (Kozak & Foa, 1997). Over 30 controlled trials from the past two decades have shown ERP to be an effective intervention for OCD in adults, with approximately two of every three treated individuals evidencing a favorable response (for reviews, see Abramowitz, 1996; Baer & Minichiello, 1998; Stanley & Turner, 1995).

ERP is often applied in conjunction with cognitive therapy. Although originally utilized in the treatment of depression (Beck, 1976), more recently cognitive therapy has also been successfully applied to the treatment of OCD (e.g., Cottraux et al., 2001; van Oppen et al., 1995; Wilhelm et al., 2005). For patients who refuse to engage in exposure tasks or for those who suffer mainly from obsessional thoughts, cognitive therapy strategies may be more effective than strictly behavioral strategies. Freeston, Rhéaume, and Ladouceur (1996), Salkovskis (1989), and van Oppen and Arntz (1994) are among those who have developed cognitive therapy tactics for adult patients with OCD.

In general, cognitive elements for treatment of patients with OCD aim to modify maladaptive beliefs and interpretations associated with OCD symptoms In the first cognitive-behavioral therapy (CBT) treatment session, the patient is educated about OCD and its treatment, and the treatment rationale is provided. Specifically, the clinician explains the rationale for exposure and response prevention techniques. For example, the patient learns that, by not engaging in compulsions, (1) the anxiety provoked by the obsessions will decrease on its own, and (2) the feared consequences (e.g., family member will be hurt if the patient does not count up to a certain number) do not come true (see Kozak & Foa, 1997). The clinician and patient create a hierarchy of all anxiety-provoking situations and stimuli, using a scale of the subjective units of distress (SUD) that they cause. Moreover, the clinician describes obsessions as ordinary intrusions everybody experiences (Rachman, 1997) and explains that the patient differs from individuals without OCD only with respect to how he or she interprets them. Furthermore, the patient's interpretations of his or her intrusions are assessed, and a treatment plan is developed. In the subsequent sessions, the clinician will design the exposure exercises. Usually the clinician starts with exposure exercises that are moderately anxiety provoking and gradually chooses more difficult ones as the patient's symptoms improve, and both the clinician and patient deem it appropriate to move up the patient's hierarchy. The patient completes homework assignments to repeat and further practice the exposure exercises between sessions.

General cognitive techniques include Socratic questioning to evaluate maladaptive thoughts, completing thought records, and identifying and evaluating the pros and cons of holding OCD-related beliefs and behaviors (see Beck, 1995). Depending on the patient's maladaptive domains of beliefs, the clinician can further choose from various cognitive techniques to identify and evaluate the interpretations of intrusions (e.g., calculating the probability of harm for overestimation of threat, or the pie technique for inflated responsibility). The clinician should never evaluate the actual intrusions but instead should focus on the maladaptive interpretations following the intrusions.

CBT for Children with OCD

In general, CBT for children with OCD follows the same principles of CBT for adults (March & Mulle, 1998; Piacentini & Langley, 2004). However, there are some important differences, depending on the developmental stage of the child (Piacentini & Bergman, 2001). For example, the younger the child is, the more difficult it can be to assess the OCD symptoms, given that clinical assessments typically include self-report questionnaires, and the child's ability for self-observation is often limited (Kozak & Foa, 1997). Moreover, it may be more difficult for children to tolerate the anxiety during the exposures. Because their coping skills for stress are limited, it may also be difficult for them to anticipate the long-term advantages of refraining from their compulsions. Thus, it is very important to spend enough time educating the child about both the OCD and the underlying treatment rationale. Furthermore, children with OCD more often report more compulsions than obsessions (e.g., Geller et al., 1998; Rettew, Swedo, Leonard, Lenane, & Rapoport, 1992; Swedo et al., 1989). Consequently, depending on the child's symptoms and his or her developmental level, the treatment may focus more on ERP than on identification and modification of maladaptive thoughts.

Another important aspect of treating children with OCD is family involvement. Children often engage their family members in their compulsions (e.g., frequently asking for reassurance or to avoid household chores). Additionally, family members often have distorted beliefs about OCD and what to expect from the child (e.g., "My child would be able to stop doing the compulsions if he only tried hard enough" or "It is all my fault that my child suffers from OCD"; Waters & Barrett, 2000). Thus, it is important to involve family members in the treatment process by educating them about the nature of OCD. It is further important to educate parents about how to coach and encourage their children to do the exposure exercises at home in order to reinforce gains made in the clinical setting (Barrett, Healy-Farrell, & March, 2004; Piacentini & Langley, 2004).

Primarily cognitive interventions have yet to be tested with children and adolescents; however, most treatment approaches for this age range now include some cognitive strategies as an adjunct to exposure-based techniques. Although fewer controlled trials have been completed for children and adolescents than adults, CBT appears similarly efficacious in this younger population (see Piacentini et al., 2006 for a review). In the two existing head-to-head trials, CBT proved equally or more efficacious for children and adolescents with OCD than medication (de Haan, Hoogduin, Buitelaar, & Keijsers, 1998; Pediatric OCD Treatment Study Team, 2004).

Recommendations for Treating TS with Comorbid OCD

The treatment of a patient with TS and comorbid OCD should entail a detailed assessment focused on the distinction between TS symptoms and OCD symptoms. Interventions for aggressive obsessions differ from treatment strategies for tics. To illustrate, a patient with violent tics (e.g., smashing the car window) should first learn to identify any premonitory urges and warning signs and how to engage in a competing response to prevent this tic from occurring. If a patient also has aggressive obsessions (e.g., "I am going to hit my child"), the clinician should introduce cognitive interventions. The interventions might include normalizing the occurrence of intrusions, learning to let intrusions come and go naturally, and challenging the maladaptive interpretations of the intrusive thoughts. The starting point for treatment is typically dictated by the need to address the most severely impairing symptoms first. Often the treatment will start with TS symptoms, especially if tics could result in harm to the patient or others, and then will focus on the OCD symptoms. This treatment strategy additionally applies to children, with greater emphasis on educating the child and family about both TS and OCD symptoms.

COMORBID ANXIETY

TS is associated with increased rates of anxiety (e.g., Comings & Comings, 1987; Pitman, Green, Jenike, & Mesulam, 1987). Pitman et al. (1987), for example, found a significantly higher lifetime prevalence of 44% for generalized anxiety disorder (GAD) in patients with TS, compared to healthy controls. Comings and Comings (1987) found high rates of panic attacks (16%) and other phobias. Interestingly, they also found that 55.1% of women with TS had three or more phobias, whereas only 25.4% of males experienced this problem. Tics may be embarrassing in social situations, which can cause substantial anxiety. Factors such as stress, anxiety, and also positive excitement have also been found to have an exacerbating effect on tics (King, Leckman, Scahill, & Cohen, 1999; Woods et al., 2005).

Treatment Approach for Anxiety Disorders

Previous studies have shown that CBT is effective in treating anxiety disorders such as GAD, panic disorder, and social phobia (for a review, see Barlow, 2001; Silverman & Berman, 2001). Specifically, CBT for anxiety disorders focuses on confronting both fears and avoidance strategies that help maintain these fears. Similar to CBT strategies for the treatment of OCD, during exposure exercises, patients learn to expose themselves to anxiety-provoking situations or stimuli and then to refrain from any avoidance behaviors or rituals. Thus, patients learn that (1) during the exposures the anxiety will eventually decrease by itself, and (2) the anticipated negative consequences do not occur (e.g., that a patient with panic disorder might have a heart attack, or that a patient with a social phobia will be ridiculed by others). Depending on the nature of the fears, the exposures may be related to social situations (for social phobia), to everyday worries (for GAD), or to somatic sensations (for panic disorder).

CBT for anxiety disorders also focuses on psychoeducation about the nature of the disorder and the vicious cycle of avoidance that helps maintain the patient's fears. Cognitive restructuring focuses on identifying and modifying cognitive errors, such as overestimation of threat (e.g., "Something bad is likely to happen"; "If my heart bounces, this means I am going to have a heart attack") and catastrophizing (e.g., "If I get panicky, people will look down on me"). The clinician identifies dysfunctional cognitions and questions the accuracy of these cognitions using Socratic questioning. Thus, patients learn to reevaluate their automatic thoughts and the negative interpretations related to their fears.

CBT for Children with Anxiety Disorders

In general, CBT for children follows the same principles as CBT for adults (Kendall & Suveg, 2006). As with children who have OCD, it is important to spend ample time assessing the child's symptoms, because clinical assessments often include self-report questionnaires, and the child's ability for self-observation is limited. Moreover, younger children may not be able to tolerate their anxiety during exposures as well as adults and may have more difficulties understanding the long-term advantages of doing the exposure exercises (Piacentini & Bergman, 2001). For this reason, behavioral reward systems designed to enhance compliance with both in- and out-of-session work are often key components of treatment in this age group (Kendall et al., 1997). Finally, CBT for children often involves training parents to assist their child in doing the exposure exercises and to identify and modify dysfunctional thoughts and attitudes they may have about their child's disorder.

Recommendations for Treating TS with Comorbid Anxiety Disorders

The initial step in treating TS with comorbid anxiety disorders is to determine the extent to which the anxiety symptoms stem from, or are independent of, the child's tic disorder. Treatment should first focus on the symptoms that cause the most distress and impairment. Usually, the treatment starts with a focus on tics, especially if they are aggressive or self-damaging. If the patient also has anxiety symptoms, the clinician should combine the strategies that are usually used for anxiety disorders with strategies that are commonly used for tics. For example, if the patient thinks "I am afraid of saying or doing something embarrassing" before entering a social situation, then the patient and therapist could engage in Socratic questioning to evaluate this thought. To name a few strategies, the patient and clinician could explore how likely it is that others would notice, how likely it would be that others would care, how embarrassing it really is to do a tic, and how important it is what others think. The patient and therapist could also focus on the patient's coping skills (e.g., learning a competing response for a tic). If the patient engages in social avoidance due to fears of tics, treatment needs to include exposure exercises (e.g., attending social gatherings). However, these should only be introduced after the patient has already gained some control over the tics, for example, with habit reversal training (HRT; Azrin & Nunn, 1973; see also Peterson, Chapter 8, this volume), and is already skilled in the cognitive exercises described above. In general, anxiety management exercises are often helpful for patients with TS, because decreased anxiety often corresponds with a decrease in tic frequency.

COMORBID DEPRESSION

Elevated rates of depression are found in children and adults with TS (e.g., Pitman et al., 1987; Wodrich, Benjamin, & Lachar, 1997). Pitman et al. (1987), for example, found a lifetime prevalence rate of 44% for unipolar depression in adult patients with TS. Similar to comorbid anxiety disorders, there are several hypotheses as to why patients with TS often report elevated levels of depression. The burden of disruptive, debilitating tics may be related to the development of depressive symptoms such as low self-esteem and hopelessness. Moreover, perceived criticism from family members or peers with respect to failing to suppress the tics may lead to further depressive symptoms.

Treatment Approach for Depression

The most commonly used cognitive-behavioral approach for treating depression is the one introduced by Beck, Rush, Shaw, and Emery in 1979. Since then, the efficacy of CBT for depression has been shown in a series of studies (e.g., Butler, Chapman, Forman, & Beck, 2006; Covi &

Lipman, 1987; Dobson, 1989; Melvin et al., 2006; Murphy, Simons, Wetzel, & Lustman, 1984). Usually, the treatment begins with psychoeducation about the nature of depressive disorders and the role of dysfunctional cognitions in influencing mood, self-perpetuating cycles of inaction, and depression (see Beck, 1995). For some patients, merely gaining knowledge about the model of depression reduces depressive symptoms and alleviates the guilt and self-blame that is often felt (Fennell & Teasdale, 1987). The treatment also focuses on identifying and modifying dysfunctional beliefs about self and the world (e.g., "I will always be a failure"). Specifically, the process of cognitive restructuring consists of becoming aware of automatic negative thoughts and interpretations. Once these dysfunctional cognitions are elicited and identified, patients are trained to treat these cognitions as hypotheses, not as facts. Hypotheses have to be evaluated in terms of the evidence. Cognitive techniques such as Socratic questioning may then guide the patient to draw his or her own conclusions about the accuracy of the dysfunctional thoughts. Other techniques involving role play, daily thought records, or metaphors are also commonly used in CBT for depression (Beck, 1995). Moreover, the treatment emphasizes the importance of scheduling positive activity, and pleasant activities the patient has experienced between sessions are reviewed.

CBT for Children with Depression

As with CBT for children with anxiety disorders, CBT for youths with depression typically follows the same general principles as CBT for adults. However, treatment often includes training in problem solving and coping skills along with cognitive restructuring and the scheduling of pleasant activities (Stark et al., 2006). This skills-based approach is based on a self-control model in which children are taught a variety of techniques they can use to achieve and/or maintain a pleasant mood (Stark et al., 2006). Psychoeducation, social skills training, and family involvement are also commonly employed adjuncts, depending on the individual needs of the depressed child (Brent, Kolko, Birmaher, Baugher, & Bridge, 1999; Clarke, Rohde, Lewinsohn, Hops, & Seeley, 1999; Rohde, Lewinsohn, & Clarke, 2005). Similar to youngsters with anxiety, however, the lack of fully developed abstract thinking abilities in children can serve to complicate therapist efforts to identify and ameliorate the cognitive biases and distortions associated with depressive symptoms (Leahy, 1988; Piacentini & Bergman, 2001). As a result, therapeutic goals typically need to include strategies for helping depressed youths to concretize targeted cognitive distortions and abstract concepts.

Recommendations for Treating TS with Comorbid Depression

As with other comorbid disorders, the clinician should focus first on the symptoms that are of primary concern. If the patient is suicidal, his or her safety has to be established. For a patient with a primary diagnosis of TS, the clinician should initially start with the implementation of HRT. If dysfunctional depressive thoughts such as "I am a loser" or "I will not succeed in this training" occur, the clinician should also use cognitive restructuring techniques to evaluate and modify these automatic thoughts. If it is difficult for a patient to complete treatment-related activities because of a lack of motivation related to symptoms of depression, the clinician should encourage him or her to schedule positive activities or activities that provide some sense of pleasure and mastery. Patients with depression are more likely than others to get discouraged with HRT treatment, especially if they experience ups and downs in tic frequency despite efforts of tic control. It important to assign homework that the patient is likely to complete successfully and to provide praise and positive feedback. In this way, the patient will be reminded of slight, moderate, and significant gains and will be more likely to continue with the treatment.

CONCLUSION

TS can be a debilitating and distressing disorder for patients and their family members. When paired with OCD, other anxiety disorders, or depression, TS can feel even more overwhelming. Individuals experiencing disruptive symptoms are encouraged to seek treatment. In the initial session, the clinician, in collaboration with the patient, needs to determine the most severe conditions. Decisions can then be made regarding which diagnosis should be approached first in treatment. If TS is a patient's primary diagnosis, HRT should be considered as the initial treatment option. However, when TS is experienced along with OCD, ADHD, other anxiety disorders, or depression, other CBT strategies, as previously reviewed in this chapter, should be considered as the starting point. Managed and treated appropriately, patients with TS and a diagnosis of a comorbid psychopathology will likely experience symptom relief.

REFERENCES

Abramowitz, J. S. (1996). Variants of exposure and response prevention in the treatment of obsessive–compulsive disorder: A meta-analysis. *Behavior Therapy, 27,* 583–600.
American Psychiatric Association. (1994). *Diagnostic and statistical manual of mental disorders* (4th ed.). Washington, DC: Author.

Azrin, N. H., & Nunn, R. G. (1973). Habit reversal: A method of eliminating nervous habits and tics. *Behaviour Research and Therapy, 11*, 619–628.

Baer, L., & Minichiello, W. E. (1998). Behavior therapy for obsessive–compulsive disorder. In M. A. Jenike, L. Baer, & W. E. Minichello (Eds.), *Obsessive–compulsive disorder: Theory and management* (3rd ed., pp. 368–399). Chicago: Mosby.

Barlow, D. H. (2001). *Clinical handbook of psychological disorders: A step by step treatment manual.* New York: Guilford Press.

Barrett, P., Healy-Farrell, L., & March, J. (2004). Cognitive-behavioral family treatment of childhood obsessive–compulsive disorder: A controlled trial. *Journal of the American Academy of Child and Adolescent Psychiatry, 43*, 46–62.

Beck, A. T. (1976). *Cognitive therapy and emotional disorder.* New York: International Universities Press.

Beck, A. T. (1995). *Cognitive therapy: Basics and beyond.* New York: Guilford Press.

Beck, A. T., Rush, A. J., Shaw, B. F., & Emery, G. (1979). *Cognitive therapy of depression.* New York: Guilford Press.

Brent, D., Kolko, D., Birmaher, B., Baugher, M., & Bridge, J. (1999). A clinical trial for adolescent depression: Predictors of additional treatment in the acute and follow-up phases of the trial. *Journal of the American Academy of Child and Adolescent Psychiatry, 38*, 263–270.

Butler, A. C., Chapman, J. E., Forman, E. M., & Beck, A. T. (2006). The empirical status of cognitive-behavioral therapy: A review of meta-analyses. *Clinical Psychology Review, 26*, 17–31.

Clarke, G. N., Rohde, P., Lewinsohn, P. M., Hops, H., & Seeley, J. R. (1999). Cognitive-behavioral treatment of adolescent depression: Efficacy of acute group treatment and booster sessions. *Journal of the American Academy of Child and Adolescent Psychiatry, 38*, 272–279.

Coffey, B. J., & Park, K. S. (1997). Behavioral and emotional aspects of Tourette syndrome. *Neurologic Clinics, 15*, 277–289.

Comings, D. E., & Comings, B. G. (1987). A controlled study of Tourette syndrome: III. Phobias and panic attacks. *American Journal of Human Genetics, 41*, 761–781.

Cottraux, J., Note, I., Yao, S. N., Lafont, S., Note, B., Mollard, E., et al. (2001). A randomized controlled trial of cognitive therapy versus intensive behavior therapy in obsessive–compulsive disorder. *Psychotherapy and Psychosomatics, 70*, 288–297.

Covi, L., & Lipman, R. S. (1987). Cognitive behavioral group psychotherapy combined with imipramine in major depression. *Psychopharmacology Bulletin, 23*, 173–176.

de Haan, E., Hoogduin, K. A., Buitelaar, J., & Keijsers, G. (1998). Behavior therapy versus clomipramine for the treatment of obsessive–compulsive disorder. *Journal of the American Academy of Child and Adolescent Psychiatry, 37*, 1022–1029.

Dobson, K. S. (1989). A meta-analysis of the efficacy of cognitive therapy for depression. *Journal of Consulting and Clinical Psychology, 57*, 414–419.

Evers, R. A. F., & van de Wetering, B. (1994). A treatment model for motor tics based on a specific tension-reduction technique. *Journal of Behavior Therapy and Experimental Psychiatry, 25*, 255–260.

Fennell, M. J. V., & Teasdale, J. D. (1987). Cognitive therapy for depression: Individual differences and the process of change. *Cognitive Therapy and Research, 11*, 253–271.

Freeston, M. H., Rhéaume, J., & Ladouceur, R. (1996). Correcting faulty appraisals of obsessional thoughts. *Behaviour Research and Therapy, 34*, 433–446.

Geller, D., Biederman, J., Jones, J., Park, K., Schwartz, S., Shapiro, S., et al. (1998). Is juvenile obsessive–compulsive disorder a developmental subtype of the disorder?: A review of the pediatric literature. *Journal of the American Academy of Child and Adolescent Psychiatry, 37*, 420–427.

Hanna, G. L.(1995). Demographic and clinical features of obsessive–compulsive disorders in children and adolescents. *Journal of the American Academy of Child and Adolescent Psychiatry, 34,* 19–27.

Hanna, G. L., Piacentini, J., Cantwell, D., Fischer, D., Himle, J., & Van Etten, M. (2002). Obsessive–compulsive disorder with and without tics in a clinical sample of children and adolescents. *Depression and Anxiety, 16,* 59–63.

Jenike, M. A. (2004). Clinical practice: Obsessive–compulsive disorder. *New England Journal of Medicine, 350,* 259–265.

Kadesjo, B., & Gillberg, C. (2000). Tourette's disorder: Epidemiology and comorbidity in primary school children. *Journal of the American Academy of Child and Adolescent Psychiatry, 39,* 548–555.

Kendall, P., Flannery-Schroeder, E., Panicelli-Mindel, S., Southam-Gerow, M., Henin, A,, & Warman, M. (1997). Therapy for youths with anxiety disorders: A second randomized clinical trial. *Journal of Consulting and Clinical Psychology, 65,* 366–380.

Kendall, P., & Suveg, C. (2006). Treating anxiety disorders in youth. *Child and adolescent therapy: Cognitive-behavioral procedures* (3rd ed., pp. 243–294). New York: Guilford Press.

King, R. A., Leckman, J. F., Scahill, L., & Cohen, D. J. (1999). Obsessive–compulsive disorder, anxiety, and depression. In J. F. Leckman & D. J. Cohen (Eds.), *Tourette's syndrome—tics, obsessions, compulsions: Developmental psychopathology and clinical care* (pp. 43–62). New York: Wiley.

Kozak, M. J., & Foa, E. B. (1997). *Mastery of obsessive–compulsive disorder: A cognitive behavioral approach.* San Antonio, TX: Psychological Corporation.

Leahy, R. L. (1988). Cognitive therapy of childhood depression: Developmental considerations. In S. R. Shirk (Ed.), *Cognitive development and child psychopathology* (pp. 187–204). New York: Plenum Press.

Leckman, J. F., McDougle, C., Pauls, D., Peterson, B., Grice, D., King, R., et al. (2000). Tic-related versus non-tic-related obsessive–compulsive disorder. In W. K. Goodman, M. V. Rudorfer, & J. D. Maser (Eds.), *Obsessive–compulsive disorder: Contemporary issues in treatment* (pp. 43–68). Mahwah, NJ: Erlbaum.

Leckman, J. F., Walker, D. E., & Cohen, D. J. (1993). Premonitory urges in Tourette's syndrome. *American Journal of Psychiatry, 150,* 98–102.

Leckman, J. F., Walker, D. E., Goodman, W. K., Pauls, D. L., & Cohen, D. J. (1994). "Just right" perceptions associated with compulsive behavior in Tourette's syndrome. *American Journal of Psychiatry, 151,* 675–680.

Mansueto, C., & Keuler, D. (2005). Tic or compulsion? It's Tourettic OCD. *Behavior Modification, 29,* 784–799.

March, J., & Mulle, K. (1998). *OCD in children and adolescents: A cognitive-behavioral treatment manual.* New York: Guilford Press.

Melvin, G. A., Tonge, B. J., King, U. J., Heyne, D., Gordon, M. S., & Klimbeit, E. (2006). A comparison of cognitive-behavioral therapy, setraline, and their combination for adolescent depression. *Journal of the American Academy of Child and Adolescent Psychiatry, 45,* 1151–1161.

Miguel, E. C., Rosário-Campos, M. C., Shavitt, R., Hounie, A., & Mercadente, M. (2001). The tic-related obsessive–compulsive disorder phenotype and treatment implications. In D. J. Cohen, J. Jankovic, & C. Goetz (Eds.), *Advances in neurology: Tourette syndrome* (Vol. 85, pp. 43–55). Philadelphia: Lippincott, William & Wilkins.

Murphy, G. E., Simons, A. D., Wetzel, R. D., & Lustman, P. J. (1984). Cognitive therapy and pharmacotherapy: Singly and together in the treatment of depression. *Archives of General Psychiatry, 41,* 33–41.

Pediatric OCD Treatment Study Team. (2004). Cognitive-behavior therapy, sertraline, and their combination for children and adolescents with obsessive–compulsive disorder. *Journal of the American Medical Association, 292,* 1969–1976.

Piacentini, J., & Bergman, R. L. (2001). Developmental issues in cognitive therapy for childhood anxiety disorders. *Journal of Cognitive Psychotherapy, 15,* 165–182.

Piacentini, J., & Langley, A. (2004). Cognitive behavior therapy for children with obsessive compulsive disorder. *In Session: Journal of Clinical Psychology, 60,* 1181–1194.

Piacentini, J., March, J., & Franklin, M. (2006). Cognitive-behavioral therapy for youngsters with obsessive–compulsive disorder. In P. Kendall (Ed.), *Child and adolescent therapy: Cognitive-behavioral procedures* (3rd ed., pp. 297–321). New York: Guilford Press.

Pitman, R. K., Green, R. C., Jenike, M. A., & Mesulam, M. M. (1987). Clinical comparison of Tourette's disorder and obsessive–compulsive disorder. *American Journal of Psychiatry, 144,* 1166–1171.

Rachman, S. (1997). A cognitive theory of obsessions. *Behaviour Research and Therapy, 35,* 793–802.

Rapoport, J., Inoff-Germain, G., Weissman, M. M., Greenwald, S., Narrow, W. E., Jensen, P. S., et al. (2000). Childhood obsessive–compulsive disorder in the NIMH MECA study: Parent versus child identification of cases. *Journal of Anxiety Disorders, 14,* 535–548.

Rasmussen, A. S., & Eisen, J. L. (1990). Epidemiology of obsessive–compulsive disorder. *Journal of Clinical Psychiatry, 51*(Suppl.), 10–13.

Regier, D., Farmer, M., Rae, D., Myers, J., Kramer, M., Robins, L., et al. (1993). One-month prevalence of mental disorders in the United States and sociodemographic characteristics: The Epidemiologic Catchment Area study. *Acta Psychiatrica Scandinavica, 88,* 35–47.

Rettew, D. C., Swedo, S. E., Leonard, H. L., Lenane, M. C., & Rapoport, J. L. (1992). Obsessions and compulsions across time in 79 children and adolescents with obsessive–compulsive disorder. *Journal of the American Academy of Child and Adolescent Psychiatry, 31,* 1050–1056.

Rohde, P., Lewinsohn, P. M., & Clarke, G. N. (2005). The adolescent coping with depression course: A cognitive-behavioral approach to the treatment of adolescent depression. In E. D. Hibbs & P. S. Jensen (Eds.), *Psychosocial treatments for child and adolescent disorders: Empirically based strategies for clinical practice* (2nd ed., pp. 219–237). Washington, DC: American Psychological Association.

Salkovskis, P. M. (1989). Cognitive-behavioural factors and the persistence of intrusive thoughts in obsessional problems. *Behaviour Research and Therapy, 27,* 677–682.

Shapiro, A. K., & Shapiro, E. (1982). An update on Tourette syndrome. *American Journal of Psychotherapy, 36,* 379–390.

Silverman, W. K., & Berman, S. L. (2001). Psychosocial interventions for anxiety disorders in children: Status and future directions. In W. K. Silverman & P. D. A. Treffers (Eds.), *Anxiety disorders in children and adolescents: Research, assessment and intervention* (pp. 313–334). New York: Cambridge University Press.

Stark, K., Hargrave, J., Sander, J., Custer, G., Schnoebelen, S., Simpson, J., & Molnar, J. (2006). Treatment of childhood depression: The ACTION Treatment Program. In P. Kendall (Ed.), *Child and adolescent therapy: Cognitive-behavioral procedures* (pp. 169–216). New York: Guilford Press.

Stanley, M. A., & Turner, S. M. (1995). Current status of pharmacological and behavioral treatment of obsessive–compulsive disorder. *Behavior Therapy, 26,* 163–186.

Swedo, S. E., Rapoport, J., Leonard, H., Lenane, M., & Cheslow, D. (1989). Obsessive–compulsive disorder in children and adolescents: Clinical phenomenology of 70 consecutive cases. *Archives of General Psychiatry, 46,* 335–341.

van Oppen, P., & Arntz, A. (1994). Cognitive therapy for obsessive–compulsive disorder. *Behaviour Research and Therapy, 32,* 79–87.

van Oppen, P., de Haan, E., van Balkom, A. J. L. M., Spinhoven, P., Hoogduin, K., & van Dick, R. (1995). Cognitive therapy and exposure in vivo in the treatment of obsessive–compulsive disorder. *Behaviour Research and Therapy, 33,* 379–390.

Waters, T., & Barrett, P. (2000). The role of the family in childhood obsessive–compulsive disorder. *Clinical Child and Family Psychology Review, 3,* 173–184.

Wilhelm, S., Steketee, G., Reilly-Harrington, N. A., Deckersbach, T., Buhlmann, U., & Baer, L. (2005). Effectiveness of cognitive therapy for obsessive–compulsive disorder: An open trial. *Journal of Cognitive Psychotherapy, 19,* 173–179.

Wodrich, D. L., Benjamin, E., & Lachar, D. (1997). Tourette's syndrome and psychopathology in a child psychiatry setting. *Journal of the American Academy of Child and Adolescent Psychiatry, 36,* 1618–1624.

Woods, D., Piacentini, J., Himle, M., & Chang, S. (2005). Initial development and psychometric properties of the Premonitory Urge for Tics Scale (PUTS) in children with Tourette syndrome. *Journal of Developmental and Behavioral Pediatrics, 26,* 1–7.

CHAPTER 10

Disruptive Behavior in Persons with Tourette Syndrome
Phenomenology, Assessment, and Treatment

DENIS G. SUKHODOLSKY
LAWRENCE SCAHILL

Tourette syndrome (TS) is a chronic neuropsychiatric disorder of childhood onset that is characterized by motor and phonic tics that vary in number, anatomic location, frequency, intensity, and complexity over time. TS often co-occurs with other psychiatric disorders, most notably obsessive–compulsive disorder (OCD) (Pauls & Leckman, 1986) and attention-deficit/hyperactivity disorder (ADHD) (Scahill, Williams, Schwab-Stone, Applegate, & Leckman, 2006). In clinical samples TS also co-occurs with mood disorders (Kerbeshian, Burd, & Klug, 1995; Robertson, Banerjee, Eapen, & Fox-Hiley, 2002), anxiety disorders other than OCD (Coffey, Biederman, Smoller, et al., 2000), pervasive developmental disorders (Marriage, Miles, Stokes, & Davey, 1993), and learning disabilities (Burd, Kauffman, & Kerbeshian, 1992; Yeates & Bornstein, 1996). The frequencies of these various conditions vary greatly across different reports, suggesting that referral biases may influence the observed rate. Historically, research and treatment efforts in TS have focused on reducing tic frequency and severity. Over the past two decades, however, there has been increasing recognition of comorbid psychiatric conditions and associated disruptive behavioral problems. In most cases, these co-occurring conditions and disruptive behavior may contribute to functional impairment (Spencer et al., 1998; Sukhodolsky et al., 2003).

Disruptive behavior, including explosive anger, physical aggression, and noncompliance, represents a considerable social and clinical problem in children. For example, when asked about their experiences with violence, 36% of adolescents reported being in a physical fight during the past 12 months (Bureau of Justice Statistics, 2000) and 10% of adolescents reported being a victim of a violent crime (Brener, Simon, Krug, & Lowry, 1999). Disruptive behavior is among the most frequent reason for outpatient mental health referrals (Armbruster, Sukhodolsky, & Michalsen, 2004), and severe aggression is the most frequent reason for psychiatric hospitalization (Rice, Woolston, Stewart, Kerker, & Horwitz, 2002). Furthermore, virtually any childhood psychiatric condition may be associated with disruptive behavior. Anger and aggression are the core symptoms of oppositional defiant and conduct disorders and are frequent associated features of ADHD (American Psychiatric Association, 2000). Irritability is a prominent feature of mood disorders (Weisbrot & Ettinger, 2002), pervasive developmental disorders (Kraijer, 2000), and mental retardation (Matson, Dixon, & Matson, 2005). This chapter reviews research literature on the phenomenology, assessment, and treatment of disruptive behavior as it is relevant to TS.

TYPES OF DISRUPTIVE BEHAVIOR

Disruptive behaviors in TS may take various forms, but most frequent problems include anger, aggression, and noncompliance. It is helpful to distinguish among these three types of disruptive behavior, even though they tend to be intercorrelated and sometimes used interchangeably in the literature. Anger is a negative affective state that may include altered physiological arousal and thoughts about harm or blame (Berkowitz, 1990; Kassinove & Sukhodolsky, 1995; Novaco, 1975). Anger is one of the basic emotions; people report that they get angry about once or twice per week and that their anger experiences last about 30 minutes, on average (Averill, 1983; Kassinove, Sukhodolsky, Tsytsarev, & Solovyova, 1997). Anger can also vary in intensity from mild annoyance to rage and fury. Factor-analytical studies distinguish between anger experience (i.e., the inner feeling) and anger expression (i.e., an individual's tendency to act on anger by showing it outwardly, suppressing it, or actively coping with it) (Spielberger, 1988). On one hand, the phenomenology of anger expression is often characterized in terms of physical and verbal aggression (Deffenbacher & Swaim, 1999; Spielberger, 1988). On the other hand, studies with healthy adults show that talking and solving the problem are the most common behaviors associated with anger (Kassinove et al., 1997).

In contrast to anger, which may be a more internal phenomenon, aggression refers to behavior that results in harm to self or others. Several subtypes of aggression (e.g., impulsive, reactive, hostile, affective) have been distinguished based on the presence of angry affect and contrasted with instrumental, proactive, or planned types of aggression that are not "fueled" by anger (Vitiello & Stoff, 1997). Other well-known classification distinguishes between the overtly confrontational antisocial behavior such as arguing and fighting and covert antisocial behaviors such as lying, stealing, and breaking rules (Achenbach, Conners, Quay, Verhulst, & Howell, 1989; Frick et al., 1993). Physical aggression was found to be a significant risk factor for early-onset conduct disorder (Lahey et al., 1998), later violence (Lipsey & Wilson, 1998), and mental health problems (Loeber, Green, Kalb, Lahey, & Loeber, 2000). Compared to physical aggression, nonaggressive antisocial behavior was shown to follow a different developmental trajectory (Maughan, Rowe, Pickles, Costello, & Angold, 2000; Nagin & Tremblay, 1999) and predict later nonviolent criminal offenses (Kjelsberg, 2002).

Children's noncompliant behavior is defined as refusal to follow instructions or established rules (Kuczynski, Kochanska, Radke-Yarrow, & Girnius-Brown, 1987; McMahon & Forehand, 2003). Noncompliance is commonly reported by parents and teachers of children in the general population, but it is more prevalent in clinic-referred children, specifically those with disruptive behavioral disorders and developmental disabilities (Benson & Aman, 1999; Keenan & Wakschlag, 2004). Noncompliance is the essential feature of oppositional defiant disorder (ODD), which involves a pattern of defiant, disobedient, and hostile behavior toward authority figures. Although noncompliance and aggression frequently co-occur, they may represent different types of disruptive behavioral problems (Kolko, 1988; Sukhodolsky, Cardona, & Martin, 2005; Van Egeren, Frank, & Paul, 1999).

PHENOMENOLOGY, PREVALENCE, AND NATURAL HISTORY OF DISRUPTIVE BEHAVIOR IN TS

Comings and Comings (1985) stressed the importance of anger in TS: "If there was a single word that best characterized the behavioral problems in TS it would be *anger*" (p. 444). Similarly, in a large-scale survey of clinicians involved in evaluation and treatment of patients with TS, history of anger control problems was noted in 37% of patients (Freeman et al., 2000). Conduct problems reported in clinical studies with children and adolescents include temper tantrums, verbal and physical aggression, acting-out behavior, and destruction of property. The term "failure of inhibition of aggression" (Cohen, 1980) was used to capture the impulsive nature and perceived lack of control over aggressive behavior reported by patients with TS. A case report of disruptive behavior in a 12-year-old boy with TS, ADHD, and OCD (Vogt & Carroll, 1999) illustrated the frequency of disruptive behavior. The boy's mother recorded her son's aggressive behavior over 4 nights for 30-minute periods; on average she noted 10 episodes of aggression, 4 instances of cruelty, and 10 episodes of defiant or noncompliant behavior. These observations translate into at least one act of aggression and one act of noncompliance every 3 minutes of family life.

Studies of clinically referred samples reveal that up to 80% of children and adolescents with TS also have co-occurring disruptive behavioral problems (Coffey, Biederman, Geller, et al., 2000; Erenberg, Cruse, & Rothner, 1986; Rosenberg, Brown, & Singer, 1995). Disruptive behavior in clinical series was characterized using one of the three methods: clinical reports of aggressive behavior, categorical DSM diagnosis of ODD or conduct disorder (CD), or as a score on a dimensional measure of aggression. Survey studies of members of local branches of the Tourette Syndrome Association also documented that anger-related problems were present in 36–67% of the respondents (Kadesjo & Gillberg, 2000; Stefl, 1984). The high rates of co-occurrence of disruptive behavioral problems with TS in clinically referred samples is difficult to interpret in terms of etiology and may simply reflect the fact that patients with several disorders are more likely to seek medical attention (Pauls, Leckman, & Cohen, 1994). The rates of disruptive behavior were somewhat lower in two community ascertained samples of children with TS. In a sample of 13- to 14-year-old children ($n = 1,012$), 7 children had TS and 3 of them (43%) also had ODD or CD (Hornsey, Banerjee, Zeitlin, & Robertson, 2001). Four recent studies demonstrated that children with tics had higher levels of disruptive behavioral problems than children without tics (Gadow, Nolan, Sprafkin, & Schwartz, 2002; Kurlan, 2002; Scahill et al., 2006; Snider et al., 2002).

Due to their intensity and unpredictability in response to minimal provocation, anger outbursts in children with TS have been described as "rage attacks" or "rage storms." The explosive and out-of-character nature of disruptive behavior in TS resembles characteristics of aggression noted in "episodic dyscontrol syndrome" (Gordon, 1999; Nunn, 1986), intermittent explosive disorder (Olvera, 2002), and "anger attacks" in depression (Fava et al., 1991). The DSM-IV criteria for intermittent explosive disorder include discrete episodes of aggression that are grossly out of proportion to provocation and result in assaultive acts or destruction of property. Anger attacks are characterized by rapid and intense anger accompanied by high levels of autonomic arousal in response to trivial provocation. Using the modified DSM-IV criteria for intermittent explosive disorder, Budman and colleagues reported recurrent rage attacks resulting in destruction of property or personal injury in 12 consecutive children with TS referred to the movement disorders center of a general hospital (Budman, Bruun, Park, & Olson, 1998). These episodes reportedly lasted from a few minutes to an hour and were usually followed by remorse. The characteristics of rage attacks were further elaborated in a sample of 48 children ages 7–17 (Budman, Rockmore, Stokes, & Sossin, 2003). In this sample, over 90% of disruptive outbursts occurred at home and were triggered by being unable to get one's way or being told to give up what one is doing. In a study of children with TS with (n = 37) or without explosive anger (n = 31), the presence of anger was associated with higher rates of ADHD and OCD (Budman & Feirman, 2001). Although anger attacks were initially described in adults with major depression, mood disorders were not significantly associated with the presence of anger outbursts in children with TS.

Anger and irritability have been noted in up to 40% of adults with TS (Freeman et al., 2000; Wand, Matazow, Shady, Furer, & Staley, 1993). However, the natural history of disruptive behavior in adults with TS has not been well studied. Follow-up investigations of clinically referred samples indicate significant decline in tics in up to 80% of the patients by late adolescence (Bloch et al., 2006; Leckman et al., 1998; Pappert, Goetz, Louis, Blasucci, & Leurgans, 2003). Comings and Comings (1987) reported that the frequency of aggressive behavior in TS decreases with age similar to the age decrease in tic severity. However, Stefl (1984) reported no difference between children and adults on the levels of severity of behavioral problems, including aggressive behavior. Similarly to the findings in child and adolescent samples, the rates of anger control problems were four times higher in adults with TS, complicated by co-occurring psychiatric conditions, compared to adults with TS only (Freeman et al., 2000). It is possible that co-occurring ADHD continues to affect the rates of anger and aggression in adults with TS (Walkup et al., 1999). The impact of anger control problems on the adaptive functioning of adults with TS remains to be investigated, but based on finding in adults without tics, an association could be expected with interpersonal, familial, and occupational maladjustment (Kassinove & Sukhodolsky, 1995).

In summary, multiple descriptive, treatment, and epidemiological studies have reported a high prevalence of anger, aggression, and noncompliance in children with TS. Whether these problems are part of TS, related to co-occurring conditions, or due to the burden of chronic illness is not clear. Nevertheless, when children and adolescents with TS are brought to clinical attention due to their conduct problems, disruptive behavior may be erroneously attributed to TS. It could be a dilemma for clinicians whether to focus treatment attention on the tics, the core characteristics of TS, or on disruptive behavioral problems. Careful evaluation of disruptive behavioral problems and associated psychopathology should be among the first steps in planning treatment for children with TS and disruptive behavior.

DISRUPTIVE BEHAVIOR AND TIC SEVERITY

Three early clinical studies reported a significant association between tic severity and behavioral disturbance (Comings & Comings, 1987; Rosenberg, Harris, & Singer, 1984; Wilson, Garron, Tanner, & Klawans, 1982), but other studies failed to find this relationship (Edell-Fisher & Motta, 1990; Erenberg et al., 1986; Stokes, Bawden, Camfield, Backman, & Dooley, 1991). When specific tics were examined, aggressive behavior was found to be associated with copropraxia and the need to touch (de Groot, Janus, & Bornstein, 1995; Robertson, Trimble, & Lees, 1988). De Groot and colleagues (1995) found that 7- to 11-year-olds with complex tics such as skin picking, tapping, and touching were more likely to have conduct problems, but those in the 12- to 18-year-old group were not. By contrast, it was reported that more severe tics were present in 12- to 16-year-olds with disruptive behavior, but not for 6- to 11-year-olds (Rosenberg et al., 1984). These contrasting findings may be related to sample differences or methods of ascertaining tic severity and disruptive behavior. For example, a low but statistically significant correlation between tic severity and behavioral problems was reported in patients with unmedicated TS, but not in the patients on medication, perhaps because of the impact of medication on tics and behavior (Rosenberg et al., 1995). Two studies (Nolan, Sverd, Gadow, & Sprafkin, 1996; Pierre, Nolan, Gadow, Sverd, & Sprafkin, 1999) suggested that tic severity made a significant contribution to the behavioral problems in children referred for ADHD. However, Spencer and colleagues reported that tic disorder had little additional impact on functional impairment in children and adults with ADHD (Spencer et al., 2001; Spencer et al., 1999).

The relationship between tic severity and behavioral problems is not clear and is difficult to study. Tics vary within individuals over time and across age. Longitudinal studies suggest that tics and tic-associated impairment decline during adolescence (Coffey et al., 2004; Leckman et al.,

1998). Furthermore, medication directed at tic reduction could complicate the relationship between tics and behavioral outcomes because some tic-suppressing medication may also decrease impulsiveness, whereas others may have little or no impact on behavior. However, if disruptive behavior is related to tics, it may be a marker for more severe forms of TS.

DISRUPTIVE BEHAVIOR IN TS WITH ADHD

ADHD is a common psychiatric disorder of childhood onset affecting 2–14% of the population and often co-occuring with OD and CD (Barkley, 1997; Pliszka, 2003; Scahill et al., 1999). Association between disruptive behavior and the presence of ADHD in children with TS has been reported in a large number of clinical studies (Budman, Bruun, Park, Lesser, & Olson, 2000; de Groot et al., 1995; Hoekstra et al., 2004; Nolan et al., 1996; Pierre et al., 1999). A growing number of controlled studies suggests that disruptive behavior in TS may be attributable to co-occurring ADHD. Two controlled studies involving participants recruited through tic disorder clinics (Carter et al., 2000; Stephens & Sandor, 1999) observed that children with TS only did not differ from normal controls, whereas those in the TS plus ADHD group scored significantly higher than normal controls on the Child Behavior Checklist subscales of aggression and delinquent behavior. The rates of ODD and CD were indistinguishable in the groups of ADHD-only and ADHD + TS children recruited through a child psychopharmacology clinic (Spencer et al., 1998). These results were recently confirmed in a well-characterized sample of 42 children with TS only compared to 52 children with TS + ADHD (Sukhodolsky et al., 2003). Both TS groups were compared to age-matched children with ADHD and unaffected controls. Children with TS-only did not differ from unaffected controls on the parent and teacher ratings of disruptive behavior. By contrast, children with TS + ADHD were significantly worse than healthy controls and similar to children with ADHD only on the measures of disruptive behavior.

The association of aggression with ADHD in children with TS suggests that anger outbursts may be related to an underlying neurobiological deficit (Leckman & Cohen, 1999). TS, ADHD, and disruptive behavioral disorders are all associated with deficits in response inhibition, that is, deficits in the deliberate suppression of predominant cognitive or behavioral reactions (Sergeant, Geurts, & Oosterlaan, 2002). The construct of response inhibition encompasses a complex set of behaviors and neuropsychological processes that are regulated by multiple cortical–subcortical neural circuits (Heyder, Suchan, & Daum, 2004; Nigg,

2003). It is possible that cortical–striatal–thalamic–cortical circuits, which are presumed to be involved in production and modulation of tics in TS (Peterson et al., 1999), also contribute to response inhibition.

Neuropsychological studies suggest that TS and ADHD may confer separate but overlapping deficits in performance on measures of inhibition and executive functioning (Channon, Pratt, & Robertson, 2003; Ozonoff, Strayer, McMahon, & Filloux, 1998). Similarly, studies that compared children with ADHD to children with ADHD and disruptive behavioral disorders suggest that executive functioning deficits were conferred by the diagnosis of ADHD and were independent from other externalizing psychopathology (Geurts, Verte, Oosterlaan, Roeyers, & Sergeant, 2004; Nigg, Hinshaw, Carte, & Treuting, 1998). By contrast, aggression was associated with higher levels of anger and poor emotion regulation in children with ADHD (Hinshaw, 2003; Melnick & Hinshaw, 2000). Taken together with studies of anger attacks in individuals with mood disorders (Dougherty et al., 2004; Fava & Rosenbaum, 1998), some form of serotonergic biology may be implied by explosive outbursts in TS. Consequently, neural and behavioral mechanisms of mood regulation may be relevant to the understanding of anger outbursts in individuals with TS (Davidson et al., 2002). Although ADHD and disruptive behavioral problems are highly correlated, the etiology of this association is not well understood. As a result, the finding of the association between ADHD and disruptive behavior in children with TS is also difficult to interpret. However, the constructs of response inhibition and mood regulation may be relevant to disentangling the roles of various comorbidities in disruptive behavior.

ASSESSMENT OF DISRUPTIVE BEHAVIOR IN TS

Clinical evaluation of TS requires assessment of tics, associated psychopathology, and adaptive functioning (Leckman et al., 1999). A detailed psychiatric interview should be conducted to evaluate the presence of co-occurring psychiatric conditions, including disruptive behavioral disorders. Research studies may require measures that reflect different aspects of disruptive behavior (e.g., aggression and noncompliance) and meet certain psychometric standards (e.g., adequate reliability and validity, availability of normative information, or sensitivity to treatment change). Although a plethora of measures of anger and aggression are available (Collett, Ohan, & Myers, 2003; Eckhardt, Norlander, & Deffenbacher, 2004), none could be considered "gold standard" at the moment. Furthermore, the expression of disruptive behaviors varies in different contexts. For example, temper tantrums and noncompliance are most likely to occur at home, and covert antisocial behaviors may take place during unsupervised time spent with peers. Consequently, parents, teachers, and children may provide different accounts of disruptive behavior, and researchers may face the challenges of integrating data from multiple informants (Kraemer et al., 2003). To provide an example, we briefly review several instruments that have been used in the ongoing investigations of disruptive behavior in children with TS at the Yale Child Study Center.

The *Child Behavior Checklist* (CBCL; Achenbach, 1991) is a 116-item parent report that asks the parent to rate overall areas of behavioral and somatic symptoms on a 0–2 Likert scale. The CBCL provides national age and gender norms, and an extensive body of research supports the scale's reliability and validity. It features both narrow-band (Aggression and Delinquency) and broad-band (Externalizing Problems) factors that are relevant to the evaluation of disruptive behavior in TS. The Aggressive behavior scale consists of 20 items that measure physical aggression, argumentativeness, and excessive anger. The scale has a high internal consistency of 0.92 in both referred and nonreferred children. The Delinquent behavior scale consists of 13 items of antisocial behaviors, including lying, stealing, truancy, vandalism, and drug use. The internal consistency of the scale ranges from 0.74 to 0.83 for younger and older children, respectively. The CBCL is probably the most commonly used behavior rating scale, and the Aggression subscale has also been used in TS populations. For example, Stokes et al. (1991) reported average Aggression subscale scores in the range of 65.8 ± 9.2, and Singer and Rosenberg (1989) reported that 40% of their sample scored in the range of two standard deviations above the mean.

The 10-item parent-rated *Swanson, Nolan, and Pelham Rating Scale–IV* (SNAP-IV; Swanson, 1992) is a measure of child irritability and noncompliance that reflects the DSM-IV criteria for ODD. Examples of relevant items on this scale include "loses temper," "argues with adults," "actively defies adult request," and "is touchy or easily annoyed." The items are scored on a 4-point Likert scale and any per-item mean of 1.5 corresponds to a clinically significant level of noncompliant behavior. This measure has adequate reliability, and it was used to measure change in disruptive behavior multimodal treatment study of ADHD sponsored by the National Institute of Mental Health (Arnold et al., 1997). A teacher-rated version of the scale is available.

The *Overt Aggression Scale* (OAS; Silver & Yudofsky, 1991; Yudofsky, Silver, Jackson, Endicott, & Williams, 1986) is a clinician-rated instrument that rates characteristics and seriousness of the incidents of aggressive behavior. The scale consists of four categories of aggression: (1) verbal aggression, (2) aggression against objects, (3) self-directed aggression, and (4) aggression against others. Each category contains four statements describing aggressive behaviors in increasing levels of severity. All statements that apply to a child's behavior during an episode of aggression are checked by the rater and assigned a weighted score. Verbal aggression is scored on a scale of 1–4; aggression against objects, 2–5; and physical aggression against self or others, 3–6. In addition to documenting the occurrence and severity of the four types of aggression, the OAS provides a global measure of aggression severity, calculated as the sum of the weighted scores of the most severe behaviors in each category (range, 0–21). The OAS has been shown to have adequate interrater and test–retest reliability coefficients. It has been also shown to be sensitive to change in clinical studies of pharmacological treatments for children with aggressive behavior (Armenteros & Lewis, 2002; Malone, Delaney, Luebbert, Cater, & Campbell, 2000).

The *Home Situations Questionnaire* (HSQ; Barkley, 1997) is a 16-item measure of noncompliance. Parents are asked to answer *yes* or *no* to items that describe typical situations within which disruptive behavior is likely to occur. Items marked *yes* are then rated on a 1 (mild) to 9 (severe) Likert scale. The HSQ yields two scores: the number of problem situations and the mean severity value (total severity score divided by the number of *yes* items). The scale has extensive normative data (DuPaul & Barkley, 1992), and it has been shown to be sensitive to stimulant drug effects and to effects of parent management training (Barkley, Edwards, Laneri, Fletcher, & Metevia, 2001). The HSQ can be presented as an interview, and a school version of the measure is available.

Child self-report may add unique information on aspects of disruptive behavior, such as subjective anger experience and covert antisocial behavior. Several instruments with extensive normative information are currently available, but only a few have been used in treatment studies. The *Children's Inventory of Anger* (ChIA; Nelson & Finch, 2000) is a 39-item measure of anger intensity in response to hypothetical provoking events (e.g., "Someone cuts in front of you in a lunch line"). The ChIA provides norms for children from 6 to 16 years. The *State–Trait Anger Expression Inventory* (STAXI; Spielberger, 1988) is a 44-item self-report measure that contains two scales of experience and three scales of anger expression. The STAXI is one of the most well-researched psychometric instruments for anger. The second edition of the test is currently available, but only the first edition of the test provides norms for 12- to 16-year-old children. The measure has been shown to be sensitive to change in anger management training for adolescents (Snyder, Kymissis, Kessler, & Snyder, 1999).

PHARMACOTHERAPY FOR TS AND IMPLICATIONS
FOR DISRUPTIVE BEHAVIOR

Three studies in TS populations have directly evaluated the impact of medication on disruptive and aggressive behaviors. In an open-label study of paroxetine, out of 45 patients (age range 6–55 years) with TS, 29 were judged to have achieved a clinically significant improvement in the number of self-reported "rage attacks" after 8 weeks of treatment (Bruun & Budman, 1998). In a retrospective chart review of twenty-eight 5- to 18-year-old children with TS treated for aggressive behavior with risperidone, more than 70% showed decrease in aggressive behavior as measured by the Clinical Global Impression Scale (Sandor & Stephens, 2000). More recently, an open-label study of olanzapine in ten 7- to 13-year-old children with TS and aggression revealed a modest reduction in the parent (16%) and teacher (11%) ratings of aggressive behavior (Stephens, Bassel, & Sandor, 2004). The results of these reports should be considered in light of limitations imposed by the open-label and retrospective designs. (See Harrison, Schneider, & Walkup, Chapter 7, this volume.)

Dopamine 2 (D2) receptor blocking agents have been the mainstay of treatment for tics (King, Scahill, Lombroso, & Leckman, 2003; Sallee, Nesbitt, Jackson, Sine, & Sethuraman, 1997; Scahill, Erenberg, & Tourette Syndrome Practice Parameter Work Group, in press; Shapiro et al., 1989). Recent placebo-controlled studies demonstrated that the atypical neuroleptics risperidone (Dion, Annable, Sandor, & Chouinard, 2002; Scahill, Leckman, Schultz, Katsovich, & Peterson, 2003) and ziprasidone (Sallee et al., 2000) were superior to placebo and resulted in a 30–60% tic reduction. The α2-adrenergic agonists clonidine (Leckman et al., 1991; Tourette's Syndrome Study Group, 2002) and guanfacine (Scahill et al., 2001) were also shown to have beneficial effects on tic reduction. Given that these classes of medications have also been used to reduce aggression (McDougle, Stigler, & Posey, 2003; Schur et al., 2003), future studies of antipsychotics and α2-adrenergic agonists for tic reduction could provide additional guidance to clinicians by including measures of aggressive behavior.

Beneficial effects of stimulants on aggressive and disruptive behavior have been well documented in children with ADHD (Connor, Glatt, Lopez, Jackson, & Melloni, 2002; MTA Cooperative Group, 1999). After a long-standing controversy regarding the use of stimulants for children with tics (Castellanos, 1999; Kurlan, 2003), recent randomized controlled studies suggest that methylphenidate (MPH) is a safe and effective treatment for ADHD in the *majority* of children with comorbid tic disorder (Gadow, Sverd, Sprafkin, Nolan, & Ezor, 1995; Tourette's

Syndrome Study Group, 2002). Gadow and colleagues also reported a significant reduction of parent- and teacher-rated oppositional behavior in children in the MPH condition (Gadow et al., 1995). Similarly, in a large placebo-controlled randomized study of MPH and clonidine in 136 children ages 7–14 years, parent ratings of oppositional defiant behavior lessened in the MPH condition (Tourette's Syndrome Study Group, 2002). (See also Harrison, Scheider, & Walkup, Chapter 7, this volume, for a detailed discussion of medication management of TS and co-occurring conditions.)

CANDIDATE PSYCHOSOCIAL INTERVENTIONS FOR DISRUPTIVE BEHAVIOR IN TS

The need for behavioral interventions to address behavioral difficulties in children with TS has been noted by several authors (e.g., Coffey & Park, 1997; King, Scahill, Findley, & Cohen, 1999). Despite the increasing recognition of anger and aggression in TS, there has been little effort to evaluate well-established psychosocial interventions for disruptive behavioral disorders in the TS population. To address this gap in clinical research, we recently completed two randomized controlled studies of psychosocial treatments for children with TS and disruptive behavior (Scahill et al., 2006; Sukhodolsky et al., in preparation). One study evaluates the effects of parent management training (PMT) for 6- to 11-year-old children, and the second study evaluates the effects of anger control training (ACT) for 12- to 16-year-old adolescents. Both PMT and ACT have been named among evidence-based treatments for children with disruptive behavior (Brestan & Eyberg, 1998; Kazdin, 2005a). These studies were still in progress during the preparation of this chapter. Thus, we provide brief descriptions of these interventions and our rationale for applying them to TS populations.

PMT is a psychosocial intervention in which parents are taught methods of reducing the child's disruptive behavior and fostering prosocial behavior by using positive and negative reinforcement (Barkley, 1997; Kazdin, 2005b). This treatment is rooted in the social learning model of aggressive behavior (Bandura, 1973; Patterson, DeBaryshe, & Ramsey, 1989), which has received extensive empirical support (Reid, Patterson, & Snyder, 2002). Specifically, aggression is viewed as reinforced through the mechanisms of escape and avoidance conditioning (negative reinforcement) in the process of coercive family interactions. For example, when parents withdraw limit setting in response to a child's temper tantrum, the child's tantrum is negatively reinforced by the removal of the unpleasant parental discipline. The advantage of this model is that it provides clear guidance for training parents to break this cycle. PMT has achieved considerable support in randomized controlled studies of children with ADHD and ODD (Barkley et al., 2001; Kazdin, Esveldt-Dawson, French, & Unis, 1987; Webster-Stratton, 1984). It has also been applied to children with internalizing disorders and developmental disabilities (Baker, Landen, & Kashima, 1991; Briesmeister & Schaefer, 1998).

Different PMT manuals share core techniques but may vary in number of sessions, content of sessions, and emphasis on particular parenting skills (Barkley, 1997; Kazdin, 2005b; McMahon & Forehand, 2003). In our study, we used Barkley's PMT manual, enhanced by two sessions of psychoeducation about TS. Briefly, this is a structured 10-session curriculum designed to teach parents about the management of noncompliant, oppositional, and hostile behavior in their children. The core skills include providing positive reinforcement for appropriate behavior, communicating directions effectively, and being consistent with consequences for disruptive behaviors. Parents also learn and practice techniques such as token economies and time out. The goals of the training are to improve parental competence in dealing with child behavior problems, to increase parental understanding of the origins of noncompliant and defiant behavior, and to improve the child's compliance with parental commands.

ACT is a form of cognitive-behavioral therapy that involves developing emotional regulation and social problem-solving skills for coping with conflicts and frustration (Feindler & Ecton, 1986; Lochman & Wells, 2004). Continuing development and evaluation of ACT has been based on several lines of research, including anger and aggression (Berkowitz, 1990), stress management (Deffenbacher, Story, Brandon, Hogg, & Hazaleus, 1988), and most notably, social information processing (Crick & Dodge, 1994; Dodge, 1980; Lochman & Dodge, 1994). The social information-processing model suggests that deficits or distortions in (1) encoding and interpretation of cues, (2) selecting action strategy, and (3) enacting behavior may result in anger or aggression. For example, people get angry when they think that they have been deliberately treated unfairly. These thoughts may be triggered not by the actual actions of another person, but by a distorted understanding of intent. This distortion in processing social information, referred to as hostile attribution bias, often leads to increased anger arousal and aggressive behavior. ACT has been evaluated in several randomized controlled studies with children and adolescents (Deffenbacher et al., 1996; Feindler, Marriott, & Iwata, 1984; Lochman, Curry, Burch, & Lampron, 1984; Omizo, Hershberger, & Omizo, 1988; Snyder et al., 1999; Sukhodolsky, Solomon, & Perine, 2000). Cognitive-behavioral anger control interventions also have been evaluated with various adult samples (DiGiuseppe & Tafrate, 2003), but have never been tested in adults with TS.

For the purposes of our study of adolescents with TS and disruptive behavior, we developed an ACT manual that consists of 10 sessions administered in the format of individual psychotherapy. The manual includes techniques and activities from Feindler and Ecton (1986), as well as other anger management resources, to increase the flexibility of the manual's application. The sessions are grouped in the modules of arousal management, cognitive restructuring, and behavioral practice. For example, as part of the cognitive restructuring module, consequential thinking skills are practiced in tasks where children have to identify and evaluate the consequences of various actions for themselves and for the others involved in hypothetical conflicts. After that, they are asked to recall a time when they were frustrated and to problem-solve and role-play behaviors that would have deescalated the problem. At the end of each session, the children are assigned particular "anger coping" skills to practice as homework, are asked to describe their experience in "hassle logs," and are told to bring their logs to the next session.

Both PMT and ACT are examples of psychosocial interventions that have been evaluated in children without tics. These treatments are also based on well-researched models of aggressive and noncompliant behavior. We reasoned that deficits in family interactions, on one hand, and in social information processing, on the other hand, may contribute to disruptive behavior in children with TS. Consequently, PMT and ACT may be relevant to treatment of disruptive behavior in children with tics.

CONCLUSION

Studies of clinically referred and population samples reveal that children with TS frequently have co-occurring disruptive behavioral problems such as explosive anger, aggression, and noncompliance. Whether these problems are part of TS, related to co-occurring conditions, or due to the burden of chronic illness is not clear. However, several controlled studies suggest that disruptive behavior in TS is associated with the presence of ADHD. Similarly to findings in children without tics, disruptive behavior in children with TS is associated with deficits in social, school, and family functioning. Therefore, evaluation of disruptive behavioral problems and associated psychopathology should be a part of comprehensive evaluation for children with TS. Clinical management of disruptive behavior in children with TS may include education, clinical monitoring, pharmacological or psychosocial treatments, and school interventions, as needed.

REFERENCES

Achenbach, T. M. (1991). *Manual for the Child Behavior Checklist/4–18 and 1991 Profile.* Burlington, VT: University of Vermont Press.

Achenbach, T. M., Conners, C. K., Quay, H. C., Verhulst, F. C., & Howell, C. T. (1989). Replication of empirically derived syndromes as a basis for taxonomy of child/adolescent psychopathology. *Journal of Abnormal Child Psychology, 17*(3), 299–323.

American Psychiatric Association. (2000). *Diagnostic and statistical manual of mental disorders* (4th ed., text rev.). Washington, DC: Author.

Armbruster, P., Sukhodolsky, D., & Michalsen, R. (2004). The impact of managed care on children's outpatient treatment: A comparison study of treatment outcome before and after managed care. *American Journal of Orthopsychiatry, 74*(1), 5–13.

Armenteros, J. L., & Lewis, J. E. (2002). Citalopram treatment for impulsive aggression in children and adolescents: An open pilot study. *Journal of the American Academy of Child and Adolescent Psychiatry, 41*(5), 522–529.

Arnold, L. E., Abikoff, H. B., Cantwell, D. P., Conners, C. K., Elliott, G., Greenhill, L. L., et al. (1997). National Institute of Mental Health collaborative multimodal treatment study of children with ADHD (the MTA). Design challenges and choices. *Archives of General Psychiatry, 54*(9), 865–870.

Averill, J. R. (1983). Studies on anger and aggression: Implications for theories of emotion. *American Psychologist, 38*(11), 1145–1160.

Baker, B. L., Landen, S. J., & Kashima, K. J. (1991). Effects of parent training on families of children with mental retardation: Increased burden or generalized benefit? *American Journal on Mental Retardation, 96*(2), 127–136.

Bandura, A. (1973). *Aggression: A social learning analysis.* Oxford, UK: Prentice-Hall.

Barkley, R. A. (1997). *Defiant children: A clinician's manual for assessment and parent training* (2nd ed.). New York: Guilford Press.

Barkley, R. A., Edwards, G., Laneri, M., Fletcher, K., & Metevia, L. (2001). The efficacy of problem-solving communication training alone, behavior management training alone, and their combination for parent–adolescent conflict in teenagers with ADHD and ODD. *Journal of Consulting and Clinical Psychology, 69*(6), 926–941.

Benson, B. A., & Aman, M. G. (1999). Disruptive behavior disorders in children with mental retardation. In H. C. Quay & A. E. Hogan (Eds.), *Handbook of disruptive behavior disorders* (pp. 559–578). Dordrecht, Netherlands: Kluwer.

Berkowitz, L. (1990). On the formation and regulation of anger and aggression: A cognitive–neoassociationistic analysis. *American Psychologist, 45*(4), 494–503.

Bloch, M. H., Scahill, L., Otka, J., Katsovich, L., Zhang, H., Leckman, J. F., et al. (2006). Adulthood outcome of tic and obsessive–compulsive symptom severity in children with Tourette syndrome. *Archives of Pediatrics and Adolescent Medicine, 160*(1), 65–69.

Brener, N. D., Simon, T. R., Krug, E. G., & Lowry, R. (1999). Recent trends in violence-related behaviors among high school students in the United States. *Journal of the American Medical Association, 282*(5), 440–446.

Brestan, E. V., & Eyberg, S. M. (1998). Effective psychosocial treatments of conduct-disordered children and adolescents: 29 years, 82 studies, and 5,272 kids. *Journal of Clinical Child Psychology, 27*(2), 180–189.

Briesmeister, J. M., & Schaefer, C. E. (Eds.). (1998). *Handbook of parent training: Parents as co-therapists for children's behavior problems* (2nd ed.). New York: Wiley.

Bruun, R. D., & Budman, C. L. (1998). Paroxetine treatment of episodic rages associated with Tourette's disorder. *Journal of Clinical Psychiatry, 59*(11), 581–584.

Budman, C. L., Bruun, R. D., Park, K. S., Lesser, M., & Olson, M. (2000). Explosive outbursts in children with Tourette's disorder. *Journal of the American Academy of Child and Adolescent Psychiatry, 39*(10), 1270–1276.

Budman, C. L., Bruun, R. D., Park, K. S., & Olson, M. E. (1998). Rage attacks in children and adolescents with Tourette's disorder: A pilot study. *Journal of Clinical Psychiatry, 59*(11), 576–580.

Budman, C. L., & Feirman, L. (2001). The relationship of Tourette's syndrome with its psychiatic comorbidities: Is there an overlap? *Psychiatric Annals, 31*(9), 541–548.

Budman, C. L., Rockmore, L., Stokes, J., & Sossin, M. (2003). Clinical phenomenology of episodic rage in children with Tourette syndrome. *Journal of Psychosomatic Research, 55*(1), 59–65.

Burd, L., Kauffman, D. W., & Kerbeshian, J. (1992). Tourette syndrome and learning disabilities. *Journal of Learning Disabilities, 25*(9), 598–604.

Bureau of Justice Statistics. (2000). *Criminal victimization in the United States.* Washington, DC: U.S. Department of Justice.

Carter, A. S., O'Donnell, D. A., Schultz, R. T., Scahill, L., Leckman, J. F., & Pauls, D. L. (2000). Social and emotional adjustment in children affected with Gilles de la Tourette's syndrome: Associations with ADHD and family functioning. *Journal of Child Psychology and Psychiatry and Allied Disciplines, 41*(2), 215–223.

Castellanos, F. X. (1999). Stimulants and tic disorders: From dogma to data. *Archives of General Psychiatry, 56*(4), 337–338.

Channon, S., Pratt, P., & Robertson, M. M. (2003). Executive function, memory, and learning in Tourette's syndrome. *Neuropsychology, 17*(2), 247–254.

Coffey, B. J., Biederman, J., Geller, D., Frazier, J., Spencer, T., Doyle, R., et al. (2004). Reexamining tic persistence and tic-associated impairment in Tourette's disorder findings from a naturalistic follow-up study. *Journal of Nervous and Mental Disease, 192*(11), 776–780.

Coffey, B. J., Biederman, J., Geller, D. A., Spencer, T. J., Kim, G. S., Bellordre, C. A., et al. (2000). Distinguishing illness severity from tic severity in children and adolescents with Tourette's disorder. *Journal of the American Academy of Child and Adolescent Psychiatry, 39*(5), 556–561.

Coffey, B. J., Biederman, J., Smoller, J. W., Geller, D. A., Sarin, P., Schwartz, S., et al. (2000). Anxiety disorders and tic severity in juveniles with Tourette's disorder. *Journal of the American Academy of Child and Adolescent Psychiatry, 39*(5), 562–568.

Coffey, B. J., & Park, K. S. (1997). Behavioral and emotional aspects of Tourette syndrome. *Neurologic Clinics, 15*(2), 277–289.

Cohen, D. J. (1980). The pathology of the self in primary childhood autism and Gilles de la Tourette syndrome. *Psychiatric Clinics of North America, 3*, 383–402.

Collett, B. R., Ohan, J. L., & Myers, K. M. (2003). Ten-year review of rating scales: VI. Scales assessing externalizing behaviors. *Journal of the American Academy of Child and Adolescent Psychiatry, 42*(10), 1143–1170.

Comings, D. E., & Comings, B. G. (1985). Tourette's syndrome: Clinical and psychological aspects of 250 cases. *American Journal of Human Genetics, 35*, 435–450.

Comings, D. E., & Comings, B. G. (1987). A controlled study of Tourette syndrome: II. Conduct. *American Journal of Human Genetics, 41*(5), 742–760.

Connor, D. F., Glatt, S. J., Lopez, I. D., Jackson, D., & Melloni, R. H., Jr. (2002). Psychopharmacology and aggression: I. A meta-analysis of stimulant effects on overt/covert aggression-related behaviors in ADHD. *Journal of the American Academy of Child and Adolescent Psychiatry, 41*(3), 253–261.

Crick, N. R., & Dodge, K. A. (1994). A review and reformulation of social information-processing mechanisms in children's social adjustment. *Psychological Bulletin, 115*(1), 74.

Davidson, R. J., Lewis, D. A., Alloy, L. B., Amaral, D. G., Bush, G., Cohen, J. D., et al. (2002).

Neural and behavioral substrates of mood and mood regulation. *Biological Psychiatry,* *52*(6), 478–502.

de Groot, C. M., Janus, M. D., & Bornstein, R. A. (1995). Clinical predictors of psychopathology in children and adolescents with Tourette syndrome. *Journal of Psychiatric Research, 29*(1), 59–70.

Deffenbacher, J. L., Oetting, E. R., Huff, M. E., Cornell, G. R., Dallager, C. J., & Deffenbacher, J. L. (1996). Evaluation of two cognitive-behavioral approaches to general anger reduction. *Cognitive Therapy and Research, 20*(6), 551–573.

Deffenbacher, J. L., Story, D. A., Brandon, A. D., Hogg, J. A., & Hazaleus, S. L. (1988). Cognitive and cognitive-relaxation treatments of anger. *Cognitive Therapy and Research, 12*(2), 167–184.

Deffenbacher, J. L., & Swaim, R. C. (1999). Anger expression in Mexican American and white non-Hispanic adolescents. *Journal of Counseling Psychology, 46*(1), 61–69.

DiGiuseppe, R., & Tafrate, R. C. (2003). Anger treatment for adults: A meta-analytic review. *Clinical Psychology: Science and Practice, 10*(1), 70–84.

Dion, Y., Annable, L., Sandor, P., & Chouinard, G. (2002). Risperidone in the treatment of Tourette syndrome: A double-blind, placebo-controlled trial. *Journal of Clinical Psychopharmacology, 22*(1), 31–39.

Dodge, K. A. (1980). Social cognition and children's aggressive behavior. *Child Development, 51*(1), 162–170.

Dougherty, D. D., Rauch, S. L., Deckersbach, T., Marci, C., Loh, R., Shin, L. M., et al. (2004). Ventromedial prefrontal cortex and amygdala dysfunction during an anger induction positron emission tomography study in patients with major depressive disorder with anger attacks. *Archives of General Psychiatry, 61*(8), 795–804.

DuPaul, G. J., & Barkley, R. A. (1992). Situational variability of attention problems: Psychometric properties of the Revised Home and School Situations Questionnaires. *Journal of Clinical Child Psychology, 21*(2), 178–188.

Eckhardt, C., Norlander, B., & Deffenbacher, J. (2004). The assessment of anger and hostility: A critical review. *Aggression and Violent Behavior, 9*(1), 17–43.

Edell-Fisher, B. H., & Motta, R. W. (1990). Tourette syndrome: Relation to children's and parents' self-concepts. *Psychological Reports, 66*(2), 539–545.

Erenberg, G., Cruse, R. P., & Rothner, A. D. (1986). Tourette syndrome: An analysis of 200 pediatric and adolescent cases. *Cleveland Clinic Quarterly, 53*(2), 127–131.

Fava, M., & Rosenbaum, J. F. (1998). Anger attacks in depression. *Depression and Anxiety, 8*(Suppl. 1), 59–63.

Fava, M., Rosenbaum, J. F., McCarthy, M., Pava, J., Steingard, R., & Bless, E. (1991). Anger attacks in depressed outpatients and their response to fluoxetine. *Psychopharmacology Bulletin, 27*(3), 275–279.

Feindler, E. L., & Ecton, R. B. (1986). *Adolescent anger control: Cognitive-behavioral techniques.* New York: Pergamon Press.

Feindler, E. L., Marriott, S. A., & Iwata, M. (1984). Group anger control training for junior high school delinquents. *Cognitive Therapy and Research, 8*(3), 299–311.

Freeman, R. D., Fast, D. K., Burd, L., Kerbeshian, J., Robertson, M. M., & Sandor, P. (2000). An international perspective on Tourette syndrome: Selected findings from 3,500 individuals in 22 countries. *Developmental Medicine and Child Neurology, 42*(7), 436–447.

Frick, P. J., Lahey, B. B., Loeber, R., Tannenbaum, L., Van Horn, Y., Christ, M. A. G., et al. (1993). Oppositional defiant disorder and conduct disorder: A meta-analytic review of factor analyses and cross-validation in a clinic sample. *Clinical Psychology Review, 13*(4), 319–340.

Gadow, K. D., Nolan, E. E., Sprafkin, J., & Schwartz, J. (2002). Tics and psychiatric comorbidity in children and adolescents. *Developmental Medicine and Child Neurology, 44*(5), 330–338.

Gadow, K. D., Sverd, J., Sprafkin, J., Nolan, E. E., & Ezor, S. N. (1995). Efficacy of methylphenidate for attention-deficit hyperactivity disorder in children with tic disorder. *Archives of General Psychiatry, 52*(6), 444–455.

Geurts, H. M., Verte, S., Oosterlaan, J., Roeyers, H., & Sergeant, J. A. (2004). How specific are executive functioning deficits in attention deficit hyperactivity disorder and autism? *Journal of Child Psychology and Psychiatry and Allied Disciplines, 45*(4), 836–854.

Gordon, N. (1999). Episodic dyscontrol syndrome. *Developmental Medicine and Child Neurology, 41*(11), 786–788.

Heyder, K., Suchan, B., & Daum, I. (2004). Cortico–subcortical contributions to executive control. *Acta Psychologica, 115*(2–3), 271–289.

Hinshaw, S. P. (2003). Impulsivity, emotion regulation, and developmental psychopathology: Specificity versus generality of linkages. *Annals of the New York Academy of Sciences, 1008*, 149–159.

Hoekstra, P. J., Steenhuis, M. P., Troost, P. W., Korf, J., Kallenberg, C. G., & Minderaa, R. B. (2004). Relative contribution of attention-deficit hyperactivity disorder, obsessive–compulsive disorder, and tic severity to social and behavioral problems in tic disorders. *Journal of Developmental and Behavioral Pediatrics, 25*(4), 272–279.

Hornsey, H., Banerjee, S., Zeitlin, H., & Robertson, M. (2001). The prevalence of Tourette syndrome in 13–14-year-olds in mainstream schools. *Journal of Child Psychology and Psychiatry and Allied Disciplines, 42*(8), 1035–1039.

Kadesjo, B., & Gillberg, C. (2000). Tourette's disorder: Epidemiology and comorbidity in primary school children. *Journal of the American Academy of Child and Adolescent Psychiatry, 39*(5), 548–555.

Kassinove, H., & Sukhodolsky, D. G. (1995). Anger disorders: Basic science and practice issues. *Issues in Comprehensive Pediatric Nursing, 18*(3), 173–205.

Kassinove, H., Sukhodolsky, D. G., Tsytsarev, S. V., & Solovyova, S. (1997). Self-reported anger episodes in Russia and America. *Journal of Social Behavior and Personality, 12*(2), 301–324.

Kazdin, A. E. (2005a). Child, parent, and family-based treatment of aggressive and antisocial child behavior. In E. D. Hibbs & P. S. Jensen (Eds.), *Psychosocial treatments for child and adolescent disorders: Empirically based strategies for clinical practice* (2nd ed., pp. 445–476). Washington, DC: American Psychological Association.

Kazdin, A. E. (2005b). *Parent management training: Treatment for oppositional, aggressive, and antisocial behavior in children and adolescents.* New York: Oxford University Press.

Kazdin, A. E., Esveldt-Dawson, K., French, N. H., & Unis, A. S. (1987). Effects of parent management training and problem-solving skills training combined in the treatment of antisocial child behavior. *Journal of the American Academy of Child and Adolescent Psychiatry, 26*(3), 416–424.

Keenan, K., & Wakschlag, L. S. (2004). Are oppositional defiant and conduct disorder symptoms normative behaviors in preschoolers?: A comparison of referred and nonreferred children. *American Journal of Psychiatry, 161*(2), 356–358.

Kerbeshian, J., Burd, L., & Klug, M. G. (1995). Comorbid Tourette's disorder and bipolar disorder: An etiologic perspective. *American Journal of Psychiatry, 152*(11), 1646–1651.

King, R. A., Scahill, L., Findley, D., & Cohen, D. J. (1999). Psychosocial and behavioral treatments. In J. F. Leckman & D. J. Cohen (Eds.), *Tourette's syndrome—tics, obsessions, compulsions: Developmental psychopathology and clinical care* (pp. 338–359). New York: Wiley.

King, R. A., Scahill, L., Lombroso, P. J., & Leckman, J. F. (2003). Tourette's syndrome and other tic disorders. In A. Martin, J. F. Leckman, D. S. Charney, & L. Scahill (Eds.), *Pediatric psychopharmacology: Principles and practice* (pp. 526–542). New York: Oxford University Press.

Kjelsberg, E. (2002). Pathways to violent and non-violent criminality in an adolescent psychiatric population. *Child Psychiatry and Human Development, 33*(1), 29–42.

Kolko, D. J. (1988). Daily ratings on a child psychiatric unit: Psychometric evaluation of the Child Behavior Rating Form. *Journal of the American Academy of Child and Adolescent Psychiatry, 27*(1), 126–132.

Kraemer, H. C., Measelle, J. R., Ablow, J. C., Essex, M. J., Boyce, W. T., & Kupfer, D. J. (2003). A new approach to integrating data from multiple informants in psychiatric assessment and research: Mixing and matching contexts and perspectives. *American Journal of Psychiatry, 160*(9), 1566–1577.

Kraijer, D. (2000). Review of adaptive behavior studies in mentally retarded persons with autism/pervasive developmental disorder. *Journal of Autism and Developmental Disorders, 30*(1), 39–47.

Kuczynski, L., Kochanska, G., Radke-Yarrow, M., & Girnius-Brown, O. (1987). A developmental interpretation of young children's noncompliance. *Developmental Psychology, 23*(6), 799–806.

Kurlan, R. (2002). Treatment of ADHD in children with tics: A randomized controlled trial. *Neurology, 58*(4), 527–536.

Kurlan, R. (2003). Tourette's syndrome: Are stimulants safe? *Current Neurology and Neuroscience Report, 3*(4), 285–288.

Lahey, B. B., Loeber, R., Quay, H. C., Applegate, B., Shaffer, D., Waldman, I., et al. (1998). Validity of DSM-IV subtypes of conduct disorder based on age of onset. *Journal of the American Academy of Child and Adolescent Psychiatry, 37*(4), 435–442.

Leckman, J. F., & Cohen, D. J. (Eds.). (1999). *Tourette's syndrome—tics, obsessions, compulsions: Developmental psychopathology and clinical care.* New York: Wiley.

Leckman, J. F., Hardin, M. T., Riddle, M. A., Stevenson, J., Ort, S. I., & Cohen, D. J. (1991). Clonidine treatment of Gilles de la Tourette's syndrome. *Archives of General Psychiatry, 48*(4), 324–328.

Leckman, J. F., King, R. A., Scahill, L., Findley, D., Ort, S. I., & Cohen, D. J. (1999). Yale approach to assessment and treatment. In J. F. Leckman & D. J. Cohen (Eds.), *Tourette's syndrome—tics, obsessions, compulsions: Developmental psychopathology and clinical care* (pp. 285–309). New York: Wiley.

Leckman, J. F., Zhang, H., Vitale, A., Lahnin, F., Lynch, K., Bondi, C., et al. (1998). Course of tic severity in Tourette syndrome: The first two decades. *Pediatrics, 102*(1, Pt. 1), 14–19.

Lipsey, M. W., & Wilson, D. B. (1998). Effective intervention for serious juvenile offenders: A synthesis of research. In R. Loeber & D. P. Farrington (Eds.), *Serious and violent juvenile offenders: Risk factors and successful interventions* (pp. 86–105). Thousand Oaks, CA: Sage.

Lochman, J. E., Curry, J. F., Burch, P. R., & Lampron, L. B. (1984). Treatment and generalization effects of cognitive-behavioral and goal-setting interventions with aggressive boys. *Journal of Consulting and Clinical Psychology, 52*(5), 915–916.

Lochman, J. E., & Dodge, K. A. (1994). Social–cognitive processes of severely violent, moderately aggressive, and nonaggressive boys. *Journal of Consulting and Clinical Psychology, 62*(2), 366–374.

Lochman, J. E., & Wells, K. C. (2004). The Coping Power Program for preadolescent aggressive boys and their parents: Outcome effects at the 1-year follow-up. *Journal of Consulting and Clinical Psychology, 72*(4), 571–578.

Loeber, R., Green, S. M., Kalb, L., Lahey, B. B., & Loeber, R. (2000). Physical fighting in childhood as a risk factor for later mental health problems. *Journal of the American Academy of Child and Adolescent Psychiatry, 39*(4), 421–428.

Malone, R. P., Delaney, M. A., Luebbert, J. F., Cater, J., & Campbell, M. (2000). A double-blind placebo-controlled study of lithium in hospitalized aggressive children and adolescents with conduct disorder. *Archives of General Psychiatry, 57*(7), 649–654.

Marriage, K., Miles, T., Stokes, D., & Davey, M. (1993). Clinical and research implications of the co-occurrence of Asperger's and Tourette syndromes. *Australian and New Zealand Journal of Psychiatry, 27*(4), 666–672.

Matson, J. L., Dixon, D. R., & Matson, M. L. (2005). Assessing and treating aggression in children and adolescents with developmental disabilities: A 20-year overview. *Educational Psychology, 25*(2–3), 151–181.

Maughan, B., Rowe, R., Pickles, A., Costello, E. J., & Angold, A. (2000). Developmental trajectories of aggressive and non-aggressive conduct problems. *Journal of Quantitative Criminology, 16*(2), 199–221.

McDougle, C. J., Stigler, K. A., & Posey, D. J. (2003). Treatment of aggression in children and adolescents with autism and conduct disorder. *Journal of Clinical Psychiatry, 64*(Suppl. 4), 16–25.

McMahon, R. J., & Forehand, R. L. (2003). *Helping the noncompliant child: Family-based treatment for oppositional behavior* (2nd ed.). New York: Guilford Press.

Melnick, S. M., & Hinshaw, S. P. (2000). Emotion regulation and parenting in AD/HD and comparison boys: Linkages with social behaviors and peer preference. *Journal of Abnormal Child Psychology, 28*(1), 73–86.

MTA Cooperative Group. (1999). A 14-month randomized clinical trial of treatment strategies for attention-deficit/hyperactivity disorder: Multimodal treatment study of children with ADHD. *Archives of General Psychiatry, 56*(12), 1073–1086.

Nagin, D., & Tremblay, R. E. (1999). Trajectories of boys' physical aggression, opposition, and hyperactivity on the path to physically violent and nonviolent juvenile delinquency. *Child Development, 70*(5), 1181–1196.

Nelson, W. M., & Finch, A. J. (2000). *Children's Inventory of Anger.* Los Angeles: Western Psychological Services.

Nigg, J. T. (2003). Response inhibition and disruptive behaviors: Toward a multiprocess conception of etiological heterogeneity for ADHD combined type and conduct disorder early-onset type. *Annals of the New York Academy of Sciences, 1008*, 170–182.

Nigg, J. T., Hinshaw, S. P., Carte, E. T., & Treuting, J. J. (1998). Neuropsychological correlates of childhood attention-deficit/hyperactivity disorder: Explainable by comorbid disruptive behavior or reading problems? *Journal of Abnormal Psychology, 107*(3), 468–480.

Nolan, E. E., Sverd, J., Gadow, K. D., & Sprafkin, J. (1996). Associated psychopathology in children with both ADHD and chronic tic disorder. *Journal of the American Academy of Child and Adolescent Psychiatry, 35*(12), 1622–1630.

Novaco, R. W. (1975). *Anger control: The development and evaluation of experimental treatment.* Lexington, MA: D. C. Health.

Nunn, K. (1986). The episodic dyscontrol syndrome in childhood. *Journal of Child Psychology and Psychiatry and Allied Disciplines, 27*(4), 439–446.

Olvera, R. L. (2002). Intermittent explosive disorder: Epidemiology, diagnosis and management. *CNS Drugs, 16*(8), 517–526.

Omizo, M. M., Hershberger, J. M., & Omizo, S. A. (1988). Teaching children to cope with anger. *Elementary School Guidance and Counseling, 22*, 241–245.

Ozonoff, S., Strayer, D. L., McMahon, W. M., & Filloux, F. (1998). Inhibitory deficits in Tourette syndrome: A function of comorbidity and symptom severity. *Journal of Child Psychology and Psychiatry and Allied Disciplines, 39*(8), 1109–1118.

Pappert, E. J., Goetz, C. G., Louis, E. D., Blasucci, L., & Leurgans, S. (2003). Objective assessments of longitudinal outcome in Gilles de la Tourette's syndrome. *Neurology, 61*(7), 936–940.

Patterson, G. R., DeBaryshe, B. D., & Ramsey, E. (1989). A developmental perspective on antisocial behavior. *American Psychologist, 44*(2), 329–335.

Pauls, D. L., & Leckman, J. F. (1986). The inheritance of Gilles de la Tourette's syndrome and associated behaviors: Evidence for autosomal dominant transmission. *New England Journal of Medicine, 315*(16), 993–997.

Pauls, D. L., Leckman, J. F., & Cohen, D. J. (1994). Evidence against a genetic relationship between Tourette's syndrome and anxiety, depression, panic and phobic disorders. *British Journal of Psychiatry, 164*(2), 215–221.

Peterson, B. S., Leckman, J. F., Arnsten, A., Anderson, G. M., Staib, L. H., Gore, J. C., et al. (1999). Neuroanatomical circuitry. In J. F. Leckman & D. J. Cohen (Eds.), *Tourette's syndrome—tics, obsessions, compulsions: Developmental psychopathology and clinical care* (pp. 230–260). New York: Wiley.

Pierre, C. B., Nolan, E. E., Gadow, K. D., Sverd, J., & Sprafkin, J. (1999). Comparison of internalizing and externalizing symptoms in children with attention-deficit hyperactivity disorder with and without comorbid tic disorder. *Journal of Developmental and Behavioral Pediatrics, 20*(3), 170–176.

Pliszka, S. R. (2003). Psychiatric comorbidities in children with attention deficit hyperactivity disorder: Implications for management. *Paediatric Drugs, 5*(11), 741–750.

Reid, J. B., Patterson, G. R., & Snyder, J. (Eds.). (2002). *Antisocial behavior in children and adolescents: A developmental analysis and model for intervention.* Washington, DC: American Psychological Association.

Rice, B. J., Woolston, J., Stewart, E., Kerker, B. D., & Horwitz, S. M. (2002). Differences in younger, middle, and older children admitted to child psychiatric inpatient services. *Child Psychiatry and Human Development, 32*(4), 241–261.

Robertson, M. M., Banerjee, S., Eapen, V., & Fox-Hiley, P. (2002). Obsessive compulsive behaviour and depressive symptoms in young people with Tourette syndrome: A controlled study. *European Child and Adolescent Psychiatry, 11*(6), 261–265.

Robertson, M. M., Trimble, M. R., & Lees, A. J. (1988). The psychopathology of the Gilles de la Tourette syndrome: A phenomenological analysis. *British Journal of Psychiatry, 152*, 383–390.

Rosenberg, L. A., Brown, J., & Singer, H. S. (1995). Behavioral problems and severity of tics. *Journal of Clinical Psychology, 51*(6), 760–767.

Rosenberg, L. A., Harris, J. C., & Singer, H. S. (1984). Relationship of the Child Behavior Checklist to an independent measure of psychopathology. *Psychological Reports, 54*(2), 427–430.

Sallee, F. R., Kurlan, R., Goetz, C. G., Singer, H., Scahill, L., Law, G., et al. (2000). Ziprasidone treatment of children and adolescents with Tourette's syndrome: A pilot study. *Journal of the American Academy of Child and Adolescent Psychiatry, 39*(3), 292–299.

Sallee, F. R., Nesbitt, L., Jackson, C., Sine, L., & Sethuraman, G. (1997). Relative efficacy of haloperidol and pimozide in children and adolescents with Tourette's disorder. *American Journal of Psychiatry, 154*(8), 1057–1062.

Sandor, P., & Stephens, R. J. (2000). Risperidone treatment of aggressive behavior in children with Tourette syndrome. *Journal of Clinical Psychopharmacology, 20*(6), 710–712.

Scahill, L., Chappell, P. B., Kim, Y. S., Schultz, R. T., Katsovich, L., Shepherd, E., et al. (2001). A placebo-controlled study of guanfacine in the treatment of children with tic disorders and attention deficit hyperactivity disorder. *American Journal of Psychiatry, 158*(7), 1067–1074.

Scahill, L., Erenberg, G., & Tourette Syndrome Practice Parameter Work Group. (in press).

Contemporary assessment and pharmacotherapy of Tourette syndrome. *Movement Disorders.*

Scahill, L., Leckman, J. F., Schultz, R. T., Katsovich, L., & Peterson, B. S. (2003). A placebo-controlled trial of risperidone in Tourette syndrome. *Neurology, 60*(7), 1130–1135.

Scahill, L., Schwab-Stone, M., Merikangas, K. R., Leckman, J. F., Zhang, H., & Kasl, S. (1999). Psychosocial and clinical correlates of ADHD in a community sample of school-age children. *Journal of the American Academy of Child and Adolescent Psychiatry, 38*(8), 976–984.

Scahill, L., Sukhodolsky, D. G., Bearss, K., Findley, D. B., Hamrin, V., Carroll, D. H., et al. (2006). A randomized trial of parent management training in children with tic disorders and disruptive behavior. *Journal of Child Neurology, 21*(8), 650–656.

Scahill, L., Williams, S. K., Schwab-Stone, M., Applegate, J. O., & Leckman, J. F. (2006). Tic disorders and disruptive behavior in a community sample. *Advances in Neurology, 99*, 184–190.

Schur, S. B., Sikich, L., Findling, R. L., Malone, R. P., Crismon, M. L., Derivan, A., et al. (2003). Treatment recommendations for the use of antipsychotics for aggressive youth (TRAAY): Part I. A review. *Journal of the American Academy of Child and Adolescent Psychiatry, 42*(2), 132–144.

Sergeant, J. A., Geurts, H., & Oosterlaan, J. (2002). How specific is a deficit of executive functioning for attention-deficit/hyperactivity disorder? *Behavior Brain Research, 130*(1–2), 3–28.

Shapiro, E., Shapiro, A. K., Fulop, G., Hubbard, M., Mandeli, J., Nordlie, J., et al. (1989). Controlled study of haloperidol, pimozide and placebo for the treatment of Gilles de la Tourette's syndrome. *Archives of General Psychiatry, 46*(8), 722–730.

Silver, J. M., & Yudofsky, S. C. (1991). The Overt Aggression Scale: Overview and guiding principles. *Journal of Neuropsychiatry and Clinical Neurosciences, 3*(2), S22–S29.

Singer, H. S., & Rosenberg, L. A. (1989). Development of behavioral and emotional problems in Tourette syndrome. *Pediatric Neurology, 5*(1), 41–44.

Snider, L. A., Seligman, L. D., Ketchen, B. R., Levitt, S. J., Bates, L. R., Garvey, M. A., et al. (2002). Tics and problem behaviors in schoolchildren: Prevalence, characterization, and associations. *Pediatrics, 110*(2, Pt. 1), 331–336.

Snyder, K. V., Kymissis, P., Kessler, K., & Snyder, K. V. (1999). Anger management for adolescents: Efficacy of brief group therapy. *Journal of the American Academy of Child and Adolescent Psychiatry, 38*(11), 1409–1416.

Spencer, T., Biederman, M., Coffey, B., Geller, D., Wilens, T., & Faraone, S. (1999). The 4-year course of tic disorders in boys with attention-deficit/hyperactivity disorder. *Archives of General Psychiatry, 56*(9), 842–847.

Spencer, T., Biederman, J., Faraone, S., Mick, E., Coffey, B., Geller, D., et al. (2001). Impact of tic disorders on ADHD outcome across the life cycle: Findings from a large group of adults with and without ADHD. *American Journal of Psychiatry, 158*(4), 611–617.

Spencer, T., Biederman, J., Harding, M., O'Donnell, D., Wilens, T., Faraone, S., et al. (1998). Disentangling the overlap between Tourette's disorder and ADHD. *Journal of Child Psychology and Psychiatry and Allied Disciplines, 39*(7), 1037–1044.

Spielberger, C. D. (1988). *Manual for the State–Trait Anger Expression Inventory (STAXI).* Odessa, FL: Psychological Assessment Resources.

Stefl, M. E. (1984). Mental health needs associated with Tourette syndrome. *American Journal of Public Health, 74*(12), 1310–1313.

Stephens, R. J., Bassel, C., & Sandor, P. (2004). Olanzapine in the treatment of aggression and tics in children with Tourette's syndrome: A pilot study. *Journal of Child and Adolescent Psychopharmacology, 14*(2), 255–266.

Stephens, R. J., & Sandor, P. (1999). Aggressive behaviour in children with Tourette syndrome and comorbid attention-deficit hyperactivity disorder and obsessive–compulsive disorder. *Canadian Journal of Psychiatry, 44*(10), 1036–1042.

Stokes, A., Bawden, H. N., Camfield, P. R., Backman, J. E., & Dooley, J. M. (1991). Peer problems in Tourette's disorder. *Pediatrics, 87*(6), 936–942.

Sukhodolsky, D. G., Cardona, L., & Martin, A. (2005). Characterizing aggressive and noncompliant behaviors in a children's psychiatric inpatient setting. *Child Psychiatry and Human Development, 36*(2), 177–193.

Sukhodolsky, D. G., Scahill, L., Vitulano, L. A., Carroll, D., Findley, D. F., & Leckman, J. F. (in preparation). *Randomized controlled study of anger control training for adolescents with Tourette syndrome and disruptive behavior.*

Sukhodolsky, D. G., Scahill, L., Zhang, H., Peterson, B. S., King, R. A., Lombroso, P. J., et al. (2003). Disruptive behavior in children with Tourette's syndrome: Association with ADHD comorbidity, tic severity, and functional impairment. *Journal of the American Academy of Child and Adolescent Psychiatry, 42*(1), 98–105.

Sukhodolsky, D. G., Solomon, R. M., & Perine, J. (2000). Cognitive-behavioral, anger-control intervention for elementary school children: A treatment outcome study. *Journal of Child and Adolescent Group Therapy, 10*(3), 159–170.

Swanson, J. M. (1992). *School-based assessments and interventions for ADD students.* Irvine, CA: K. C. Publishing.

Tourette's Syndrome Study Group. (2002). Treatment of ADHD in children with tics: A randomized controlled trial. *Neurology, 58*(4), 527–536.

Van Egeren, L. A., Frank, S. J., & Paul, J. S. (1999). Daily behavior ratings among child and adolescent inpatients: The Abbreviated Child Behavior Rating Form. *Journal of the American Academy of Child and Adolescent Psychiatry, 38*(11), 1417–1425.

Vitiello, B., & Stoff, D. M. (1997). Subtypes of aggression and their relevance to child psychiatry. *Journal of the American Academy of Child and Adolescent Psychiatry, 36*(3), 307–315.

Vogt, A., & Carroll, A. (1999). The variation and variability of Tourette syndrome: A single case study approach. *Clinical Child Psychology and Psychiatry, 4*, 247–264.

Walkup, J. T., Khan, S., Schuerholz, L., Paik, Y.-S., Leckman, J. F., & Schultz, R. T. (1999). Phenomenology and natural history of tic-related ADHD and learning disabilities. In J. F. Leckman & D. J. Cohen (Eds.), *Tourette's syndrome—tics, obsessions, compulsions: Developmental psychopathology and clinical care* (pp. 63–79). New York: Wiley.

Wand, R. R., Matazow, G. S., Shady, G. A., Furer, P., & Staley, D. (1993). Tourette syndrome: Associated symptoms and most disabling features. *Neuroscience and Biobehavioral Reviews, 17*(3), 271–275.

Webster-Stratton, C. (1984). Randomized trial of two parent-training programs for families with conduct-disordered children. *Journal of Consulting and Clinical Psychology, 52*(4), 666–678.

Weisbrot, D. M., & Ettinger, A. B. (2002). Aggression and violence in mood disorders. *Child and Adolescent Psychiatric Clinics of North America, 11*(3), 649–671.

Wilson, R. S., Garron, D. C., Tanner, C. M., & Klawans, H. L. (1982). Behavior disturbance in children with Tourette syndrome. *Advances in Neurology, 35*, 329–333.

Yeates, K. O., & Bornstein, R. A. (1996). Neuropsychological correlates of learning disability subtypes in children with Tourette's syndrome. *Journal of the International Neuropsychological Society, 2*(5), 375–382.

Yudofsky, S. C., Silver, J. M., Jackson, W., Endicott, J., & Williams, D. (1986). The Overt Aggression Scale for the objective rating of verbal and physical aggression. *American Journal of Psychiatry, 143*(1), 35–39.

PART III

Clinical Management
of Secondary Problems

CHAPTER 11

Management of Familial Issues in Persons with Tourette Syndrome

GOLDA S. GINSBURG
JULIE NEWMAN KINGERY

As reviewed elsewhere in this text, Tourette's syndrome (TS) is associated with impairment in children's familial, social, and academic functioning. A growing literature has identified effective treatments that reduce the symptoms of TS and improve the lives of affected individuals. However, most of these treatments are individually focused and offer little guidance for families in how to manage TS and its related disorders. This omission is unfortunate because the lives of family members are directly impacted by TS. In this chapter we suggest that a critical component of any treatment plan is guidance for family members who, along with the affected individual, often struggle with how to cope with TS. Parenting a child with TS is further complicated by high rates of comorbid disorders, such as attention-deficit/hyperactivity disorder (ADHD), obsessive–compulsive disorder (OCD), and learning disorders (see Piacentini et al., Chapters 2, and Scahill et al., Chapter 4, this volume). In this connection, we discuss how the specific symptoms of TS and its comorbid conditions affect families, and we provide suggestions for managing these very challenging issues.

225

FAMILY DIFFICULTIES AND MANAGEMENT OF TS

Because the symptoms of TS almost always begin in childhood, family members such as parents and siblings tend to be most directly affected by this disorder. Several key areas of potential family difficulty have been identified in relation to TS, including:

1. Parents' initial reactions to the diagnosis of TS.
2. Family members' responses to tics.
3. Parenting a child with TS.
4. Increased conflict in sibling relations.
5. Strains on the marital relationship.

The difficulties encountered in each of these domains often create a stressful home environment that can exacerbate TS symptoms. Consequently, optimal treatment for TS should include all family members and address each of these family issues in order to minimize the negative impact of TS. Below we discuss the difficulties routinely encountered by families when a child has a tic disorder.

Reactions to the Initial Diagnosis

Parents' initial reaction to their child's diagnosis may be one of relief at finally receiving a diagnosis. However, parents may also experience feelings such as guilt about the causes of the illness, worry about their child's future, doubts about their competence to parent a child with TS, and embarrassment or shame when their child's illness is evident to others (Scahill, Ort, & Hardin, 1993). Indeed, one study comparing parents' self-concepts found that mothers of children with TS had significantly lower self-concepts than mothers of matched controls who did not have a neurological or psychiatric disorder (Edell-Fischer & Motta, 1990). The authors of this study concluded that parents are negatively affected by their child's diagnosis and that parents' reaction to their child's illness is an important issue to address in treatment. They suggest that parents of children with TS may require increased emotional support to cope with the needs of the child and family.

After receiving a diagnosis of TS, it is important for parents to acknowledge the various emotions that they are experiencing (e.g., anger, guilt, despair) and take steps to cope with these feelings by seeking extra emotional support from a friend or family member, talking with a professional or religious counselor, or focusing on a hobby or special interest (Haerle, 2002). Second, it is important for parents to "get the facts" about the symptoms and course of TS. Parents can access information about TS in a number of ways, including talking with a doctor who is knowledgeable about TS, contacting the national Tourette Syndrome Association (TSA) for informational pamphlets and videos (*www.tsa-usa.org*), joining a local TSA support group to connect with other parents who have a child with TS, and reading books and articles about TS. Once parents and other family members have accepted the diagnosis and have facts about the illness, they must learn how to respond to their child's tics and the challenges associated with parenting a child with TS on a daily basis.

Responding to Tics

Involving all family members in the treatment of TS is beneficial because they are often unsure about how to respond to tics. The manner in which parents and siblings respond to tics can have a significant impact both on the child and the family environment. Obviously, it is important for parents and other family members to restrain themselves from blaming or shaming the child when they tic. In an effort to be helpful, however, family members may fall into the habit of pointing out tics or unnecessarily comforting the child when tics occur. It is generally recommended that parents and other family members ignore tics as much as possible. Continually pointing out or making comments when a child tics can lead to an increase in stress and a subsequent worsening of the tics (Haerle, 2002). In contrast, ignoring the tics typically leads to reductions in their frequency and severity. Given that the task of ignoring tics is difficult, it may be helpful for parents to develop methods of distracting themselves and turning their focus to other tasks. If a child has a socially unacceptable tic that is nearly impossible to ignore (e.g., spitting at others), the parents could instruct their child to substitute a more socially acceptable tic (e.g., swallowing rather than spitting).

Functional analysis—that involves the identification of specific antecedents (i.e., what may trigger the tics) and consequences (i.e., how others respond or what happens after the child tics)—is a potentially useful strategy for identifying and ameliorating environmental factors that may be impacting tic expression (see Peterson, Chapter 8, this volume). An initial period of observing and recording this type of information on a simple chart is helpful in identifying exactly how people in the family are responding to tics. For instance, a child with an arm jerking tic may notice that this tic is most likely to occur at home after school, while watching TV or playing video games. When the tics occur, the child's mother comforts him, his brother tells him to stop it, and a fight might ensue. To minimize the tics, Mom should no longer comfort the child but rather allow him some time alone after school to unwind. Specific instructions should also be given to the brother to ignore the tics and leave the room if they bother him instead of teasing or fighting. This strategy requires careful attention and monitoring of how family members respond to tics but can help remove or reduce unhelpful consequences or reactions to tics that often go unidentified.

Parenting a Child with TS

One of the most difficult aspects of having a child with TS is the challenge placed upon parenting (Scahill et al., 1993; Walkup, 1999; Walkup & Riddle, 1997). Indeed, it is not uncommon for parents of children with TS to be more concerned about their child's disruptive behaviors than their tics. Research indicates that children with TS are more difficult to parent, and are therefore at a greater risk for developing behavior problems (Fava, 1997; Sukhodolsky & Scahill, Chapter 10, this volume). In trying to manage their child's behavior, parents of children with TS often implement a number of different parenting strategies and tend to give up when these strategies do not appear to be effective (Walkup, 1999). Unfortunately, it is difficult for these parents to implement behavior management strategies, such as applying rewards and/or punishment, consistently. One reason parents struggle with applying consistent parenting practices is because they are unclear about which behaviors their child can control versus those that are uncontrollable and tic related (Walkup, 1999). Parents may also feel guilty about disciplining their child with TS, whom they feel has to suffer through so many other challenges in his or her life. Consequently, parents tend to comfort their children when they tic or after they have exhibited a problem behavior, thereby reinforcing these behaviors and increasing the likelihood that they will occur again in the future. In light of the fact that stressful situations tend to exacerbate TS symptoms, parents may also attempt to intervene to protect their children when a problem has occurred (Scahill et al., 1993). When parents are overprotective, their children do not learn to take responsibility for their own behaviors or develop their own problem-solving skills. Thus, parents should be encouraged to allow their children to resolve developmentally appropriate conflicts and manage the typical stressors of childhood, thereby facilitating the development of problem-solving skills. These problem-solving skills will then transfer to managing the symptoms of TS.

In addition to ignoring tics as much as possible, it is crucial for parents to provide structure, consistency, and routine for children with TS (Kaplan, 1992). Having a daily routine (e.g., child gets up at the same time each day, has a certain sequence of activities after school through bedtime) helps to reduce unpredictable surprises that can exacerbate tics. As discussed later in this chapter, establishing a consistent structure is especially important for youngsters also suffering from comorbid ADHD or other behavioral problems. During the summer, parents can maintain a structured schedule by enrolling children in camp or other summer activities. Parents should also enforce clear rules and guidelines for acceptable behavior by consistently providing consequences when children do not follow these rules. Being consistent means that situations should be handled the same way each time (e.g., every time a child fights with a sibling, the same consequence is provided), and parents should be on the "same page" (i.e., parents handle situations in the same way). Writing expectations for the child on a chart and monitoring his or her progress can help parents improve their consistency, because written charts often serve as reminders for all family members and reduce conflict associated with ambiguous expectations.

A number of established and evidence-based parent training programs are available (e.g., Barkley, 1997; Barkley & Benton, 1998). In addition to developing new parenting skills and strategies, it is important for parents to remain optimistic, not catastrophize (e.g., always thinking the worst about a child's symptoms and the long-term course of TS), and to model coping skills for their child with TS. Parents can also take steps to boost their child's self-esteem. For instance, as noted above, parents should resist the temptation to be overprotective (e.g., rushing to a child's side to intervene when an interpersonal problem occurs). When children are allowed to face their own problems, they develop coping skills that can lead to increases in self-esteem and a sense of self-competence. Because so many aspects of TS are unpredictable, it is important for parents to allow their children to have a sense of mastery and control by making their own choices in as many areas as possible on a daily basis (e.g., what to wear). It is also crucial for families of children with TS to engage in normal family activities, such as going to the park, shopping, restaurants, and movies. Not only does this allow family members to spend quality time together, but it also provides opportunities for parents to model appropriate coping skills when tics occur in public places. When parents and siblings model an attitude of acceptance, the child with TS will also learn to accept his or her illness and gradually feel more comfortable with the diagnosis. Finally, it is important for parents to focus on their child's unique talents and abilities (Kaplan, 1992). Participating in sports or other group activities, such as Boy Scouts or Girl Scouts, could increase social skills and boost a child's self-esteem. Similarly, children who excel in art, music, or computer skills should be encouraged to develop these skills. Children with TS often are very aware of other reactions to their tics, which can have a negative impact on their self-esteem. Therefore, providing opportunities for children to nurture special talents is strongly recommended.

Sibling Relations

Another area of family life affected by TS is its toll on siblings and the sibling relationship. In the context of the family, siblings may experience differential treatment given to the child with TS and feel rejected or neglected. In response, siblings may become resentful and begin to display their own behavior problems, thereby increasing overall family distress and conflict in the home. Thus, strategies to manage sibling reactions are important to incorporate in the management of familial issues. Another common sibling reaction is embarrassment about the TS symptoms as the sibling may engage in tics when others are around, eliciting stares or comments. One consequence is that siblings may discourage friends from coming over to their family's house or refuse to attend family activities in public (Hansen, 1992). Embarrassment about TS becomes a particularly salient issue once siblings reach adolescence, when feelings of self-consciousness typically increase. Sibling relationships may also become strained. When children with TS display tics in public, their siblings may exhibit verbal or physical aggression in an effort to try to correct this behavior (Hansen, 1992). If a child has tics that involve inappropriate language or aggressive behavior (e.g., pinching, kicking, slapping) that is directed toward siblings, then siblings may retaliate aggressively.

In addition to the recommendations outlined in previous paragraphs regarding the best approaches for responding to tics, there are several ways in which parents can assist siblings of children with TS. Particularly after a child is first diagnosed, it is important for parents to explain the facts about TS to siblings. In discussing TS with the sibling, parents should emphasize that TS is not something that the child with TS can control (e.g., "like a hiccup") and that TS is not contagious (e.g., "not like the cold or flu"). Siblings should be instructed to ignore the tics whenever possible (Hansen, 1992). Because it is common for siblings to develop feelings of anger and jealousy because the child with TS receives a great deal of attention, it is essential for parents to set aside "special time" for the siblings, in which the parent and siblings engage in an enjoyable activity together. Also to reduce feelings of resentment, parents should distribute chores and other household responsibilities as evenly as possible between the child with TS and his or her sibling(s). It may also be helpful if parents arrange for the sibling to get to know other children who have a sibling with TS. To help the sibling cope with feelings of embarrassment, parents can engage the sibling in a discussion about his or her feelings surrounding TS, model coping with embarrassment in public, explain to the sibling that some individuals make fun of things that they do not understand, and emphasize that the sibling with TS is not deliberately trying to do things to embarrass family members. If a sibling is being victimized by the tics of the child with TS, it is important for parents to intervene to stop this behavior. If ignoring tics is difficult for the sibling, parents can provide a quiet place for the sibling to have time alone. Finally, because all children benefit from a structured and predictable routine, many of the general parenting tips for managing the behavior of children with TS would also apply to the other children in the family.

Marital Strain

Another family challenge associated with having a child with TS is its potential negative impact on the parents' marriage. For instance, parents may disagree about how best to respond to tics or upon the most appropriate parenting strategy. To reduce this negative impact, Hansen (1992) suggests that parents try to work together as a team as much as possible, sharing the day-to-day responsibilities of caring for the child with TS. Parents should also communicate openly with each other (e.g., express feelings, listen carefully to each other, talk about individual needs of each spouse). Finally, it is crucial for parents of children with TS to spend quality time together without their children (Haerle, 1992). In most cases, parents will have to deliberately schedule this time in advance to ensure that it actually occurs. It may be necessary for some couples to consult a professional (e.g., psychologist, social worker, marriage and family therapist) for assistance in working through their marital difficulties.

Taken together, there are several ways that living with a child who has TS can negatively impact on family functioning. Thus, even when children have only mild tics and no behavioral difficulties, psychoeducation about the disorder and guidance for family members can reduce the potential negative impact of TS (Petersen & Cohen, 1998). However, when youths with TS have comorbid behavior problems, additional interventions may be necessary. These issues are discussed next.

FAMILY DIFFICULTIES AND THE MANAGEMENT OF TS AND COMORBID CONDITIONS

Children with TS often present with a number of difficult to manage comorbid psychiatric and behavioral difficulties. The psychiatric disorders that most commonly co-occur with TS are attention-deficit/hyperactivity disorder (ADHD), oppositional defiant disorder (ODD), and obsessive–compulsive disorder (OCD; Dykens et al., 1990; Walkup, Scahill, & Riddle, 1995; see also Scahill et al., Chapter 4; Harrison et al., Chapter 7; Buhlmann et al., Chapter 9, this volume). Children with these comorbid conditions evidence high rates of impulsivity, aggression, anxiety, attentional difficulties, and obsessive–compulsive behaviors (e.g., Rosenberg, Brown, & Singer, 1995). In contrast to tic severity, which generally peaks between ages 9 and 14 (Leckman et al., 1998), these comorbid conditions are often chronic and associated with disability that may increase over the lifespan. Children who present with TS and these comorbid conditions experience greater impairments in their self-perceptions, academic performance, and peer relations than youths with TS only (e.g., Bawden, Stokes, Camfield, Camfield, & Salisbury, 1998; Dykens et al., 1990; Edell-Risher & Motta, 1990; Stokes, Bawden, Camfield, Backman, & Dooley, 1991). Conflicted family relationships are also a more common occurrence in these families, because comorbidity exacerbates the challenges that parents of children with TS encounter in their daily lives (Carter et al., 2000; Sukhodolsky et al., 2003). In fact, the comorbid psychiatric diagnoses, behavioral problems, and psychosocial difficulties that co-occur with TS are usually more disabling than the tics and are often the reason that parents initially seek professional attention for their child.

Impact of TS and Comorbid Conditions

Current understanding of the impact of TS and comorbid conditions on family members' adjustment and family functioning is based largely on clinical experience. However, the small numbers of studies that have empirically evaluated this topic indicate that TS complicated by comorbid disorders has a greater negative impact on family functioning than TS alone. Carter and colleagues (2000) compared the social–emotional and family functioning of children with TS alone, children with a dual diagnosis of TS and ADHD, and control children with no psychiatric diagnosis. Various aspects of children's behavioral and social–emotional adjustment were assessed, and information about the quality of the parents' marital relationship and family functioning (e.g., extent of support, conflict, emotional expression within the family) was obtained. Relevant here were results that children with poorer social–emotional adjustment had poorer quality of family relations and that children with TS and comborbid ADHD reported the poorest adjustment. In similar fashion, Sukhodolsky et al. (2003) compared the relationship between disruptive behavior and family functioning in children with TS only, children with

TS and comorbid ADHD, children with ADHD only, and control children. In terms of family functioning, the families of children with TS and comorbid ADHD did not differ from those of children with ADHD only. However, both of these groups had significantly more family conflict and less cohesion than the control families. The children with TS only did not differ from controls on family functioning variables. These researchers concluded that the presence of comorbid disruptive behavior problems in children with TS places an extra strain on family functioning. It is likely that this relationship is reciprocal. The more behavior problems a child has, the poorer the family functioning, and the poorer the family functioning, the more likely the child is to develop behavior problems.

Clinical experience also bears out findings from empirical research. Family relations of children with TS and comorbid disruptive behaviors tend to be strained and conflicted. Frequently, a pattern of negative and coercive parent–child interactions develops. Parents spend so much of their time trying to manage their child's noncompliant or disruptive behavior that they have little time or energy for positive parent–child interactions, such as providing praise or engaging in enjoyable activities with their child. As noted above, child behavior problems can also negatively impact on the parents' relationship. One source of potential marital conflict is differences in child behavior management styles between parents, especially if the parents' strategies are ineffective. In one study, marital satisfaction was significantly negatively correlated with these comorbid child externalizing behaviors (Carter et al., 2000).

Overall, it appears that a child with TS that is complicated by comorbid psychopathology has a greater impact on family functioning than a child with TS alone (see also Wilkinson et al., 2001). This information underscores the importance of identifying and treating these comorbid conditions in children with TS. It is even more critical for parents and other family members to equip themselves with the knowledge and skills necessary to be as helpful as possible in response to these related disorders and seek professional assistance when needed. Below we discuss specific parenting skills that might be helpful for families when their child has TS and comorbid disruptive behavior problems.

Behavior Management Programs

A substantial literature indicates that the skills taught in parent–child behavior management interventions are effective in reducing the types of comorbid disruptive behavior problems present in children with TS (see Taylor & Biglan, 1998; Brestan & Eyberg, 1998, for reviews). Across numerous studies, parent–child behavior management programs have produced improvements in child behavior, with both short- and long-term maintenance of treatment gains (Taylor & Biglan, 1998). Given the broad utility of parent–child behavior management programs and the strong research support for their use, it is surprising that researchers are only now beginning to evaluate the effectiveness of using these programs for comorbid behavior difficulties in children with TS (Scahill et al., 2006).

Compounding the limited research on parent–child behavior management programs for youths with TS is the fact that these programs are not frequently employed by clinicians involved in the treatment of children with TS—neither as an adjunctive strategy to medications or as a "front-line" approach. In part, this omission occurs because most medical professionals who treat children with TS (i.e., neurologists and psychiatrists) receive little or no training in these important interventions. In light of the short- and long-term impairment caused by these comorbid behavior problems and the effectiveness of established psychosocial treatments in other child populations, they are presented here as a tool for parents to use in managing disruptive behaviors that often co-occur with TS.

A parent–child behavior management program for children with TS should be specifically tailored to include (1) education about TS and why children with TS are more difficult to parent; (2) how children with and without TS tend to develop behavioral difficulties; and (3) parent–child behavior management skills that recognize the unique role of TS in the day-to-day life of the child and family. Parents of children with TS should also be taught to modify their own negative attributions for their child's behaviors (e.g., that children are faking symptoms, being manipulative, or cannot control their noncompliant behavior because they have a neurological disorder).

The skills taught in parent–child behavior management programs are based primarily upon social learning and behavioral principles. In this connection, parents are taught how patterns of child noncompliance develop or are learned over time. More specifically, and as noted earlier, children's behavior is greatly influenced by how parents and others respond to their behavior or the consequences of behaviors. When a child's behavior (including tics) is followed by reinforcement either by a parent or another person or event (e.g., praise, privileges, a special activity, escape from an aversive activity), the reinforced behavior is more likely to occur in the future. Alternatively, parents can unintentionally reinforce children's defiant or aggressive behavior by making this behavior the focus of their attention. Parents' attention, even in the form of yelling, can unintentionally reinforce inappropriate behaviors (Taylor &

Biglan, 1998). Thus, rather than attending to inappropriate behavior, parents can learn to remove children from any reinforcement or attention (e.g., by ignoring a minor tantrum) for a brief period of time after misbehavior occurs, thereby reducing the likelihood that the child's inappropriate behavior will occur in the future. With this approach children "learn" that their misbehavior will no longer get a reward, parents' attention, or escape from something aversive (e.g., cleaning their room).

Another goal of parent–child behavior management is to disrupt coercive interactions. That is, families of children with behavior problems tend to develop coercive patterns of interaction that seem effective in the short term but do not lead to reductions in problematic child behaviors in the long term (Patterson, 1982). For example, a parent may yell to try to convince a child to clean his or her room, and the child may respond with whining and complaining. If the parent eventually stops insisting that the child complete this task (because he or she can no longer stand the whining and complaining), the child's complaining behavior and noncompliance are reinforced (negatively) by the *removal* of the parent's yelling. The parent's behavior of removing the request is also reinforced (negatively) by the fact that the child stopped complaining. As a result, the child's whining or complaining and the parent's removal of the request are both more likely to occur again in the future (Patterson, 1982). Alternatively, if the child complies after the repeated yelling, the parent's yelling is reinforced and more likely to occur as a first-line approach in the future. With each similar interaction, the potential for escalating conflict increases (e.g., parent yells louder, child whines louder/longer). Parent–child behavior management programs aim to modify these coercive interaction patterns, of which children and parents are often unaware and which usually escalate over time.

Monitoring Systems

Once parents have a better understanding of how these coercive interactions develop and how they can modify their child's behavior through reinforcement (or the removal of reinforcement), additional skills may be useful. Application of all skills should begin with the use of a monitoring system. Monitoring systems such as charts or calendars help parents and children identify the frequency of problematic behaviors and times of the day when those disruptive behaviors are most likely to occur. A monitoring system also allows parents to track progress and change over time. In addition, written monitoring systems can reduce conflict between children and parents over expectations or consequences and how they will be implemented. Moreover, they increase parents' consistency, force parents to be proactive about rewards and consequences, provide explicit instructions to children, and help establish a structured schedule at home in which activities can be carefully planned and scheduled based on the child's behavior. Finally, written and explicit monitoring systems can increase children's self-control skills as they learn to manage and monitor their own behaviors on a day-to-day basis.

Selective Attending

Another useful skill is that of selective attending. Using this skill, the parent carefully watches for moments when the child is behaving appropriately and provides specific verbal praise or rewards during these times. Arranging a daily "special time" in which parents and children engage in 10–15 minutes of quality time together (e.g., playing with Legos, coloring, playing a game) often provides a good opportunity for parents to apply this skill (Hembree-Kigin & McNeil, 1995). During this time, parents should follow the child's lead, allow them to choose the activity, use few requests or commands, and look for opportunities to praise or positively reinforce the child's appropriate behavior.

Delivery of Commands

In addition to attending to children's positive behaviors, parents can reduce problematic child behaviors, such as noncompliance, by improving their delivery of commands. Reducing unnecessary commands, making commands more specific and direct, providing a clear consequence if a child does not comply with the parent's request, and consistently following through with the stated consequence if a child does not comply are all aspects of effective delivery. More specifically, parents are instructed not to provide a command unless they are willing to "follow through" and provide a consequence (e.g., removal of a privilege) if a child does not comply. Parents are encouraged to provide commands in the form of direct statements that are very specific (e.g., "Please hang up your coat on this hook right here"), rather than general questions (e.g., "Can you pick up your things by the door?"). Parents are also taught to provide single commands (e.g., "Please take your plate to the counter"), rather than commands that include many different tasks ("Please clean up your plate, put it in the dishwasher, wipe the table, and then sweep the floor"), and to allow an adequate amount of time for the child to complete each task before delivering a new command. Other effective command-giving skills that parents learn include making eye contact with their child, reducing distractions in the environment when giving a command, and having the child repeat the command to make sure that he or she understood it. Most parent–child behavior management programs incorporate "compliance training periods" in which parents schedule two to three 3- to 5-minute time periods per day in which they deliver a series of simple commands for the child to complete (e.g., Barkley, 1997; Hembree-Kigin & McNeil, 1995).

Point System

Although selective attending with verbal praise and effective delivery of commands will lead to increases in compliance, a point or token system with concrete rewards typically produces greater change in children's behavior. To develop a point system to use at home, parents and children begin by creating lists of daily, weekly, and long-term rewards and privileges (Anastopoulos, 1998). Parents and children also work together to create a list of chores (e.g., making bed, doing homework) and other "target" behaviors (e.g., sharing with a sibling) and assign a point value to each item on this list. Children earn the predetermined number of points for completing the tasks or demonstrating the behaviors that are on the list. Parents can also provide "bonus points" for chores that are done particularly well or behaviors that a child exhibits without a parental reminder. Younger children (under 8 years old) respond well to a tangible reminder of points earned, such as plastic poker chips that can be deposited into a special container (Barkley, 1997). Older children can record points on a chart or in a notebook that is kept in a visible place at home. After a point system is implemented for a week or two, parents may need to make adjustments to the point values and may choose to gradually add additional target behaviors to the list. Given that establishing and maintaining an effective point system can be quite complicated, parents may find it helpful to consult with a psychologist or other professional with expertise in child behavior management strategies.

During the first few weeks of a point system, parents are typically instructed to use the program only for rewarding appropriate behavior (rather than deducting points for noncompliance). Once the point system is working smoothly, parents can expand it to include *response cost*—that is, deducting points for noncompliance with tasks or disruptive behavior. Parents begin this phase of the strategy by choosing one or two items on the list and letting children know that they will lose points or chips from their "bank" if they fail to complete these tasks. The number of points or chips that a child loses for noncompliance is equal to the number of points that he or she would have earned for completing the task (Anastopoulos, 1998). Adding response cost to the point system often leads to a higher level of compliance because children become highly motivated about not losing points that they have already earned. When using response cost, parents are cautioned not to take away so many points that a child has a negative number of points in his or her bank. If a child is repeatedly noncompliant, rather than continuing to take away large amounts of points, parents may have to rely on a secondary method of discipline, such as time out from specific activities. If a parent is not using a point system, then response cost can involve removing privileges or special activities (e.g., 30 minutes less computer time).

Time Out

In addition to response cost, many parent–child behavior management programs incorporate a time-out strategy. Although most noncompliant or disruptive behavior will be addressed through response cost, there may be a few more severe behaviors (e.g., hitting) for which parents will need to use time out (Anastopoulos, 1998). Many parents report that they have tried time out with little success. However, the time-out strategies that parents learn in a structured parent–child behavior management program are usually much different from what they have tried at home in the past. Skilled clinicians work very closely with parents to plan how time out will be implemented, including where the time-out area will be located and what back-up strategies parents can use if the child leaves time out (e.g., early bed time for older children, safe physical restraint for younger children). The exact time-out procedure varies slightly across parent–child behavior management programs, but the following procedure is generally followed: (1) The child must spend a minimum number of minutes in time out (e.g., 1 minute for each year of age); (2) after the minimum amount of time, parents may approach the time-out area only if the child is quiet; (3) after sitting in time out, the child must complete the original request (e.g., "Please pick up your toy"). The time-out procedure is repeated until compliance occurs. Similar to developing and refining a point system, consultation with a skilled clinician is advised for parents who are interested in developing a discipline program that includes time out.

Public Places and Transitions

Once parents have successfully implemented the point system, response cost, and time-out procedures at home, they are ready to learn about managing their child's behavior in public places (e.g., grocery stores, restaurants) and during transitions from one activity to the next. In this component of parent–child behavior management programs, parents learn to anticipate potential behavior problems before they actually occur and develop a plan for dealing with this behavior (Barkley, 1997). For example, just before entering a public place such as a store, parents can stop and spend a few minutes reviewing the rules that a child is expected to follow (e.g., "Stand close to me, don't touch anything") and then ask the child to repeat these rules back to the parent. Next, parents inform the child that he or she will earn a certain number of points for complying with the rules. Parents should also clearly state the consequence for not following the rules. Finally, parents can occupy a child's attention and reduce the likelihood of misbehavior by giving the child an activity to complete (e.g., checking items off of a list, helping the parent find specific foods). The procedure mentioned here can also be used to ease transitions from one activity to the next. For example, before a relative comes to visit, parents can spend a few minutes discussing rules, an incentive for good behavior, consequences for misbehavior, and then assigning an activity for the child to complete (e.g., making a welcome sign for the front door or place cards for the dinner table). Other key transition times include before a friend comes over to play, when shifting from playtime to homework time, or before a child goes outside to play. By planning ahead, parents can greatly reduce, and sometimes even prevent, the occurrence of misbehavior (Barkley, 1997).

Over the course of parent–child behavior management programs, therapists also often assist parents in setting developmentally appropriate expectations and consequences for their child's behavior, extending the family's behavior management plan into the school setting through a daily behavior report card that teachers can complete, and helping children and parents to develop and utilize effective problem-solving skills. All of these strategies are designed to reduce child disruptive behaviors and foster more positive parent–child relations.

SUMMARY AND CONCLUSIONS

TS and related tic disorders directly affect the lives of all family members. Specifically, family members often have difficulty adjusting to the diagnosis and responding to tics. Conflicts may arise among siblings or within the coparenting relationship. Parenting a child with TS, particularly when comorbid disruptive behavior disorders are present, is especially challenging. In light of the difficulties experienced by family members, treatments should address these issues by providing support, information, and instruction to all family members. This chapter discussed the specific challenges that family members face and provided specific guidelines to assist in improving family functioning.

REFERENCES

American Psychiatric Association. (1994). *Diagnostic and statistical manual of mental disorders* (4th ed.). Washington, DC: Author.

Anastopoulos, A. D. (1998). A training program for parents of children with attention-deficit/hyperactivity disorder. In J. M. Briesmeister & C. E. Schaefer (Eds.), *Handbook of parent training: Parents as co-therapists for children's behavior problems* (pp. 27–60). New York: Wiley.

Barkley, R. A. (1997). *Defiant children: A clinician's manual for assessment and parent training* (2nd ed.). New York: Guilford Press.

Barkley, R. A., & Benton, C. M. (1998). *Your defiant child: Eight steps to better behavior.* New York: Guilford Press.

Bawden, H. N., Stokes, A., Camfield, C. S., Camfield, P. R., & Salisbury, S. (1998). Peer relationship problems in children with Tourette's disorder or diabetes mellitus. *Journal of Child Psychology and Psychiatry, 39,* 663–668.

Brestan, E. V., & Eyberg, S. M. (1998). Effective psychosocial treatments of conduct-disordered children and adolescents: 29 years, 82 studies, and 5, 272 kids. *Journal of Clinical Child Psychology, 27,* 180–189.

Carter, A. S., O'Donnell, D. A., Schultz, R. T., Scahill, L., Leckman, J. F., & Pauls, D. L. (2000). Social and emotional adjustment in children affected with Gilles de la Tourette's syndrome: Associations with ADHD and family functioning. *Journal of Child Psychology and Psychiatry, 41,* 215–223.

Dykens, E. M., Leckman, J. F., Riddle, M. A., Hardin, M. T., Schwartz, S., & Cohen, D. J. (1990). Intellectual, academic, and adaptive functioning of Tourette syndrome children with and without attention deficit disorder. *Journal of Abnormal Child Psychology, 18,* 607–615.

Edell-Fischer, B. H., & Motta, R. W. (1990). Tourette syndrome: Relation to children's and parents' self-concepts. *Psychological Reports, 66,* 539–545.

Fava, M. (1997). Psychopharmacologic treatment of pathologic aggression. *Psychiatric Clinics of North America, 20,* 427–451.

Haerle, T. (1992). Adjusting to your child's diagnosis. In T. Hearle (Ed.), *Children with Tourette syndrome: A parents' guide* (pp. 27–52). Rockville, MD: Woodbine House.

Hansen, C. R. (1992). Children with Tourette syndrome and their families. In T. Hearle (Ed.), *Children with Tourette syndrome: A parents' guide* (pp. 113–138). Rockville, MD: Woodbine House.

Hembree-Kigin, T. L., & McNeil, C. B. (1995). *Parent–child interaction therapy.* New York: Plenum Press.

Kaplan, M. (1992). Daily life with your child. In T. Hearle (Ed.), *Children with Tourette syndrome: A parents' guide* (pp. 71–111). Rockville, MD: Woodbine House.

Leckman, J. F., Zhang, H., Vitale, A., Lahnin, F., Lynch, K., Bondi, C., et al. (1998). Trajectories of tic severity in Tourette's syndrome: The first two decades. *Pediatrics, 102,* 14–19.

Patterson, G. (1982). *Coercive family process.* Eugene, OR: Castalia.

Peterson, B. S., & Cohen, D. J. (1998). The treatment of Tourette's syndrome: Multimodal, developmental intervention. *Journal of Clinical Psychiatry, 59*(Suppl. 1), 62–72.

Rosenberg, L. A., Brown, J., & Singer, H. S. (1995). Behavioral problems and severity of tics. *Journal of Clinical Psychology, 51,* 760–767.

Scahill, L., Ort, S. I., & Hardin, M. T. (1993). Tourette's syndrome: Part II. Contemporary approaches to assessment and treatment. *Archives of Psychiatric Nursing, 7,* 209–216.

Scahill, L., Sukhodolsky, D. G., Bearss, K., Findley, D., Hamrin, V., Carroll, D. H., & Rains, A. L. (2006). Randomized trial of parent management training in children with tic disorders and disruptive behavior. *Journal of Child Neurology, 21,* 650–656.

Stokes, A., Bawden, H. N., Camfield, P. R., Backman, J. E., & Dooley, J. M. (1991). Peer problems in Tourette's disorder. *Pediatrics, 87,* 936–942.

Sukhodolsky, D. G., Scahill, L., Zhang, H., Peterson, B. S., King, R. A., Lombroso, P. J., et al. (2003). Disruptive behavior in children with Tourette's syndrome: Association with ADHD comorbidity, tic severity, and functional impairment. *Journal of the American Academy of Child and Adolescent Psychiatry, 42,* 98–105.

Taylor, T. K., & Biglan, A. (1998). Behavioral family interventions for improving child-rearing: A review of the literature for clinicians and policy makers. *Clinical Child and Family Psychology Review, 1,* 41–60.

Walkup, J. T. (1999). The psychiatry of Tourette syndrome. *CNS Spectrums, 4,* 54–61.

Walkup, J. T., & Riddle, M. A. (1997). Tic disorders. In A. Tasman, J. Kay, & J. Lieberman (Eds.), *Psychiatry* (pp. 702–719). Philadelphia: Saunders.

Walkup, J. T., Scahill, L., & Riddle, M. A. (1995). Disruptive behavior, hyperactivity and learning disabilities in children with Tourette's syndrome. In W. J. Weiner & A. E. Lang (Eds.), *Advances in neurology* (Vol. 65, pp. 259–272). New York: Raven Press.

Wilkinson, B. J., Newman, M. B., Shytle, R. D., Silver, A. A., Sanberg, P. R., & Sheehan, D. (2001). Family impact of Tourette's syndrome. *Journal of Child and Family Studies, 10,* 477–483.

World Health Organization. (1993). *The ICD-10 classification of mental and behavioural disorders: Diagnostic criteria for research.* Geneva, Switzerland: Author.

CHAPTER 12

Management of Learning and School Difficulties in Children with Tourette Syndrome

HAYDEN O. KEPLEY
SUSAN CONNERS

One of the more difficult facets of coping with Tourette syndrome (TS) may be developing and implementing an educational plan for a child with TS. There are a number of complicating factors about TS that can present a challenging situation for parents and educators. Although there are some similarities across children with TS and chronic tic disorders, each child will present with a unique clinical and educational history. Although some children with the disorder can be quite disruptive and require significant accommodations in their educational environment, school personnel may be unaware that other children have the disorder. Not only does TS manifest in presentations that range from mild to severe, it is further complicated by tics that wax and wane. Thus there are times when tics will appear more severe and may be more disruptive in the school environment, and at other times, the child may appear symptom free. Additionally, we know that children with TS reflect the normal intelligence curve, with most possessing average intelligence (Chappell, Leckman, & Riddle, 1995; Hagin, Beecher, Pagano, & Kreeger, 1982). Some will be exceptional students, others will be athletes, and others will express their talents artistically or musically. Indeed, children with TS are just like other children with the exception that they carry the additional burden of a neurological disorder (Walter & Carter, 1997). Given the variance of tics, assessment and treatment of TS at school may be challenging—a situation that underscores the importance of educating school personnel about the disorder. School professionals will play a critical role in the evaluation and implementation of a treatment plan. Although the percentage of children with TS is small and those children requiring intervention at school is even smaller, their behaviors in the classroom do have the potential to be quite disruptive. Thus school professionals should be well informed about recent research on TS and how this research may guide intervention strategies.

WHEN TO INTERVENE

Not all children and teenagers with TS will require school intervention or specialized education plans. In fact, the majority will not require services. Others may simply need a supportive and accepting environment in order to function well. Specific intervention and advocacy, however, are indicated when (1) there is a significant decline in grades or the child is falling behind; (2) the student evidences increased frustration; (3) the student evidences significant problems with self-esteem; (4) the student has no friends or is having problems with peer acceptance; (5) the student evidences a negative change in attitude regarding school or teachers; (6) behavioral problems at school interfere in some manner; and (7) the student evidences an increase in tics or TS symptoms that interfere with his or her ability to learn or participate in class activities (Cohen, 1990; Giordano, 2004; Packer, 2005). Sometimes parents may fear that their child will be "labeled" if they inform the school or teacher that the child has a diagnosis of TS. The assumptions behind this type of fear are typically unfounded and may do more to hinder the child if the parents fail to advocate for him or her (Giordano, 2004). If the symptoms are serious enough for parents to seek professional guidance and receive a diagnosis, they are most likely causing some difficulty at school. Early advocacy for the child can prevent failing grades, school refusal, school suspensions, and considerable school-related stress. There are many ways in which a teacher or other school professionals may be helpful to a child with TS without requiring special education services. However, this ability to help will always be predicated upon the teacher's (or other school personnel) awareness of the tics as well as an understanding of the complexities of TS. Raising awareness is always the first step when advocating for a child.

TEACHER AND SCHOOL TRAINING

The academic success of children with TS not only depends on awareness of school personnel and good documentation (to be explained later) but also on the willingness of teachers, classroom aides, and school psychologists to actively engage in working with the students identified as having TS. School administrators must also be involved and interested in the identification and intervention process for students with TS and its related difficulties. Further, the teacher's knowledge of TS (its complexities and changing presentation) and his or her attitude will be critical. When teachers do not understand the causes, course, and outcome of this disorder, the behavioral manifestations will be misattributed, and little will be gained when trying to implement behavioral interventions in the classroom. On the other hand, when there is a positive teacher–student relationship, based on an understanding of the student and the disorder, the potential for academic and social gains in the classroom is much stronger. Teachers should be aware of the following facts about TS and chronic tic disorders:

- TS is neurobiological in nature. It is a chronic disorder that is treatable but not curable. It is an educational disability. Interventions in the classroom can have a profound and positive impact because the disorder, as well as its common comorbid conditions, are very sensitive to the environment.
- Tics are purposeless and meaningless motor movements and vocalizations that may range from simple to complex. Motor tics vary from simple eye blinking and facial grimacing to more complex tapping, touching, and kicking. Vocal tics also range from simple sniffing, coughing, and throat clearing to complex words and phrases. Although coprolalia (verbalizing obscenities) is one of the more publicized and recognized vocal tics, it is actually quite rare.
- Although tics are involuntary, children are typically able to suppress them for certain periods of time. Tic suppression should not be confused or misunderstood as intentional control of the occurrence of tics. Suppression often takes great effort and also has the strange effect of increasing the urge to tic as well as decreasing the child's attention to the task at hand (Scahill, Ort, & Hardin, 1993). Schoolwork may be adversely affected as a result of suppression. A child who appears to be well behaved and is sitting quietly may actually be focused on suppressing his or her tics. On the other hand, if the child concentrates on schoolwork and does not suppress the tics, he or she runs the risk of being viewed as a disruptive behavior problem by the teacher as well as being teased by classmates (Stokes, Bawden, Camfield, Backman, & Dooley, 1991).

• Tics wax and wane over time. Not only may the teacher observe periods of relatively tic-free intervals, but also periods when the tics occur in intense bouts. A further complication of the situation is that tics change over time. Some tics may gradually disappear over time, and new tics may emerge. Thus, not only do the frequency and intensity of tics vary during the day and weeks, but the expression of the tics changes over time. Every child with TS will display a unique and changing presentation of the disorder.

Education about tic disorders can be gained from in-service presentations and by providing school personnel with brief reading materials or videos. Numerous educational materials are available from the Tourette Syndrome Association. Many educational professionals may need training about the disorder because it is not as common as disruptive behavior disorders such as attention-deficit/hyperactivity disorder (ADHD) and internalizing disorders such as anxiety. All teachers who have contact with a child with TS should have at least a basic understanding of the disorder so that they can interact with the child in a supportive way. Those school professionals who have teaching responsibilities with the children will need more training in order to implement effective behavioral programs in their classroom. Pfiffner, Barkley, and DuPaul (2006) describe how schools can educate their staff members on how to implement these strategies. Briefly, although 1–day in-service programs may be sufficient for imparting knowledge about the disorder, they are not adequate to cover behavioral modification programs. To overcome this problem, some schools have sponsored ongoing consultation with behavioral experts following an in-service training. Other schools have begun collaborative consultation models wherein a behavioral consultant or school psychologist works with general and special education teachers to assess specific student needs and to design and implement interventions (Shapiro et al., 1996).

MANAGING CLASSROOM BEHAVIOR

Special education teachers who have small class sizes and prior experience with behavioral management programs may have little difficulty when implementing these programs in their classroom. General education teachers, however, who have 25 or more children in their class may find that these programs are not feasible because they demand increased record keeping, closer monitoring of the child, and the dispensing of rewards/consequences. Without this kind of systematic intervention, symptoms of TS and its co-occurring disorders are more likely to emerge. In general, TS symptoms are much less problematic when the child is engaged in schoolwork at a pace that does not add increased pressure or stress. To the extent that these conditions can be achieved in the classroom, children often perform more successfully. For this reason, consideration should be given to incorporating the following motivational strategies:

1. When children with TS become upset, anxious (Silva, Munoz, Barickman, & Friedhoff, 1995), or stressed (Surwillo, Shafii, & Barrett, 1978), they are more prone to tic; therefore, it is often necessary to provide them with a nurturing and supportive environment, which may include giving them more supportive feedback about their performance. Teachers should consider providing relatively more feedback, particularly positive, than would be the case for other children in the classroom. Additionally, acceptance and support in the classroom—by ignoring the majority of nondisruptive tics and not expressing frustration when tics do occur—will be the key to managing a child with tics. Modeling acceptance and support will also demonstrate to classmates how they should respond to a child with tics.

2. For children with disruptive behaviors (e.g., hyperactivity/ impulsivity) and disruptive tics, incentives should be incorporated into the school programming as much as possible. Such incentives or rewards should be meaningful to the children and delivered in a frequent, immediate, and consistent manner. To reduce the possibility that children will become bored with this type of programming, target behaviors and consequences should be modified periodically. Rewards may include helping the teacher, stickers, verbal praise, and any other rewards upon which both child and teacher agree. The emphasis should be on frequency and consistency in order to help modify the behavior in the classroom. In addition, efforts should be made to notice and reward the child's appropriate behavior at least as much as punishing inappropriate behavior. One caveat to note is that when managing tic behaviors in the classroom, there is empirical support for only positive consequences to be utilized (i.e., reward for use of a competing response or modified tic), because negative and/or neutral consequences, such as punishing tic occurrence, are likely to have negative outcomes (i.e., increased ticcing; Packer, 2005).

3. Although classroom applications of behavior management programs are highly desirable, they are often difficult to incorporate for only one child in a regular classroom setting. Thus, it is usually necessary to consider alternative approaches for children with TS or associated disorders. One such alternative is to incorporate a daily report card system. In this system, teachers monitor various classroom behaviors by

providing ratings on an index card, which is sent home on a daily basis. Parents then convert these ratings into either positive or negative consequences (e.g., loss of television privileges), which for many children are more meaningful and effective than those readily available in school. The child's caretaker and teachers should discuss which specific behaviors need to be targeted and develop a list of several measurable behaviors to work on each week.

Parents may be unfortunately confronted with the teacher who is unwilling to implement behavioral modifications in the classroom or unwilling to work with children who have TS for "theoretical" reasons. In such cases where there is poor teacher motivation or when teacher philosophy comes into conflict with the interventions necessary to affect a TS student's academic success, parents should be encouraged to strongly advocate for their child by appealing to school administrators for greater teacher accountability or a transfer to another classroom or school. Children with TS who have an Individualized Education Plan (IEP) or Section 504 plan may have certain legal protections, which are explained later.

PARENT–SCHOOL COLLABORATION

The academic success of a child, whether he or she is diagnosed with TS, any other disorder, or has no psychiatric history, will depend on the relationship between the school and the parents. A collaborative relationship between the parents and school personnel is going to be necessary for effective evaluation and treatment. When the parents and teachers are knowledgeable about TS and tics in general, have realistic expectations, and are motivated to work with the child who has TS, then a strong partnership will easily develop (Carter et al., 1999; Pfiffner et al., 2006). In other situations, conflicts between the home and school can be crippling and ultimately hinder the child's academic progress. In these cases, parents may blame the school for their child's difficulties and feel that the school system is not responding to their child's needs. Teachers may feel that the child's troubles in school are caused from problems in the family and that medication be used instead of classroom accommodations (federal guidelines prohibit schools from insisting that a child be medicated in order to remain in school). These types of parent–school conflicts have escalated in recent years, as seen by the number of lawsuits filed against school districts and other involvement with the legal system and child advocates when attempting to determine a child's appropriate educational placement (Pfiffner et al., 2006). Some of the difficulty may arise from misconceptions about the disorder, which can be addressed through education about TS or consultation with a school psychologist or other mental health professional. Another source of difficulty may arise from the reluctance of school districts to provide specialized services. If the ultimate aim of the school and the parents is truly the welfare of the child, however, then both sides will need to set aside blame and work toward creating an environment that will maximize the child's learning both at home and at school.

There is also a need to establish generally consistent and complementary behavioral interventions in all settings where problems occur. Use of behavioral systems such as the daily report card (DRC) can help establish similar programs at school and home. Additionally, the DRC helps to facilitate ongoing communication between the school and parents, which is essential when planning and tailoring educational interventions. This shared knowledge of the child's strengths, educational needs, and changes in specific target behaviors will greatly enhance the academic planning and behavioral strategies. Further, behavioral changes in one setting rarely generalize to other settings unless interventions are in place at all affected settings (Pfiffner et al., 2006). This need for consistent interventions underscores the importance of both parents and teachers working together.

CO-OCCURRING DISORDERS

The good news about TS is that most children with this disorder do not need formal modifications to their education plan, although it is still a good idea to educate teachers and other school professionals about TS and common comorbid conditions such as obsessive–compulsive disorder (OCD) and ADHD. Learning disabilities (LD) are also quite common in children with ADHD, and formal testing may be needed to assess for these. Children with these co-occurring disorders will most likely require more specific educational modifications, including special education services received through an IEP or Section 504 plan. When this is the case, and as stated previously, complementary behavioral modification programs at home and school will be most beneficial for the child. To date there are no formal studies examining the best approaches to educational modifications or structured programs for a child with TS. For ADHD, however, we do know that token economies and use of behavioral modification programs in school and at home have solid empirical support (Pfiffner et al., 2006). We also know that these strategies also work well for children with TS. Additionally, recommendations and guidelines for strategies are recommended by advocacy groups such as the Tourette Syndrome Association (TSA), the Obsessive Compulsive Foundation (OCF), and Children and Adults with Attention Deficit Disorders (CHADD). These organizations provide support, guidance, and education for individuals and families affected by these disorders. They can be valuable resources for parents struggling with school and home difficulties because they provide valuable information designed for use by educators and parents (e.g., pamphlets, videos, books). Given that research and empirical support for specific strategies are still forthcoming, parents and educators will find it helpful in the interim to consult school psychologists when designing behavioral management programs for the classroom and the home. Good behavioral programs will require careful planning, selection of target behaviors, collection of baseline data, monitoring of the child's progress, and evaluation of the program when interventions are introduced. The evaluation and monitoring components are particularly important in any behavioral intervention because they inform parents and school professionals if they are headed in the right direction. Poorly implemented programs or inappropriate selection of target behaviors can have the opposite effect of that desired; hence, the importance of involving individuals with experience in behavioral management programs, such as the school psychologist, becomes apparent. The next sections describe how to begin the process of receiving services in the school as well as approaches that have been found useful in structuring the child's school and home environments.

RECEIVING HELP AT SCHOOL

The most difficult challenge a parent may face with a newly diagnosed child is working with the school system. The parent will first want to educate school professionals, particularly the child's teacher, about TS (see previous section about what a teacher should know about TS). The next step is to begin the process of obtaining special education services, if they are necessary. Whereas it may be possible to implement informal arrangements with a cooperative teacher and school if the child has a mild case of TS that is generally not disruptive, other cases will probably require some kind of formal services. Parents might want to consider requesting a parent–teacher conference or a meeting with their child's guidance counselor. If a parent has never met with school personnel, then this is a good time to meet them in person. Any issues or concerns can be discussed at that meeting and planning can begin for special services if that is necessary. For parents who have never had to advocate for their child in an educational setting, this task can be daunting and extremely stressful. Furthermore, parents run the risk of feeling guilty if they are not successful. For these reasons, Packer (1997) recommends that parents learn when to turn to an educational advocate for assistance. In this manner, parents can navigate the law on education and avoid additional frustration and guilt that can come from school bureaucracy. Some local chapters of the TSA provide these services, and the national TSA has valuable information on its website. For parents or others wishing to become familiar with laws regulating special education in the public schools, brief descriptions of these follow.

There are two laws regulating how children in public schools receive special services. The first is the Americans with Disabilities Act (ADA), which provides for a Section 504 plan, and the second is the Individuals with Disabilities Education Act (IDEA). The two routes to receiving services in the public schools are through an IEP and the Section 504 plan. The TSA has noted that more and more schools are denying parental requests for the classification of children under the IDEA, which would make them eligible for an IEP (Conners, n.d.). Instead, schools are opting to provide a Section 504 accommodation plan. There are distinct differences between these two types of plans in terms of rights and protections provided to children. Additionally, IDEA was renewed in December 2004 with changes implemented in July 2005. These changes affect most children with an IEP. Some fundamental definitions and the key school resources in special education are reviewed first.

The Child Study Team (CST) consists of educators at the child's local school and meets regularly to discuss children who have been referred to them by parents, teachers, or other school staff because these children are experiencing difficulties. Although this team attempts to resolve the problems within the school, they often refer the child for further testing and classification by the Committee on Special Education (CSE). The CSE is comprised of various educators throughout a school district and includes a special education teacher, a regular education teacher, a school psychologist, a parent representative, a school system representative (who usually chairs the committee), the child's parents, the student (when appropriate), and other representatives with knowledge or special expertise about the child. The parents of the child may also bring an advocate, a medical doctor, an outside psychologist, and/or a legal representative to the meeting. This committee meets to establish the classification, placement, appropriate services, and to write the IEP.

As mentioned earlier, the two routes to receiving special services are the IEP and a Section 504 Plan. The differences between a 504 Plan and an IEP are discussed first. Section 504 is a federal civil rights law. The purpose of this law is to provide protections to persons with disabilities from discrimination based on their disability. Unlike IDEA, Section 504 does not guarantee that a child with a disability will receive an IEP. Eligibility for protections under Section 504 depends on the child having a physical or mental impairment that significantly limits at least one major life activity. Major life activities may include walking, seeing, hearing, speaking, breathing, learning, reading, writing, performing math calculations, and caring for oneself. The special education team at the child's school will assess whether the child has an impairment that is significantly limiting any of their major life activities. Section 504 requires that students with disabilities be provided with appropriate education services that are designed to meet the individual needs of the student. Examples of an appropriate education could include education in the regular classrooms, education in regular classes with supplementary services, and/or special education services. The 504 plan does not require an IEP but does provide for classroom modifications and/or related services such as occupational or speech therapy. These accommodations and modifications are not available to students who are not disabled; however, they are also available to students under IDEA. Modifications for children with TS and associated disorders under a 504 plan may include tests taken in a separate location with time limits waived or extended, education of other students who come into contact with the child who has TS, use of a computer if there are fine motor skills deficits, orally administered tests, modified assignments, help with class notes, preferential seating in the classroom, and a DRC. The TSA has noted that children with milder cases of TS may function well with a 504 plan, but children with more severe cases will probably require an IEP to meet their needs (Conners, n.d.).

The specific rights and services a child receives are dependent on how he or she is classified by the school system and whether the child receives services under an IEP or a Section 504 plan. There is the mistaken belief that if a child is classified under IDEA, then he or she is automatically placed in a special education class. Likewise, if a child has a 504 plan, he or she would remain in the regular classroom. Those parents desiring to have their child remain in regular classes might reach the conclusion that the 504 plan is more desirable, given these assumptions. This scenario is actually inaccurate. IDEA is the law governing how school systems manage special education. The IEP will determine placement; classification of a child under IDEA does not mean placement. It does mean that the child has been identified as having unique education needs related to his or her disability and is entitled to an IEP to meet those needs. Additionally, a child who receives services under a 504 plan has fewer rights than the child who receives special education services under an IDEA (Conners, n.d.). The child receiving special education services under IDEA is automatically protected under Section 504, a law that guarantees that children with disabilities will not be discriminated against because of their disability. However, certain procedural protections that are specified under IDEA will not be available to students who are not classified under this law. In other words, a student who has a 504 plan will not have the same protections as a child who has an IEP, because the child with the IEP has the additional protections that are afforded in IDEA. For example, a child with a 504 plan who misbehaves in school may be subject to permanent expulsion. Under IDEA, the child has the right to a fair and appropriate education even if he or she is expelled. IDEA also includes a system of procedural safeguards designed to protect the student and parents. These procedures include the requirement of a prior written notice before any change in placement can take place and the right to an independent educational evaluation at public expense.

When IDEA was recently renewed (IDEA 2004), TS was added to the list of conditions eligible for the other health impaired (OHI) category. This does not mean that every child with TS automatically qualifies for an IEP, but it does mean they will be considered in the context of OHI. In other words, when a child with TS has been identified by the school system under IDEA and is eligible for an IEP, the appropriate classification for him or her is the Other Health Impaired OHI category ("The New IDEA," 2006). This is the same classification used for children with ADHD. If a child has a comorbid LD, then the Learning Disabled (LD) classification can be used to receive services for both the learning disability and TS. A learning disability, however, does not have to be present for classification under OHI. After classification has been determined, the specific accommodations and educational plan will be discussed and approved at the IEP meeting. It is important to note that a child's parents are equal voting members at this meeting. Parents should be prepared for this meeting because it could have a major impact on the child's future. They should also become knowledgeable about TS and associated disorders, particularly since school professionals may not be. Parents may invite their child's psychologist or physician to the meeting, which may be helpful when discussing the complexities of TS. A good idea for parents is either to talk over the phone or meet with their child's guidance counselor or school psychologist prior to the IEP meeting. Ideally, any agenda items or concerns should be discussed prior to the IEP meeting, and this is a good opportunity to discuss those items. Schools as well as parents will not appreciate surprises at the IEP meeting. A prior meeting will give parents the chance to add any items to the IEP meeting agenda they would like discussed, and this will also give the school a chance to be accommodating. Parents may receive a copy of their child's current IEP or learn about the options that may be available to accommodate their child's specific needs. In this manner, parents arrive at the IEP meeting already prepared and knowledgeable about what issues will be discussed. Although this entire process can be extremely frustrating for parents, they should try to arrive at these meetings with positive attitudes and behave appropriately. Schools do not respond well to lists of demands or to parents who threaten them. A good working relationship will be the best way to accomplish everyone's goals.

CLASSROOM STRATEGIES FOR TICS

Whether or not a child has an IEP or 504 plan, the child's regular teacher (in the majority of cases) will have the most contact with him or her. Thus this teacher's reaction to tics may be the most important element in a specialized education plan or even when implementing informal changes in the classroom. As stated before, this means that the teacher will need to be familiar with tic disorders. A good starting place is the four points mentioned earlier in the chapter. Additionally, teachers will benefit from information and support that can be provided by the child's parents, a TSA representative or advocate, or the school psychologist. Parents should contact TSA in order to receive literature that may be helpful to classroom teachers or educators. Although tics may be annoying and somewhat disturbing in the classroom, reactions from the teacher that include anger, frustration, or disappointment will not be effective in helping the child to stop ticcing. Further, instructing a child not to tic usually has the opposite of the desired effect. When attention is called to the tic behavior, particularly when this attention is combined with negative affect, the child will feel anxiety and pressure to suppress future tic behaviors. This anxiety and added stress have the effect of actually increasing the urge to tic, thereby further increasing the child's frustration and anxiety—as well as the tic behaviors. We know that tics are increased when a child becomes anxious (Silva et al., 1995) or when a negative social reaction occurs (Watson & Sterling, 1998). Both of these situations are likely to occur as a result of a teacher's reaction to the tics at school. Thus negative attention in response to the tic can lead to a cycle of increased tic behaviors and further disruption for the class.

On the other hand, children with TS and tic disorders respond well to a calm, supportive environment. Teachers and classmates who are well informed about TS and generally ignore tics in their classroom will find that this strategy alone may be very successful. In fact, a recent study found that parents rate this strategy as the single most important classroom modification (Packer, 2005). Although there are no studies evaluating the effectiveness of ignoring tics, there is evidence that talking to children about their tics may lead to tic exacerbation (Woods, Watson, Wolfe, Twohig, & Friman, 2001). Thus, even though ignoring tics may not prevent tics from occurring, the parent reports may be accurate in that it is a useful strategy in preventing a worsening of tics (Packer, 2005).

EDUCATING PEERS

In terms of educating about TS and tics, classmates may be somewhat more problematic—if education of classmates is determined to be the best course of action. Parents should work closely with their school psychologist and teacher before attempting to educate classmates of the child with TS. In fact, it may take months to plan and coordinate a good program to educate other students about this disorder. Classmates who know little or nothing about tic disorders may have exaggerated responses to the tics that take the form of teasing or avoidance. Children may quickly discover that teasing the child with tics has the effect of making the tics much worse and will continue to tease or bully the child with TS. Alternately, children may have a fearful reaction and wonder if the tics are contagious. These types of reactions are based on ignorance of TS and tic disorders. The idea is that educating classmates about tic disorders will change their reaction. Although most students become more empathic toward the student with TS once they know more about it, there is the chance that an outlying student may take this information and use it against the affected child. This undesirable situation underscores the importance of working closely with the classroom teacher and school psychologist before presenting information to an entire class.

Other times the student with TS may not want classmates to know he or she has a disorder, particularly if the tics are relatively mild or are not disruptive at school. In these cases in particular (and all others), the teacher will serve as the best role model for students. When students observe the teacher ignoring the tics, they will usually follow that lead. Also, teachers may present information on tic disorders in the context of other chronic illnesses that are biological in nature and not contagious. This type of presentation may be less stigmatizing for a student with the disorder and, at the same time, removes the mystery of it for other students, allowing them to be empathic. The level of involvement of the student with TS will depend on how comfortable he or she feels discussing the disorder. Depending on the child's age, maturity level, and comfort level discussing the tics, teachers may want his or her input when devising strategies for dealing with tics in the classroom as well as for any class presentation on tic disorders.

There is mixed evidence regarding the effectiveness of peer education in reducing peer teasing and/or peer rejection. Packer (2005) reported that of nine cases in which peer education programs were utilized, three participants indicated that the programs were effective, five reported that the programs were somewhat helpful, and one reported that it was not helpful. The author's previous experiences with peer education (Packer, 1997) as well as another study's (Friedrich, Morgan, & Devine, 1996) indicate that these programs may be of some benefit. However, no study to date has objective data showing the benefit of peer education programs; thus, no firm conclusions can be stated as to whether these programs make significant reductions in classroom teasing or peer rejection. For parents considering this option, careful planning and coordination with the child's teacher and guidance counselor or school psychologist will be very important to increase the likelihood of a desired outcome.

MANAGING SEVERE TICS

More severe forms of tic behaviors and their management in the classroom present a greater challenge to teachers. The difficulty for teachers who have students with severe tics comes in the form of balancing the needs of the student with tics with possible disruptions to the class. The best strategy is to ignore as many tics as possible. The teacher and classmates need to be educated about TS and given support as well. Because many tics may wane or disappear within a matter of weeks, implementing behavioral strategies may not be required in most cases. Support for the child, teacher, and peers in accepting the situation and working around the tic may be the most effective strategy, particularly with children who are more resilient (Packer, 2005). However, when tics become severe to the point that they are disruptive to the class, teachers will need to determine what is reasonable to tolerate and when other action is necessary. Tics tend to occur in bouts, and inevitably, they will occur at the most inconvenient of times. The best option for managing moderate to severe tics in the classroom—and the one most likely to achieve a good outcome—is habit reversal therapy (HRT). Use of HRT combined with positive reinforcement for performing a competing response or modifying a tic has the most empirical support of all behavioral strategies. There are studies showing HRT is significantly effective for tic reduction both in and out of the classroom. (For a review of the evidence for HRT, see Piacentini & Chang [2006]; for treatment utilizing HRT, see Woods [2001]; see also Peterson, Chapter 8, this volume.) Packer (2005) has shown that modifying tic behaviors in the classroom in combination with positive consequences was the only intervention to show a positive outcome.

Briefly, HRT consists of awareness training and teaching the child a competing response, which the child performs whenever he or she feels the urge to tic. When a competing response is performed, the child is not able to tic at the same time. Ideally, the competing response is inconspicuous and something the child can do while still performing other tasks, such as listening to the teacher, reading, or taking notes in class. This behavioral strategy is ideal for classroom settings because the child can remain in the classroom, the competing responses are not disturbing to others, and the responses are not noticeable so the child can perform them without fear of being teased. Additionally, the HRT strategy allows the child much control over the tics, and because they are remaining in class, there is no risk of falling behind from missed course work, and they will appear like every other student (i.e., no stigma will be associated with HRT).

Another option that is described in many articles (e.g., Carter et al., 1999; Conners, 2004; Packer, 1997, 2005) is to allow the child to ask permission to leave the class for a brief period of time until the bout of tics has subsided. This strategy still allows the child some control in managing the tics, which will reduce anxiety about them (less anxiety about tics = fewer tics), create a sense of greater self-efficacy, and will help to minimize class disruptions. When this strategy works well, the affected child is able to remain on task more often because he or she is not worrying about the negative social consequences of ticcing, and he or she may be less stigmatized by the tics, allowing for greater peer acceptance. When selecting a place for the student to go when leaving the classroom, the principal's office should be avoided because this may be perceived as punishment to the child.

A variation on this plan is to allow the student frequent breaks from the classroom in order for him or her to release the tics in a less embarrassing environment. For example, the child may be allowed to go to the water fountain, the bathroom, or run an errand for the teacher. The student may also be given a laminated pass to allow him or her to leave the room, when needed, for a quick break. Again, careful and collaborative planning by the teacher, school psychologist, and parents will ensure that accommodations such as these are not used by the child to avoid classroom instruction. To help avoid this situation, if it is a concern, selected periods of separation may be more beneficial. In this circumstance, short breaks could be scheduled throughout the day rather than occurring on an as-needed basis. In the rarer circumstances when tics are socially inappropriate (e.g., spitting swearing, touching people), it will be necessary to brainstorm different solutions. As an example, one solution for a spitting tic may be to give the child a tissue into which to spit (Conners, 2004).

Although these strategies remain somewhat consistent with behavioral theory, in that the child retains some control in the situation and there is less chance of being stigmatized by classmates, they are also associated with potential risks. As noted earlier, the child who leaves the classroom whenever he or she tics misses classroom instruction, and the tics may develop an escape function (e.g., relief from a noxious situation). The potential for the child's tics to develop into an escape function can be a serious consequence, so determining how the child leaves the classroom and the context in which the leaving is sanctioned is important. Whereas the escape function may serve to reduce tics or classroom disruption in the short term, missing class time may lead to the child's falling behind in course work, which in turn may increase his or her anxiety surrounding school—thus increasing the frequency and severity of the tics. Additionally, the potential for stigma remains with this strategy because classmates may wonder why this student is allowed to leave class frequently. There is no research showing that leaving the classroom is effective for tic reduction; instead, this strategy has been recommended in the past based on the clinical experience and wisdom of practitioners working with children who have TS. Therefore, given these significant disadvantages, the HRT strategy appears superior and should be utilized before attempting limited time away from class.

Additional strategies may also be implemented by the regular classroom teacher in the absence of a formal intervention plan. These strategies have been cited elsewhere (i.e., Carter et al., 1999; Conners, 2004; Packer, 1997) and are recommended as potentially helpful for students with TS, although there are no formal studies showing their effectiveness. For students who engage in tics during tests, making it difficult to complete the tests within a specified time period, extended time or waived time limits are often beneficial. Additionally, tests taken in a separate location may reduce anxiety for the affected student, which will help reduce ticcing during testing. For students with motor tics that make it difficult to write or make handwriting illegible, use of a word processor or computer for taking classroom notes or taking tests is helpful. A change in seating assignment will also allow for less classroom disruption. Never seat a child with TS in the center front of the class where the tics will be more noticeable and embarrassing. Instead, a seat in the front on the side is ideal so that the teacher can help the child remain on task. With regard to the student's work productivity, the teacher should focus on gradually increasing completion of assignments rather than just rewarding on-task performance. This strategy is also helpful for students with comorbid ADHD. The goal of these strategies is to maximize the child's productivity and learning. Any modifications should be tailored to the specific child and his or her needs.

Because tics change over time, modifications for students with tics may need to be made frequently to continually meet their needs. Teachers may also wish to consult with the child's parents when planning tic management strategies to try in the classroom. Parents may be able to offer suggestions that have worked for them at home, and these ideas may be easy and inexpensive to implement. Teachers should also consult with the school psychologist when possible. School psychologists with experience in implementing behavioral programs can be an invaluable resource to the teacher.

Tic disorders and related behaviors, including the more serious tics, are not justification for removing a child from regular education classes. All of the classroom modifications discussed to this point can be implemented in a regular classroom by the child's regular teacher. Further, allowing the child to take breaks either when needed or on a more scheduled basis should not be misconstrued by any school personnel as indicating that this child needs to be in a special education classroom. In fact, under IDEA, children must be maintained in the least restrictive educational setting (Office of Education, 1990), and Section 504 requires that children with disabilities not be unfairly treated because of their disability. Parents with a child who has just received a diagnosis of TS or a chronic tic disorder may want to consult with a child advocate from TSA in order to understand and implement modifications under the federal and state laws governing special education.

STRATEGY EFFECTIVENESS

When accommodations are provided to a student with TS, it is important that they be evaluated for effectiveness, even if they have been empirically validated for groups of children. Currently, there are no data showing that schools objectively determine whether an accommodation is needed or effective for a given student (Packer, 2005). This issue is not specific to children with TS and applies to any child with a disability, 504 plan, IEP, or who is receiving a specialized educational program. Similarly, another problem may arise when ineffective strategies or accommodations that are no longer needed continue to be provided. This problem is particularly salient for children with TS, because tics change rapidly over time. It is possible that the more accommodations provided to a child, the more the child and his or her peers may view the accommodations or the child him- or herself as different. This situation may contribute to peer rejection, isolation, and/or poor self-regard. Thus, when considering strategies for children in school settings, it is important to weigh the potential benefits with these risks and to continually monitor their usefulness.

STRATEGIES FOR COMORBID ATTENTION DIFFICULTIES

ADHD is the most common co-occurring condition with TS, with rates between 50 and 90% of children with TS also having ADHD (Walkup et al., 1999). Fortunately for teachers, children with both TS and ADHD will benefit from the same strategies that are helpful for children who have ADHD without TS (Walter & Carter, 1997). However, educators and parents should keep in mind that strategies aimed at reducing attentional problems and hyperactive behaviors do not appear to influence the rate of tic behaviors (Nolan, Gadow, & Sverd, 1994). There are already numerous sources of information available describing how to manage ADHD behaviors in schools and at home (e.g., Barkley, 2006; Silver, 1999; Swanson, 1992). In general, teachers and parents should keep the following in mind (as recommended by Pfiffner et al., 2006) when planning interventions for children with both ADHD and TS:

- Effective behavioral management programs directly target the areas in which change is desired and focus on teaching children a set of skills. For example, to address organizational difficulties, the child may be asked to write down all homework assignments in a single notebook. When adaptive behaviors are not taught and only problem behaviors are targeted for intervention, children may replace one problem behavior with another.
- Effective programs target academic performance (e.g., amount of work completed accurately) rather than just on-task behavior. A student who is sitting quietly may not complete his or her work any better than when he or she was fidgety and inattentive. Improvement in classroom behavior does not necessarily lead to improvement in academic functioning.
- Consider very simple programs targeting the brief transitions of the day (between classes, activities, lunch, recess) because these times may be very problematic for a child with ADHD.
- Consider using a functional behavioral assessment as an effective method for linking the selection of target behaviors with the intervention. Every child and classroom are different; thus, the unique needs of the individual must be taken into consideration. Implementing generic interventions may be counterproductive if the specific needs of the child and the context in which the behavior occurs are not considered.

STRATEGIES FOR COMORBID OCD

Obsessive–compulsive symptoms are also quite common in children with tics. Approximately 30% of adults with tics have symptoms sufficiently severe to meet criteria for OCD (King, Leckman, Scahill, & Cohen, 1999). In children, OCD symptoms may not be visible or disruptive to classmates or teachers. On the other hand, behavioral compulsions can be quite distracting for the affected student as well as others in the classroom. They may appear as bizarre behaviors to others and have the potential for misdiagnosis when incomplete information is used for classification. OCD is a potentially debilitating disorder whose seriousness underscores the importance of a comprehensive evaluation by a licensed psychologist or psychiatrist as well as a functional behavioral analysis in the classroom. When a teacher suspects that a child has obsessive or compulsive symptoms, he or she should alert the parents and school psychologist. Teachers are advised not to confront a student with these types of symptoms because this situation will often result in denial by the student (due to embarrassment) and has the potential to make the anxiety symptoms worse in the short term. Like tics, OCD symptoms may wax and wane over time; therefore, ongoing communication among school personnel, parents, and outside clinicians will be necessary.

Teachers should understand that compulsions are very hard to resist; it is not simply a matter of willpower on the affected student's part. This knowledge can have a positive effect on the manner in which teachers and school personnel respond to the child. There are a number of classroom modifications that may be helpful to children whose obsessions and compulsions inhibit their academic performance. Children with OCD may need help with note taking, with time limits on tests, and with short breaks from the classroom. Switching tasks, transitioning, and finishing a task may be particularly difficult for a child with OCD, because he or she may not be able to understand when a task is finished. The student may need positive reinforcement and encouragement to complete tasks or to continue working on a task if he or she gets stuck. As with any child, modifications in the classroom should be tailored for the individual and the classroom. Treating clinicians may want to consult March and Mulle (1998) for a comprehensive overview of the empirically supported treatment for this disorder.

NEW DIRECTIONS IN RESEARCH

Clarke, Bray, Kehle, and Truscott (2001) examined the effects of a two-component treatment package consisting of habit reversal and self-modeling to reduce the frequency of tics in a school setting. The authors used a multiple baseline design with four students diagnosed with TS. This protocol outlined a treatment consisting of 13 sessions (20 minutes in duration) over the course of 20 days. Sessions were held in the school psychologist's office. Each participant had to describe his or her tics and reliably detect occurrences of the tics. All participants were then taught a competing response that was incompatible with their tic. Students were videotaped in their classrooms and instructed to behave as they normally would. Videotapes were edited and students viewed the tapes in a random order for six or seven treatment sessions. Throughout treatment, students practiced the competing responses at home and at school. Results indicated that three of four students showed substantial decreases in tics that were maintained at follow-up. No changes were made to the students' academic programs while participating in this study. Although small, this study is promising in that it demonstrates that this type of treatment can be effectively carried out in a school setting without disruption to the student's day-to-day schedule. A new national multisite study, funded by the National Institutes of Health and conducted by the TSA Behavioral Sciences Consortium, is currently examining a similar HRT-based treatment package for children and adolescents with chronic tic disorders.

Another recent study focusing on school accommodations also examined many issues discussed to this point. The results from Packer (2005), which are based on survey data and not experimental manipulation, indicated that school personnel tried to ignore and/or attempted to accommodate for tics in most cases. This was the most helpful strategy cited by parents of these children with TS. Other strategies used frequently in the schools studied and that parents perceived as important included allowing for extended time on tests, preferential seating, reduced homework, and allowing the child to leave the classroom. Peer education programs and in-school counseling by guidance counselors or school psychologists were not usually provided. Attempts to modify children's tics with behavioral interventions and aversive consequences were either unsuccessful or counterproductive. However, when the attempts to modify tics (i.e., HRT) were utilized with positive consequences (i.e., giving the children rewards), then those strategies met with success.

CONCLUSIONS

TS is a neurobiological disorder that can impact a child's school performance. Educators working with children who have TS should be aware of the etiology, presentation, and course of the illness. Awareness of these aspects of TS allows teachers and school personnel to implement effective strategies to manage classroom behavior thereby allowing the child to maximize his or her learning potential. Specific interventions such as medication, behavioral modification, and classroom accommodations are determined on an individual basis, because every child with TS has a unique presentation. Further, because of the rapidly changing nature of the disorder, flexibility and frequent reevaluation of school interventions are necessary to continue effective management. For more severe and troublesome tics, classroom strategies with the most success and empirical support involve use of habit reversal techniques along with positive consequences or rewards; otherwise, ignoring tics appears to work best. More research in the area of school strategies for tics and their effectiveness is certainly needed. What we do know and what will not change is that parents and teachers working in a collaborative manner, with the student's best interests in mind, will find that they have a profound positive impact on his or her academic success and development.

REFERENCES

Barkley, R. A. (2006). *Attention-deficit/hyperactivity disorder: A handbook for diagnosis and treatment* (3rd ed.). New York: Guilford Press.

Carter, A. S., Fredine, N. J., Findley, D., Scahill, L., Zimmerman, L., & Sparrow, S. S. (1999). Recommendations for teachers. In J. F. Leckman & D. J. Cohen (Eds.), *Tourette's syndrome—tics, obsessions, compulsions: Developmental psychopathology and clinical care* (pp. 360–368). New York: Wiley.

Chapell, P. B., Leckman, J. F., & Riddle, M. A. (1995). The pharmacologic treatment of tic disorders. In M. Lewis & M. Riddle (Eds.), *Child and adolescent psychiatric clinics of North America: Pediatric psychopharmacology* (Vol. 4, pp. 197–215). Philadelphia: Saunders.

Clarke, M. A., Bray, M. A., Kehle, T. J., & Truscott, S. D. (2001). A school-based intervention designed to reduce the frequency of tics in children with Tourette's syndrome. *School Psychology Review, 30,* 11–22.

Cohen, D. J. (1990). *Tourette's syndrome: Developmental psychopathology of a model psychiatric disorder of childhood* (Strecker Monograph Series No. 27). Philadelphia: Institute of Pennsylvania Hospital.

Conners, S. (2004). *Catalog of accommodations for students with Tourette syndrome, attention deficit hyperactivity disorder and obsessive compulsive disorder.* New York: Tourette Syndrome Association.

Conners, S. (n.d.). *Section 504, the Americans with Disabilities Act (ADA) vs. the Individuals with Disabilities Education Act (IDEA): What is the difference?* Retrieved January 26, 2005, from *www.tsa-usa.org.*

Friedrich, S., Morgan, S. B., & Devine, C. (1996). Children's attitudes and behavioral intentions toward a peer with Tourette syndrome. *Journal of Pediatric Psychology, 21,* 307–319.

Giordano, K. (2004). *Educational advocacy manual.* New York: Tourette Syndrome Association.

Hagin, R. A., Beecher, R., Pagano, G., & Kreeger, H. (1982). Effects of Tourette syndrome on learning. *Advances in Neurology, 35,* 323–328.

King, R. A., Leckman, J. F., Scahill, L., & Cohen, D. J. (1999). Obsessive–compulsive disorder, anxiety, and depression. In J. F. Leckman & D. J. Cohen (Eds.), *Tourette's syndrome—tics, obsessions, compulsions: Developmental psychopathology and clinical care* (pp. 43–62). New York: Wiley.

March, J. S., & Mulle, K. (1998). *OCD in children and adolescents: A cognitive-behavioral treatment manual.* New York: Guilford Press.

The New IDEA: A user's manual. (2006, Winter). *Tourette Syndrome Association Newsletter, 34*(3), 7–10.

Nolan, E. E., Gadow, K. D., & Sverd, J. (1994). Observations and ratings of tics in school settings. *Journal of Abnormal Child Psychology, 22,* 579–593.

Office of Education. (1990). *Individuals with Disabilities Education Act (IDEA).* 20 U.S.C. 1401(1) (15).

Packer, L. E. (1997). Social and educational resources for patients with Tourette syndrome. In J. Jankovic (Ed.), *Neurologic clinics: Vol. 15. Tourette syndrome* (pp. 457–473). Philadelphia: Saunders.

Packer, L. E. (2005). Tic-related school problems: Impact on functioning, accommodations, and interventions. *Behavior Modification, 29,* 876–899.

Pfiffner, L. J., Barkley, R. A., & DuPaul, G. J. (2006). Treatment of ADHD in school settings. In R. A. Barkley (Ed.), *Attention-deficit/hyperactivity disorder: A handbook for diagnosis and treatment* (3rd ed., pp. 547–589). New York: Guilford Press.

Piacentini, J., & Chang, S. (2006). Behavioral treatments for tic suppression: Habit reversal therapy, In J. Walkup, J. Mink, & P. Hollenbeck (Eds.), *Advances in neurology: Tourette syndrome* (pp. 227–233). Philadelphia: Lippincott, Williams & Wilkins.

Scahill, L., Ort, S. I., & Hardin, M. T. (1993). Tourette's syndrome: Part I. Definition and diagnosis. *Archives of Psychiatric Nursing, 7,* 203–208.

Shapiro, E. S., DuPaul, G. J., Bradley, K. L., & Bailey, L. T. (1996). A school-based consultation program for service delivery to middle school students with attention deficit hyperactivity disorder. *Journal of Emotional and Behavioral Disorders, 4*(2), 73–81.

Silva, R. R., Munoz, D. M., Barickman, J., & Friedhoff, A. J. (1995). Environmental factors and related fluctuation of symptoms in children and adolescents with Tourette's disorder. *Journal of Child Psychology and Psychiatry and Applied Disciplines, 36,* 305–312.

Silver, L. B. (1999). *Attention-deficit/hyperactivity disorders: A clinical guide to diagnosis and treatment for health and mental health professionals* (2nd ed.). Washington, DC: American Psychiatric Association.

Stokes, A., Bawden, H. N., Camfield, P. R., Backman, J. E., & Dooley, M. B. (1991). Peer problems in Tourette's disorder. *Pediatrics, 87,* 936–942.

Surwillo, W. W., Shafii, M., & Barrett, C. L. (1978). Gilles de la Tourette syndrome. *Journal of Nervous and Mental Disease, 166,* 812–816.

Swanson, J. M. (1992). *School-based assessments and interventions for ADD students.* Irvine, CA: K. C. Publishing.

Walkup, J. T., Khan, S., Schuerholz, L., Paik, Y., Leckman, J. F., & Schultz, R. T. (1999). Phenomenology and natural history of tic-related ADHD and learning disabilities. In J. F. Leckman & D. J. Cohen (Eds.), *Tourette's syndrome—tics, obsessions, compulsions: Developmental psychopathology and clinical care* (pp. 63–79). New York: Wiley.

Walter, A. L., & Carter, A. S. (1997). Gilles de la Tourette's syndrome in childhood: A guide for school professionals. *School Psychology Review, 26,* 28–46.

Watson, T. S., & Sterling, H. E. (1998). Habits and tics. In T. S. Watson & F. M. Gresham

(Eds.), *Handbook of child behavior therapy* (pp. 431–450). New York: Plenum Press.

Woods, D. W. (2001). Habit reversal treatment manual for tic disorders. In D. W. Woods & R. G. Miltenberger (Eds.), *Tic disorders, trichotillomania, and other repetitive behavior disorders: Behavioral approaches to analysis and treatment* (pp. 97–132). Norwell, MA: Kluwer.

Woods, D. W., Watson, T. S., Wolfe, E., Twohig, M. P., & Friman, P. C. (2001). Analyzing the influence of tic-related talk on vocal and motor tics in children with Tourette's syndrome. *Journal of Applied Behavior Analysis, 34,* 353–356.

CHAPTER 13

Management of Social and Occupational Difficulties in Persons with Tourette Syndrome

Douglas W. Woods
Brook A. Marcks
Christopher A. Flessner

The physical manifestations of Tourette syndrome (TS) are the most salient characteristics of the disorder, but those with TS frequently suffer from various social and occupational difficulties. Throughout this chapter, we provide a brief review of these difficulties and examine potential strategies for their management.

SOCIAL DIFFICULTIES

A wide range of research has examined some of the social and occupational difficulties experienced by those with TS, including decreased social acceptability (Boudjouk, Woods, Miltenberger, & Long, 2000; Friedrich, Morgan, & Devine, 1996; Long, Woods, Miltenberger, Fuqua, & Boudjouk, 1999; Woods, 2002; Woods, Fuqua, & Outman, 1999; Woods, Koch, & Miltenberger, 2003), peer relationship problems (Bawden, Stokes, Camfield, Camfield, & Salisbury, 1998; Burd, Kerbeshian,

Cook, Bornhoeft, & Fisher, 1988; Champion, Fulton, & Shady, 1988; Hubka, Fulton, Shady, Champion, & Wand, 1988; Kurlan et al., 1996), poor self-concept (Stefl, 1984; Thibert, Day, & Sandor, 1995), poor academics, criminality, psychopathology (Parker & Asher, 1987), and disrupted family functioning (Champion et al., 1988; Hubka et al., 1988; Woods, Himle, & Osmon, 2005). Below we discuss each of these difficulties in more detail.

Social Acceptability

A growing body of research has developed over the past 10 years examining the social acceptability of individuals with chronic tic disorders (e.g., motor or vocal) and TS. Much of this research has been done in controlled settings by comparing acceptability ratings of actors exhibiting displays of tics to actors not displaying tics. Although limited in generalizability, this research suggests that individuals with tics are viewed as less socially acceptable by their peers than individuals with no tics (e.g., Budjouk et al., 2000; Friedrich et al., 1996; Long et al., 1999; Woods et al., 1999, 2003; Woods, 2002). For example, Friedrich et al. (1996) recruited a fourth-grade boy (e.g., actor) to display tics in one condition (e.g., neck, shoulder, and head-jerking movements) and to act "normally" (i.e., tic free) in a separate condition. Results indicated that peers (i.e., children enrolled in third through fifth grades) rated the TS condition less positively than the "normal" condition. Woods et al. (1999) extended this research to examine the effects that intensity (i.e., the form each tic takes) and frequency of tics (i.e., the number of tics an individual exhibits) had on the social acceptability of persons with TS. Participants were asked to rate the social acceptability of male and female actors exhibiting motor tics, vocal tics, or a combination of both (i.e., TS). Tics varied in both intensity (i.e., mild and severe) and frequency (i.e., high and low frequency). Woods et al. found that men displaying tics were seen as less socially acceptable than women displaying tics, and motor tics were viewed as more acceptable than vocal tics. Additionally, those displaying low-frequency and mild tics were seen as more socially acceptable than those with high-frequency and severe tics.

Despite the research described above, questions remain with regard to the effects of tics on social acceptability. For example, the role of frequency, severity, and topography of tics in influencing social acceptability remains understudied. Likewise, replications of the social acceptability studies, using different age groups and persons with actual tic disorders would improve the external validity of the findings.

Peer Relationship Problems

Not only has research demonstrated that those with TS may be perceived as less socially acceptable than those without tics, but there is some evidence that others' negative perceptions may translate into impaired social relationships. A number of articles has suggested that persons with TS may have difficulties making and keeping friends (Bawden et al., 1998; Burd et al., 1988; Carter et al., 2000; Hubka et al., 1988). Often, individuals with TS report ridicule or rejection by peers and feelings of isolation as a result of their tics (Champion et al., 1988; Comings & Comings, 1985; Hagin, Beecher, Pagano, & Kreeger, 1982). In fact, some research has suggested that children with TS are significantly more withdrawn and less popular than their peers (Stokes, Bawden, Camfield, Backman, & Dooley, 1991). Difficulties with dating situations and lower marriage rates are additional difficulties faced by individuals with TS (Champion et al., 1988; Shapiro, Shapiro, & Wayne, 1972).

Burd et al. (1988) conducted a study of 39 individuals with TS and had participants complete a detailed questionnaire about their social experiences. The results demonstrated a number of alarming trends. School-age children and adolescents reported being teased by classmates because of their tics, having few (if any) friends, and feeling as though they were unfairly treated by their teachers. An important limitation to this study, however, was the failure of the authors to compare individuals with TS to another group (e.g., individuals with no prior psychiatric diagnosis). Bawden et al. (1998) addressed this research question by examining how peer relationships in children with TS compared to peer relationships in children with another chronic disease (e.g., diabetes mellitus). The authors found that children with TS were at a significantly higher risk for peer relationship problems when compared to children with diabetes mellitus. Results of the study also showed that children with a comorbid diagnosis such as attention-deficit/hyperactivity disorder (ADHD) were at an even greater risk of developing poor peer relationships.

Self-Concept

Relatively little research has been conducted on the effects of TS on self-concept. Evidence is equivocal with regard to deficits or strengths commonly found in those with TS (Edell-Fisher & Motta, 1990; Stefl, 1984; Stokes et al., 1991; Thibert et al., 1995). Stefl (1984) compared individuals from the general population to those diagnosed with TS and found that persons with TS exhibit significantly lower and increasingly negative self-perceptions.

In contrast, Edell-Fisher and Motta (1990) compared children with TS to age-matched controls and found no difference in self-concept ratings. Similar results have been found in subsequent research studies (Stokes et al., 1991; Thibert et al., 1995). For example, Stokes et al. (1991) found that although children with TS had significant difficulties in their relationships with peers, they displayed no significant difference with regard to self-esteem levels. In fact, self-reports indicated that these children displayed relatively positive self-esteem.

Academics, Criminality, and Psychopathology

Parker and Asher (1987) conducted a review of literature examining peer acceptance and development during later stages of life. It was discovered that poorly accepted children stood a greater chance of developing difficulties in later life when compared to children who had adequate levels of peer acceptance. Research indicates that low peer status is a good predictor of an individual's likelihood to drop out of school. Evidence also suggests that adolescents and young adults with pervasive and persistent histories of peer rejection problems are more likely to engage in criminal activity and to be psychologically troubled (Parker & Asher, 1987).

Unfortunately, little research of the type described above has been conducted specifically with a TS population. Research that has been conducted shows that children and adolescents with TS often experience feelings of alienation or social withdrawal (Bawden et al., 1998; Champion et al., 1988; Singer & Rosenberg, 1989; Stokes et al., 1991). These feelings of alienation and withdrawal can prevent individuals from pursuing school-related activities and add to their dislike of school (Comings & Comings, 1985; Stokes et al., 1991; Thibert et al., 1995). To our knowledge, no research in TS has examined the role social difficulties may play in the later development of criminality.

Research has begun to examine whether the social difficulties experienced by children with TS play a role in the development of adult psychopathology (Carter, Pauls, Leckman, & Cohen, 1994). Some researchers have postulated that these difficulties may lead to the development or exacerbation of psychiatric conditions (Boudjouk et al., 2000; Woods et al., 1999), but there are few studies to actually support such claims.

Given the dearth of research in the realms of academic success, criminality, and the development of psychopathology in the TS population, it should become quite apparent that more research within these areas is needed. In particular, research is needed to determine if TS-related social difficulties in childhood impact the development of criminal behavior or psychiatric functioning later in life.

Family Functioning

A possible combination of factors, including TS symptoms themselves and social difficulties, may have a detrimental effect on family functioning. Hubka et al. (1988) found that approximately 21% of their sample reported marital difficulties since their child was diagnosed with TS. These families also noted either alcohol or drug problems developing in either the parent or affected child in approximately 10% of respondents.

Subsequent research has found that as many as 85% of persons with TS and/or their families report greater levels of distress than the general public, and the peer and behavioral problems often associated with this disorder further exacerbate these stress levels (Champion et al., 1988; Woods et al., 2005). Also, increased stress within the family may lead to the development of psychopathology as the child becomes an adult (Carter et al., 1994). Additional research has shown that lower family functioning is often associated with poorer social and emotional adjustment in children and adolescents with TS, although the exact direction of this correlation is impossible to determine (Carter et al., 2000). (See Gingsburg and Newman Kingery, Chapter 11, this volume, for a detailed discussion of family issues.)

Psychiatric Disorders: The Impact on Social Problems Experienced by Those with TS

Children, adolescents, and adults with TS may face considerable hurdles in forming and maintaining solid peer relationships, but even more distressing is the fact that these individuals often face additional hurdles with regard to comorbid psychiatric conditions. Most research examining the role of comorbid diagnoses in social problems has focused on a distinct range of psychiatric disorders (e.g., obsessive–compulsive disorder [OCD], ADHD, and learning disabilities), which may contribute significantly to socialization problems (Bawden et al., 1998; Burd et al., 1998; Carter et al., 2000; Dykens et al., 1990; Shady, Broder, Staley, Furer, Brezden-Papadopolos, 1995; Stokes et al., 1991). For example, Carter et al. (2000) examined behavior problems and social adaptation difficulties in children with TS, children with TS and ADHD, and nonpsychiatric control children. Results showed that children diagnosed with both TS and ADHD demonstrated significantly more behavioral problems and poorer social adaptation than either children with TS alone or controls. These results are similar to those observed previously by Bawden et al. (1998), which indicated that individuals with TS and ADHD were at an increased risk for poorer peer relationships. Additionally, Woods et al. (2005) found that the influence of internalizing problems and ADHD-related behaviors had a greater impact on the family than the impact of tic severity alone, suggesting that the tics themselves may not significantly contribute to impairment in family functioning. However, there exists a body of previous research contradicting these findings.

Dykens et al. (1990) examined differences between children with TS and children diagnosed with both TS and ADHD on measures of intellectual, academic, and adaptive functioning. Significant differences were found between the groups with regard to intelligence, but not in academic or adaptive functioning. Both groups showed relative weaknesses in socialization skills (e.g., their use of playtime, interpersonal relationships, and coping skills). These results are similar to those found by other researchers finding few differences, with regard to socialization or adaptive skills, between children with TS and children with TS + ADHD (Shapiro & Shapiro, 1982; Singer & Rosenberg, 1989).

Although research is still inconclusive regarding the impact of comorbid disorders on socialization difficulties in children and adolescents with TS, findings suggests that individuals with TS, regardless of comorbid diagnoses, are at risk for social difficulties. Future research is necessary to determine the separate impact TS and various comorbid diagnoses have on individuals with TS.

It is apparent that individuals with tic disorders may exhibit a number of social difficulties. They have been found to be less socially acceptable than peers (Friedrich et al., 1996) and often experience significant problems with regard to peer relationship difficulties (Burd et al., 1988). In addition, children and adolescents diagnosed with TS often experience a variety of emotional problems (e.g., ADHD, OCD) and potential difficulties developing a positive self-concept (Edell-Fisher & Motta, 1990). As noted, social difficulties such as these often lead to additional problems with academics, criminality, and the possible development or exacerbation of psychopathology (Parker & Asher, 1987) in children and adolescents, although little research has examined these trends in a TS population (Siponmaa, Kristiansson, Johnson, Nyden, & Gillberg, 2001). In many instances these social difficulties can also lead to problems in family functioning (Hubka et al., 1988). Although it is obvious to most researchers that the problems described above are serious and warrant more study, questions still remain regarding whether the difficulties individuals with TS experience are a result of the tics or are better explained by the comorbid psychiatric disorders that often accompany a diagnosis of TS. (For detailed discussions of disorders that are commonly comorbid with TS, see Scahill et al., Chapter 4; Harrison et al., Chapter 7; Buhlmann et al., Chapter 9, this volume.) With this question in mind, we turn away from the social difficulties and their possible ramifications and turn to an area that has been studied considerably less among individuals with TS: occupational impairment.

OCCUPATIONAL DIFFICULTIES

Relatively little information is available about employment difficulties experienced by those with TS. Shady et al. (1995) surveyed persons with TS and found that nearly 50% of responders indicated that TS influenced their job choice "greatly" or "to some degree." Twenty-one percent indicated they had been dismissed or fired from a job because of their TS, and 30% said they had been denied a job, promotion, or pay increase because of TS.

In a survey of patients with TS, Meyers (1988) reported that 48% were unemployed compared to a 12.8% unemployment rate in the general population at the time of the study. Similar unemployment rates have been found in subsequent research (Elstner, Selai, Trimble, & Robertson, 2001). Approximately 46.5% of respondents in the study reported by Meyers indicated they had graduated from college or completed some form of graduate study. These findings, in combination with a relatively high unemployment rate, point to a considerable level of underemployment among individuals with TS. In addition, the survey showed that approximately 40% of respondents reported job discrimination, and only 8.9% reported that their employers made any form of special accommodation for them due to their difficulties. Although limited research has been conducted on the topic, evidence suggests that an individual's level of social functioning may have a significant effect on his or her ability to gain employment and function well within their respective career (Elstner et al., 2001; Shady et al., 1995).

Future research in this area will need to focus on providing more detailed information about the occupational difficulties experienced by persons with TS. Questions still remain with regard to the relationship between lower levels of employment and social functioning among individuals with TS. For example, do lower levels of employment result in impaired social functioning, or do lower levels of social functioning result in decreased levels of employment? In addition, research has suggested that the social toll of a TS diagnosis may strain individuals' coping resources, making it difficult for these individuals to attain economic and occupational independence (Shapiro et al., 1972), but this hypothesis needs to be examined further. Finally, research is needed to determine the aspects of TS (e.g., frequency of tics, severity of tics, comorbid diagnoses) that most powerfully impact employment rates and why there appear to be such high levels of underemployment among individuals with TS.

Not only is it important to understand the social difficulties faced by those with TS, but it is important to understand the strategies used to prevent or cope with these difficulties. In the remaining sections, we discuss the legal protections afforded persons with TS as well as specific environmental modifications that may be of assistance.

LEGAL PROTECTIONS FOR PERSONS WITH TS

Individuals with disabilities, including persons with TS, are afforded certain legal protection under Section 504, the American with Disabilities Act (ADA). This civil rights law protects against discrimination related to one's disability and is typically relevant in educational and occupational settings. In order to be protected under the ADA, one must have a physical or mental impairment that limits at least one major area of functioning, such as walking, speaking, hearing, seeing, breathing, learning, reading, writing, performing math, working, performing manual tasks, or caring for oneself. An in-depth discussion of the ADA and its implications for those with TS is described by Kepley and Conners (Chapter 12, this volume).

ENVIRONMENTAL MANAGEMENT OF SOCIAL AND OCCUPATIONAL DIFFICULTIES

In the following section, we describe a number of different settings in which modifications may be made to prevent or cope with the functional impairments associated with TS.

Addressing Social Difficulties

As described above, individuals with TS may encounter a number of social difficulties ranging from decreased social acceptability and negatively impacted peer relationships to poor self-concept, academic difficulties, and negative family functioning. In the following section, we describe potential modifications/interventions that may be made to improve the lives of those experiencing such difficulties.

Improving Social Acceptability

A growing body of research suggests that negative perceptions of those with TS can be significantly altered by education about the syndrome. Woods (2002) showed that adults without TS who watched a 10-minute educational video about TS had more positive social impressions about persons with TS than those who did not receive the educational intervention. These results have been replicated and extended. Woods et al. (2003) found that the beneficial effects of TS education were greater for those with a severe TS presentation and for females with the disorder. In addition, Woods and Marcks (2005) demonstrated that the content of the educational material needed to be specific to TS as opposed to a broader educational video sensitizing individuals to the impact of psychiatric illness. A study by Marcks, Berlin, Woods, and Davies (2003) also showed that preventively disclosing one's TS produced a broad reduction in negative perceptions, and reduced negative attributions about the tics. A large body of TS-related educational material is available from the national Tourette Syndrome Association (*www.tsa-usa.org*).

In addition to educating others about the disorder, other strategies may be useful in fostering social acceptability of persons with TS. One such strategy is mere exposure. The greater number of opportunities peers have to engage in group activities with those who have TS, the more likely the tics will be overlooked and healthy attitudes toward the person will develop. In our clinical experience, those with severe tics are not necessarily cursed with a negative social prognosis. Those who succeed socially are those who do not let their tics interfere with their daily lives or who find ways to work around the tics to participate fully in their social experience.

Improving Peer Relationships

A number of additional strategies exist to improve peer relationships, in addition to those strategies described above. Given that a significant body of research exists to suggest that comborbid diagnoses, and not tics, negatively impact peer relationships, the first strategy in improving peer relationships is to treat the comorbid psychopathology. In addition, providing structured interaction times with peers or social skills training may help to improve peer relationships, as may the education of peers, described above.

Improving Self-Concept

Virtually no research exists to guide the recommendations for improving the self-concept of persons with TS. Nevertheless, treatment strategies that lead the person with TS to (1) perceive greater control over his or her environment, (2) experience success in meaningful daily activities, and (3) begin to function independently, should all contribute to improved self-concept. Specific strategies for improving self-concept in those with TS may include providing education about the etiology and prognosis of TS, teaching independence in solving problems and completion of daily activities, and encouraging the person with TS to initiate new, and develop existing, areas of interest (e.g., sports, arts, music).

Improving Academic/Family Functioning

Strategies for improving family and academic functioning are described fully in Ginsburg and Newman Kingery (Chapter 11, this volume) and 13 Kepley and Conners (Chapter 12, this volume). Readers interested in more detailed suggestions for addressing these difficulties should read these chapters carefully.

Addressing Occupational Difficulties

As with each area of functioning, modifications for the workplace environment may be helpful in aiding persons with TS to manage social and occupational difficulties. It is important to note that even though TS may lead to work-related difficulties, there is no evidence suggesting that simply having a diagnosis of TS prevents one from being able to pursue certain careers. In the vast majority of the cases, persons with TS are capable of succeeding in their given careers, if provided with the opportunity and necessary accommodations (Taubert, 1999).

As discussed earlier, persons with TS may experience a number of job-related difficulties, including discrimination, unequal opportunities, or reluctance by employers to provide the necessary accommodations needed for the individual to succeed. Consequently, guidelines have been proposed to ameliorate these issues, including modifications related to the employer, coworkers, or individual with the disorder (Shady et al., 1995). Several suggestions focus on the employer. First, many employers have little to no knowledge or misinformation about TS. If this is the case, the first step is to provide educational material to the employer— the responsibility for which often falls to the employee with TS. The employer may need to look at his or her own assumptions and beliefs regarding TS to determine whether they are accurate; if they are inaccurate, they may need to be modified. Additionally, employers should enlist the help of their employees with TS in making decisions regarding their employment. For example, the employer should not make decisions regarding assigned tasks or other aspects of the job without the input of the employee with TS. In addition, the employer should not make assumptions about the employee's skills or capabilities, because such assumptions are often inaccurate and not in the best interest of the employee.

Other modifications focus on coworkers and the employees with TS. Just as providing education to the employer is important, it is also recommended that persons with TS offer information (e.g., pamphlets, informational sheets) to coworkers about the disorder (Shady et al., 1995). It may also be useful to answer any questions coworkers have about the disorder to further demystify it. Should a coworker react negatively to the tics, the employee with TS has a number of options for dealing with the situation: ignoring the situation, discussing the issue with the coworker, reporting the negative response to a supervisor, or working out specific management strategies with the employee's supervisor.

A number of structural and organizational changes can also be made in a workplace to help persons with TS cope with occupational difficulties. With the passage of the ADA, more employers are becoming aware of the need to provide adequate accommodations for employees with disabilities, including TS. Although employers are more aware of the need, however, they are often unsure what type of accommodations might be needed. Although the types of accommodations needed vary by individual, these accommodations could include modifying tasks or types of responsibilities, breaking tasks into more manageable or structured parts, allowing flexibility in deadlines, permitting time alone, allowing more breaks, or modifying environmental factors such as the noise level (some persons with vocal tics prefer working in louder environments to make the tics less noticeable). Although such changes may indeed be warranted and beneficial in some cases, not all persons with TS would necessarily need any of these modifications. Simply stated, modifications need to be developed on an individual basis.

Efficacy of Modification Programs

Although many guidelines identifying components to include in environmental modification programs have been proposed, little to no research has examined the efficacy of such programs. Because empirical support for these types of modifications has not been gathered, it is important to monitor the efficacy of individualized home, school, or workplace modifications that are developed and implemented. Without such monitoring, there is no way to assess whether the modifications are beneficial to the individual or whether changes to the current modifications are warranted. Thus, it is essential for parents, school personnel, and employers, as well as the individuals with TS, to evaluate such factors on an ongoing basis. Clearly, research is needed on the efficacy of such modification programs in order to improve the management of the social and occupational difficulties experienced with TS.

REFERENCES

Bawden, H. N., Stokes, A., Camfield, C. S., Camfield, P. R., & Salisbury, S. (1998). Peer relationship problems in children with Tourette's disorder and diabetes mellitus. *Journal of Child Psychology and Psychiatry, 39*(5), 663–668.

Boudjouk, P. J., Woods, D. W., Miltenberger, R. G., & Long, E. S. (2000). Negative peer evaluation in adolescents: Effects of tic disorders and trichotillomania. *Child and Family Behavior Therapy, 22*(1), 17–28.

Burd, L., Kerbeshian, J., Cook, J., Bornhoeft, D. M., & Fisher, W. (1988). Tourette disorder in North Dakota. *Neuroscience and Biobehavioral Reviews, 12,* 223–228.

Carter, A. S., O'Donnell, D. A., Schultz, R. T., Scahill, L., Leckman, J. F., & Pauls, D. L. (2000). Social and emotional adjustment in children affected with Gilles de la Tourette's syndrome: Associations with ADHD and family functioning. *Journal of Child Psychology and Psychiatry, 41*(2), 215–223.

Carter, A. S., Pauls, D. L., Leckman, J. F., & Cohen, D. J. (1994). A prospective longitudinal study of Gilles de la Tourette syndrome. *Journal of the American Academy of Child and Adolescent Psychiatry, 33*(3), 377–385.

Champion, L. M., Fulton, W. A., & Shady, G. A. (1988). Tourette syndrome and social functioning in a Canadian population. *Neuroscience and Biobehavioral Reviews, 12,* 255–257.

Comings, D. E., & Comings, B. G. (1985). Tourette syndrome: Clinical and psychological abstracts of 250 cases. *American Journal of Human Genetics, 37,* 435–450.

Dykens, E., Leckman, J., Riddle, M., Hardin, M., Schwartz, S., & Cohen, D. (1990). Intellectual, academic, and adaptive functioning of Tourette syndrome children with and without attention deficit disorder. *Journal of Abnormal Child Psychology, 18*(6), 607–615.

Edell-Fisher, B. H., & Motta, R. W. (1990). Tourette syndrome: Relation to children's and parents self-concepts. *Psychological Reports, 66,* 539–545.

Elstner, K., Selai, C. E., Trimble, M. R., & Robertson, M. M. (2001). Quality of life (QOL) of patients with Gilles de la Tourette's syndrome. *Acta Psychiatrica Scandinavica, 103,* 52–59.

Friedrich, S., Morgan, S. B., & Devine, C. (1996). Children's attitudes and behavioral intentions toward a peer with Tourette's syndrome. *Journal of Pediatric Psychology, 21*(3), 307–319.

Hagin, R. A., Beecher, R., Pagano, G., & Kreeger, H. (1982). Effects of Tourette syndrome on learning. In A. J. Friedoff & T. N. Chase (Eds.), *Gilles de la Tourette syndrome* (pp. 323–328). New York: Raven Press.

Hubka, G. B., Fulton, W. A., Shady, G. A., Champion, L. M., & Wand, R. (1988). Tourette syndrome: Impact on Canadian family functioning. *Neuroscience and Biobehavioral Reviews, 12,* 259–261.

Kurlan, R., Daragjati, C., Como, P. G., McDermott, M. P., Roddy, S., Brower, C. A., & Robertson, M. M. (1996). Non-obscene complex socially inappropriate behavior in Tourette's syndrome. *Journal of Neuropsychiatry and Clinical Neuroscience, 8,* 311–317.

Long, E. S., Woods, D. W., Miltenberger, R. G., Fuqua, R. W., & Boudjouk, P. J. (1999). Examining the social effects of habit behaviors exhibited by individuals with mental retardation. *Journal of Developmental and Physical Disabilities, 11*(4), 295–312.

Marcks, B. A., Berlin, K. S., Woods, D. W., & Davies, W. H. (2003, November). *Impact of Tourette's syndrome disclosure on peer perceptions and social functioning.* Poster session presented at the annual meeting of the Association for the Advancement of Behavior Therapy, Boston.

Meyers, A. S. (1988). Social issues of Tourette's syndrome. In D. J. Cohen, R. D. Bruun, & J.

F. Leckman (Eds.), *Tourette's syndrome and tic disorders: Clinical understanding and treatment* (pp. 257–264). New York: Wiley-Interscience.

Parker, J. G., & Asher, S. R. (1987). Peer relations and later personal adjustment: Are low-accepted children at risk? *Psychological Bulletin, 102*(3), 357–389.

Shady, G., Broder, R., Staley, D., Furer, P., & Brezden-Papadopolos, R. (1995). Tourette syndrome and employment: Descriptors, predictors, and problems. *Psychiatric Rehabilitation Journal, 19*(1), 35–42.

Shapiro, A. K., & Shapiro, E. (1982). An update on Tourette syndrome. *American Journal of Psychotherapy, 36*(3), 379–390.

Shaprio, A. K., Shapiro, E., & Wayne, H. (1972). Birth, developmental, and family histories and Demographic information in Tourette's syndrome. *Journal of Nervous and Mental Disease, 155*(5), 335–344.

Singer, H. S., & Rosenberg, L. A. (1989). Development of behavioral and emotional functioning problems in Tourette syndrome. *Pediatric Neurology, 5*, 41–44.

Siponmaa, L., Kristiansson, M., Jonson, C., Nyden, A., & Gillberg, C. (2001). Juvenile and young adult mentally disordered offenders: The role of child neuropsychiatric disorders. *Journal of the American Academy of Psychiatry and the Law, 29*, 420–426.

Stefl, M. E. (1984). Mental health needs associated with Tourette syndrome. *American Journal of Public Health, 74*(12), 1310–1313.

Stokes, A., Bawden, H. N., Camfield, P. R., Backman, J. E., & Dooley, J. M. (1991). Peer problems in Tourette's disorder. *Pediatrics, 87*(6), 936–942.

Taubert, K. A. (1999). Role of voluntary organizations in clinical care, research, and public policy. In D. J. Cohen, R. D. Bruun, & J. F. Leckman (Eds.), *Tic and tic disorders: Clinical understanding and treatment* (pp. 399–413). New York: Wiley.

Thibert, A. L., Day, H. I., & Sandor, P. (1995). Self-concept and self-consciousness in adults with Tourette's syndrome. *Canadian Journal of Psychiatry, 40*, 35–39.

Woods, D. W. (2002). The effect of video-based peer education on the social acceptability of adults with Tourette's syndrome. *Journal of Developmental and Physical Disabilities, 14*(1), 51–62.

Woods, D. W., Fuqua, R. W., & Outman, R. C. (1999). Evaluating the social acceptability of persons with habit disorders: The effects of topography, frequency, and gender manipulation. *Journal of Psychopathology and Behavioral Assessment, 21*(1), 1–18.

Woods, D. W., Himle, M. B., & Osmon, D. C. (2005). Use of the Impact on Family Scale in children with tic disorders: Descriptive data, validity, and tic severity impact. *Child and Family Behavior Therapy, 27*, 11–21.

Woods, D. W., Koch, M., & Miltenberger, R. G. (2003). The impact of tic severity on the effects of peer education about Tourette's syndrome. *Journal of Developmental and Physical Disabilities, 15*(1), 67–78.

Woods, D. W., & Marcks, B. A. (2005). Controlled evaluation of an educational intervention used to modify peer attitudes and behavior toward persons with Tourette's syndrome. *Behavior Modification, 29*, 900–912.

Index

Page numbers followed by a *t* or *f* indicate tables or figures.